Asthma
SOURCEBOOK

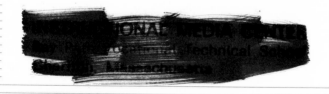

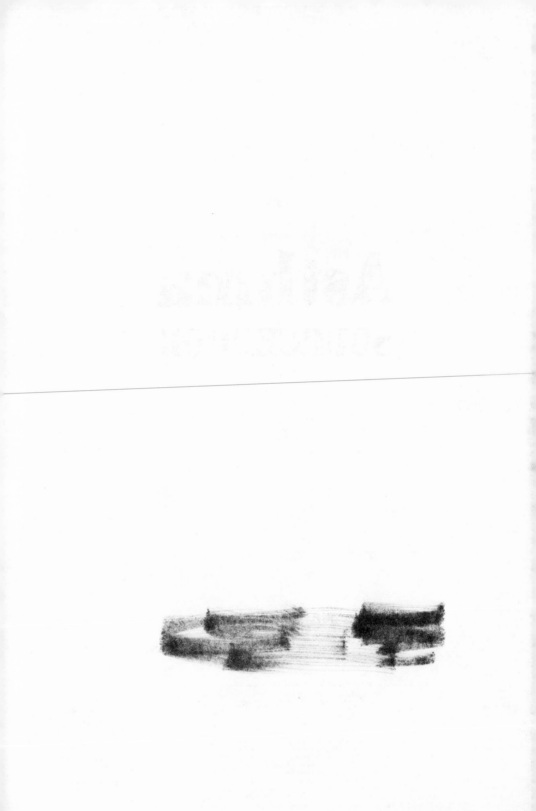

Health Reference Series

First Edition

Asthma
SOCRCEBOOK

Basic Consumer Health Information about Asthma, Including Symptoms, Traditional and Nontraditional Remedies, Treatment Advances, Quality-of-Life Aids, Medical Research Updates, and the Role of Allergies, Exercise, Age, the Environment, and Genetics in the Development of Asthma

Along with Statistical Data, a Glossary, and Directories of Support Groups, and Other Resources for Further Information

Edited by
Annemarie S. Muth

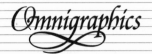

Omnigraphics

615 Griswold Street • Detroit, MI 48226

Bibliographic Note

Because this page cannot legibly accommodate all the copyright notices, the Bibliographic Note portion of the Preface constitutes an extension of the copyright notice.

Each new volume of the *Health Reference Series* is individually titled and called a "First Edition." Subsequent updates will carry sequential edition numbers. To help avoid confusion and to provide maximum flexibility in our ability to respond to informational needs, the practice of consecutively numbering each volume will be discontinued.

Edited by Annemarie S. Muth

Health Reference Series

Karen Bellenir, *Series Editor*
Peter D. Dresser, *Managing Editor*
Joan Margeson, *Research Associate*
Dawn Matthews, *Verification Assistant*
Jenifer Swanson, *Research Associate*

EdIndex, Services for Publishers, *Indexers*

Omnigraphics, Inc.

Matthew P. Barbour, *Vice President, Operations*
Laurie Lanzen Harris, *Vice President, Editorial Director*
Kevin Hayes, *Production Coordinator*
Thomas J. Murphy, *Vice President, Finance and Comptroller*
Peter E. Ruffner, *Senior Vice President*
Jane J. Steele, *Marketing Consultant*

Frederick G. Ruffner, Jr., Publisher

© 2000, Omnigraphics, Inc.

Library of Congress Cataloging-in-Publication Data

Asthma sourcebook : basic consumer health information about asthma, including symptoms, traditional and nontraditional remedies ... / edited by Annemarie S. Muth.-- 1st ed.
    p. cm. -- (Health reference series)
    Includes bibliographical references and index.
    ISBN 0-7808-0381-7 (lib. bdg. : acid-free paper)
    1. Asthma--Popular works. I. Muth, Annemarie. II. Health reference series (Unnumbered)

RC591 .A84 2000
616.2'38--dc21
                                       00-063716

∞

Printed in the United States

Table of Contents

Preface ix

Part I: The Nature of Asthma and Related Ailments

Chapter 1—What Is Asthma? 3
Chapter 2—Practical and Effective Asthma Care 9
Chapter 3—Exercise-Induced Asthma 15
Chapter 4—Sinusitis 25
Chapter 5—Rhinitis Update: A Guide to Diagnosis and
            Treatment 29
Chapter 6—Cardiac Asthma and Emphysema 43
Chapter 7—Chronic Obstructive Pulmonary Disease 45
Chapter 8—Gastroesophageal Reflux: A Common Factor
            in Adult Asthma 53
Chapter 9—Vocal Cord Dysfunction 65
Chapter 10—Chronic Cough 69

Part II: Asthma Statistics

Chapter 11—Asthma Surveillance and Intervention
            Programs 83
Chapter 12—Asthma by Race, Sex, Age, and State 97
Chapter 13—Forecasted Estimates of Self-Reported
            Asthma Prevalence by State 131

Chapter 14—Seasonal Variation of Hospitalizations for
            Asthma, Bronchitis, and Emphysema 137
Chapter 15—Asthma by Family Income and Age 147
Chapter 16—Missing the Mark: U.S. Not Meeting
            Asthma Goals 151
Chapter 17—Mortality and Markers of Risk of Asthma
            Death 155
Chapter 18—Asthma Symptom Differences by Age
            and Sex 169
Chapter 19—Asthma in the Workplace 187

Part III: Theories about the Causes of Asthma

Chapter 20—Genetics of Asthma 195
Chapter 21—Environmental Genome Project 203
Chapter 22—Asthma Clinical Genetics Network 209
Chapter 23—Asthma and Race 213
Chapter 24—Interleukin-11 and Asthma 217
Chapter 25—Infectious Asthma 221

Part IV: Triggers and Risk Factors Associated with Asthma

Chapter 26—Targeting Asthma Triggers 235
Chapter 27—Nitrogen Dioxide and Allergic Asthma 245
Chapter 28—Ozone and Your Health 249
Chapter 29—How Energy Policies Affect Public
            Health 265
Chapter 30—Noncancer Respiratory Health Effects of
            Passive Smoking 285
Chapter 31—Fragrances and Health 297
Chapter 32—Cockroach Antigens 301
Chapter 33—Occupational Asthma... 307
Chapter 34—Agricultural Allergens and Irritants 317
Chapter 35—Latex Allergy 329
Chapter 36—Food and Asthma 337
Chapter 37—Risk Factors Associated with Fatal Asthma
            Attacks in Children.................................. 343
Chapter 38—Access to Asthma Health Care by African
            American Families 345

Part V: Diagnosis and Treatments

Chapter 39—Asthma Assessment and Diagnosis 365
Chapter 40—Asthma Medications 371
Chapter 41—Pediatric and Geriatric Drug Safety................. 379
Chapter 42—Corticosteroids: Benefits and Risks 387
Chapter 43—Update on Theophylline 397
Chapter 44—Asthma Inhalation Therapy 399
Chapter 45—Your Metered-Dose Inhaler and
        Chlorofluorocarbons 405
Chapter 46—Adrenergic Bronchodilators 411
Chapter 47—Stepwise Management of Symptoms 415
Chapter 48—How to Use Your Inhaler Effectively 429
Chapter 49—Immunotherapy (Allergy Shots) 433
Chapter 50—Asthma and the Leukotriene Receptor:
        New Options for Therapy 437

Part VI: Asthma Management

Chapter 51—Role of the Allergist in Cost-Effective
        Treatment of Asthma... 443
Chapter 52—Role of the Pharmacist in Asthma Care 461
Chapter 53—Peak Flow Monitoring 473
Chapter 54—Chronotherapy: Controlling Nocturnal
        Breathing Problems 477
Chapter 55—Managing Asthma in the Child Care Setting 481
Chapter 56—Managing Asthma at School 485
Chapter 57—Controlling Asthma Exacerbations at Home,
        in the Emergency Department, and in the
        Hospital 489
Chapter 58—Asthma and Pregnancy 501
Chapter 59—Asthma and Aging 507

Part VII: Other Aids to Wellness and Prevention

Chapter 60—Home Air Cleaners: Preventative Therapy
        for Asthma 513
Chapter 61—Vitamin Supplements: Aid for Asthmatics
        against Air Pollution... 517
Chapter 62—Vitamin C's Role in Controlling Asthma 519

Chapter 63—Who Should Get the Flu Vaccine 523
Chapter 64—Estrogen Fluctuation and Asthma
              Severity 529
Chapter 65—Breathing Method Reduces Asthma
              Attacks 533
Chapter 66—Exercise for Asthma Patients............................. 537

Part VIII: Additional Help and Information

Chapter 67—Glossary 549
Chapter 68—Resources 573

Index 585

Preface

About This Book

Despite major advancements in its treatment, asthma cases and deaths are on the increase in the United States and in many other Western countries. This rise has made asthma an especially important public health issue because it comes at a time when deaths from most other causes are on the decline. In 1993, an estimated 13.7 million persons in the United States reported having asthma, a 75% increase since 1980. By 1998, that number had jumped to an estimated 17.3 million.

This *Sourcebook* brings together current information on the reasons for the rise, including better diagnosis of the disease, increased exposure to environmental allergens and irritants, increased exposure of children to parents' tobacco smoke, and psychosocial and socioeconomic factors. In addition, statistical data, reports on research and prevention measures, and new treatment programs are presented. A comprehensive glossary and directory of organizations and online resources provide guidance to readers seeking further help and information.

How to Use This Book

This book is divided into parts and chapters. Parts focus on broad areas of interest. Chapters are devoted to single topics within a part.

Part I: The Nature of Asthma and Related Ailments provides basic information about asthma and its symptoms. It also describes diseases related to asthma, such as rhinitis and chronic obstructive pulmonary disease, and diseases often mistaken for asthma, such as emphysema.

Part II: Asthma Statistics gives an overview of asthma prevalence in the United States, including the number of state asthma surveillance programs, the annual number of asthma office visits, hospitalizations, and deaths by race, sex, age, state, and family income. Additionally, it lists occupational respiratory illnesses by industry, and summarizes the findings of a survey on asthma care in the United States as compared with the goals set by the National Heart, Lung, and Blood Institute (NHLBI).

Part III: Theories about the Causes of Asthma describes government and private sector research into the genetic predisposition for asthma and the possible connection between asthma and related infectious diseases such as pneumonia, bronchitis, and respiratory syncytial virus (RSV).

Part IV: Triggers and Risk Factors Associated with Asthma lists environmental allergens, irritants, and foods that may provoke an asthma attack and how to avoid them. Additionally, it examines certain socioeconomic factors, including poverty and the lack of access to health care, as predictors of asthma.

Part V: Diagnosis and Treatments describes the medical tests used for diagnosing asthma; lists currently accepted asthma medications plus information on a new class of antiasthma drugs; provides an update on the use of theophylline and advisories concerning recent FDA regulations on pediatric and geriatric asthma drug testing and labeling; offers instructions on the correct use of asthma inhalers and correct dosage for inhaled steroids; and discusses the efficacy and safety of immunotherapy (allergy shots).

Part VI: Asthma Management looks at how a working relationship among allergist, pharmacist, and patient can control asthma in various environments and at various stages of life—at home, day care, school, hospital, during the night, during pregnancy, in the elderly—with the aid of counseling on proper medication and peak flow monitoring.

Part VII: Other Aids to Wellness and Prevention highlights the benefits of home air cleaners, vitamin supplements, flu shots, estrogen (in women), breathing perception training, and exercise.

Part VIII: Additional Help and Information provides a glossary of medical terminology related to asthma and a list of government and private agencies, support groups, and online sites that may be contacted for further information.

Bibliographic Note

This volume contains documents and excerpts from publications issued by the following U.S. government agencies: Centers for Disease Control and Prevention (CDC), Food and Drug Administration (FDA), National Center for Health Statistics (NCHS), National Heart, Lung, and Blood Institute (NHLBI), National Institute for Occupational Safety and Health (NIOSH), National Institute of Allergy and Infectious Diseases (NIAID), National Institute of Environmental Health Sciences (NIEHS), National Institutes of Health (NIH), U.S. Department of Health and Human Services (DHHS), and U.S. Environmental Protection Agency (EPA).

In addition, this volume contains copyrighted documents from the following organizations and individuals: Allergy and Asthma Network—Mothers of Asthmatics, Inc. (AANMA); Louise H. Bethea, M.D., P.A.; Center for Complementary & Alternative Medicine Research in Asthma (CAMRA); Glaxo Wellcome, Inc.; International Food Information Council Foundation; National Jewish Medical and Research Center. Copyrighted articles from *Air Conditioning, Heating & Refrigeration News, Allergy and Asthma Magazine, American Family Physician, American Journal of Respiratory and Critical Care Medicine, Chest, Consultant, Family and Community Health, Journal of Family Practice, The Lancet, Medical Sciences Bulletin, The Nurse Practitioner, Occupational Hazards, Patient Care, Pediatrics for Parents, The Physician and Sportsmedicine,* and *Tufts University Diet & Nutrition Letter,* are also included.

Full citation information is provided on the first page of each chapter. Every effort has been made to secure all necessary rights to reprint the copyrighted material. If any omissions have been made, please contact Omnigraphics to make corrections for future editions.

Acknowledgements

In addition to the many organizations and agencies that contributed the material included in this book, thanks go to Joan Margeson for her tireless efforts in tracking down documents and Dawn Matthews for her verification assistance.

Note from the Editor

This book is part of Omnigraphics' *Health Reference Series*. The series provides basic information about a broad range of medical concerns. It is not intended to serve as a tool for diagnosing illness, in prescribing treatments, or as a substitute for the physician/patient relationship. All persons concerned about medical symptoms or the possibility of disease are encouraged to seek professional care from an appropriate health care provider.

Our Advisory Board

The *Health Reference Series* is reviewed by an Advisory Board comprised of librarians from public, academic, and medical libraries. We would like to thank the following board members for providing guidance to the development of this series:

Dr. Lynda Baker,
Associate Professor of Library and Information Science,
Wayne State University, Detroit, MI

Nancy Bulgarelli,
William Beaumont Hospital Library, Royal Oak, MI

Karen Imarasio,
Bloomfield Township Public Library, Bloomfield Township, MI

Karen Morgan,
Mardigian Library, University of Michigan-Dearborn,
Dearborn, MI

Rosemary Orlando,
St. Clair Shores Public Library, St. Clair Shores, MI

Health Reference Series *Update Policy*

The inaugural book in the *Health Reference Series* was the first edition of *Cancer Sourcebook* published in 1992. Since then, the *Series* has been enthusiastically received by librarians and in the medical community. In order to maintain the standard of providing high-quality health information for the lay person, the editorial staff at Omnigraphics felt it was necessary to implement a policy of updating volumes when warranted.

Medical researchers have been making tremendous strides, and it is the purpose of the *Health Reference Series* to stay current with the most recent advances. Each decision to update a volume will be made on an individual basis. Some of the considerations will include how much new information is available and the feedback we receive from people who use the books. If there is a topic you would like to see added to the update list, or an area of medical concern you feel has not been adequately addressed, please write to:

Editor
Health Reference Series
Omnigraphics, Inc.
615 Griswold
Detroit, MI 48226

The commitment to providing on-going coverage of important medical developments has also led to some format changes in the *Health Reference Series*. Each new volume on a topic is individually titled and called a "First Edition." Subsequent updates will carry sequential edition numbers. To help avoid confusion and to provide maximum flexibility in our ability to respond to informational needs, the practice of consecutively numbering each volume has been discontinued.

Part One

The Nature of Asthma and Related Ailments

Chapter 1

What Is Asthma?

Think of someone—a child or an adult—racked by uncontrolled coughing. With a heaving, distended chest, neck muscles straining, and eyes showing alarm verging on panic, the person can utter only a few brief words between rasping, wheezing, frantic efforts to breathe.

The person puts a tubelike device in his or her mouth and inhales twice. Within minutes, remarkably it seems, the crisis is over. Breathing returns to normal. The person can go back to school or work or even jogging—until the next attack, which might be hours or months away.

Asthma attacks are often milder than this description—just a shortness of breath that soon passes without treatment. But they can also be much, much worse, requiring a hurried trip to the hospital for emergency—sometimes lifesaving—care. Even in severe cases, hospital treatment usually enables asthma patients to regain near-normal breathing. But not always. Almost 5,000 asthma deaths were reported in the United States in 1992, according to the American Lung Association (1992 is the most recent year for which statistics are available). Most of the deaths occurred in patients who misjudged the severity of symptoms or failed to reach a hospital or clinic in time to prevent respiratory failure.

From "Controlling Asthma," by Ken Flieger, in *FDA Consumer* [Online] November 1996. Available: http://www.fda.gov. Produced by the U.S. Food and Drug Administration. For complete contact information, please refer to Chapter 68, "Resources."

Although African-Americans make up approximately 12 percent of the U.S. population, they account for 21 percent of deaths due to asthma, according to the American Lung Association.

For reasons that are not well understood, the number of newly diagnosed cases of asthma in the United States is rising sharply, up 56.7 percent between 1982 and 1992. Asthma deaths, too, are climbing—4,964 in 1992 compared with 2,598 in 1979. Lack of necessary health care, especially among the urban poor, is thought to play an important role in the rising asthma death rate.

Ironically, these increases are taking place at a time when some things believed to be associated with asthma—such as air pollution, dust, molds, and tobacco smoke—are better understood and often under better control than they once were. The reason for the increases remains a mystery, but some investigators think one contributing factor is modern, tightly sealed homes and workplaces that trap and recirculate contaminants, increasing exposure to them in the air we breathe.

Inflamed Airways

Most of America's 12 million to 14 million people with asthma, of whom more than 4 million are under age 18, have a relatively mild illness. About a quarter of asthmatic children seem to "outgrow" their disease in their teen years or as young adults. It's not certain, however, that they are completely free of asthma. Studies of people with late-onset asthma—asthma that first shows up in the fifth or sixth decade of life or even later—have found that many of them experienced asthma-like breathing difficulties as children.

There is no known cure, but most asthma can be controlled by a strategy aimed at preventing acute episodes and halting those that do occur.

This two-pronged attack is increasingly effective because scientists are piecing together a more comprehensive picture of the nature of asthma and gaining new insights into the cause, prevention, and management of acute asthma attacks. New information is changing the way practicing physicians and the Food and Drug Administration view the role of drugs in asthma treatment and prevention.

Changing Theories

Until the 1970s and early 1980s, asthma was understood to result from over-responsiveness of the tubes (bronchi and bronchioles) that carry air to and from the lungs. People with hypersensitive airways, when exposed to certain irritants called "triggers"—such as household dust, tobacco smoke, cat fur (dander), cockroach droppings, air pollutants, even vigorous exercise or cold air—would experience "bronchospasm," a narrowing of the airways caused by contraction of the muscles that encircle the bronchial tubes.

Asthmatics also tend to produce thick, sticky mucus and have inflamed, damaged airways, both of which worsen the breathing restriction caused by bronchospasm. During an acute attack, asthmatics seem to have a hard time getting their breath. Actually they are struggling to push air out of over-inflated lungs through constricted airways.

That understanding of asthma led to treatments aimed primarily at opening up the bronchial tubes by using drugs that cause the bronchial muscles to relax their grip on air passages. Bronchodilators are still a mainstay of asthma therapy. But Robert Meyer, M.D., of FDA's Center for Drug Evaluation and Research, notes that scientists' understanding of asthma has changed significantly over the last decade or so.

He points out that since the early 1980s, increasing scientific evidence shows that inflammation is as much responsible for bronchospasm as anything else. Today, Meyer says, putting primary emphasis on controlling bronchospasm rather than chronic airway inflammation "looks like putting the cart before the horse."

The evidence Meyer refers to strongly indicates that asthma is a chronic inflammatory disease that usually develops within the first few years of life. Much of this evidence is discussed by H.W. Kelly of the University of New Mexico College of Pharmacy in the October 1992 issue of the *Journal of Clinical Pharmacology and Therapeutics.*

In people with asthma, whether mild or severe—even in asthmatics whose first acute attack occurs long after childhood—the air passages are continuously inflamed, causing them to be swollen and to react strongly to inhaled irritants. But because patients may not be aware of any symptoms, this inflammation is sometimes called "the quiet part" of asthma.

People with chronically inflamed airways may show no outward signs of asthma until the first acute attack requires urgent medical attention, often at a hospital emergency department. Emergency care physicians and nurses—who are all too familiar with acute asthma—are able to administer powerful drugs to open the patient's air passages and restore virtually normal breathing. They are likely to recommend the patient be seen by an asthma specialist, who can devise a combination of treatment and prevention measures aimed at avoiding or minimizing further acute asthma attacks. The first step in that process is an accurate diagnosis.

Diagnosing Asthma

The diagnosis of asthma is based on repeated, careful measurements of how efficiently the patient can force air out of the lungs and on a thorough medical history and laboratory tests to find out what "triggers" the patient's acute attacks.

People with asthma react to external irritants in a way that non-asthmatics don't. Many but not all asthmatics have allergies that cause their bodies to produce an abnormal array of chemicals in response to environmental allergens. In that sense, asthma is akin to pollen allergies, hives, and eczema. But in asthma, the allergic reaction contributes to inflammation of the airways rather than of skin, eyes, or nose and throat. An acute asthma attack may come on rapidly after exposure to an irritant or develop slowly over several days or weeks, which can complicate the job of identifying a patient's asthma "triggers."

Which drugs asthma patients need, when to use them, and how much to use depend largely on the character of their illness, as shown by the degree of breathing impairment, and the frequency and severity of acute attacks. Asthma experts agree, however, that the first line of defense is avoidance of whatever brings on an acute asthma episode. Though for most patients "triggers"—there are often more than one—are likely to be common allergens or air pollutants. In some asthmatics, attacks can be brought on by strenuous exercise, exposure to cold outdoor air, industrial or household chemicals (cleaning fluids, for example), and food additives such as sulfites. In other cases, the triggers cannot be identified, even after a thorough investigation.

Asthma Drugs

Knowing what provokes an asthma attack is critically important in prevention, but it's often difficult or impractical to avoid contact with triggering irritants. Today, however, physicians can prescribe drugs to lessen the risk of acute attacks after exposure to an offending irritant, as well as halt attacks that can't be prevented.

The drugs used to treat asthma fall into two broad categories: controllers to prevent acute attacks and relievers that check acute symptoms when they occur. Some drugs do both.

In light of mounting evidence that asthma is fundamentally an inflammatory disease, asthma authorities today regard inhaled corticosteroids—marketed under numerous brand names, including Aerobid, Azmacort, Vanceril, Flovent, and Pulmicort—as the most effective agents for controlling airway inflammation and thus preventing acute asthma attacks. Corticosteroids in pill or tablet form (such as Medrol) and in liquid form for children (such as Pediapred and Prelone) are prescribed for some patients with severe asthma.

Other inhaled anti-inflammatory controller drugs include Intal (cromolyn sodium), which is useful in preventing asthma brought on by exercise, and Tilade (nedrocromil sodium).

A new class of oral anti-inflammatory controller drugs acts by blocking a certain part of the inflammation pathway. This class of "anti-leukotriene" drugs include Zyflo (zileuton), Accolate (zafirlukast) and Singulair (montelukast). Long-acting inhaled bronchodilators, such as Serevent (salmeterol), and long-acting oral bronchodilators, such as Alupent (metaproterenol), Proventil (albuterol sulfate), Theo-24 (theophylline anhydrous), and many others, are often used in conjunction with anti-inflammatory agents to control symptoms. They don't provide immediate relief of symptoms, but their preventive action persists for many hours, which makes them useful in controlling attacks that might occur during hours of sleep.

Drugs to bring quick relief in acute asthma attacks are chiefly short-acting inhaled bronchodilators that act rapidly but for a relatively brief time to relax bronchial constriction. There are many short-acting bronchodilators to chose from, including Alupent or Metaprel (metaproterenol), Brethaire (terbutaline), and Ventolin or Proventil (albuterol). Although these drugs are effective in treating asthma, there is some controversy about their safety, especially when they are overused. Scientific debate makes it clear, however, that an increasing need for inhaled bronchodilators, or a decreasing response to each dose, is a signal that the patient's asthma is not being adequately controlled. Patients who have an increasing need for short-acting inhaled bronchodilators should be reevaluated promptly by their physicians.

Nonprescription Products

Both prescription and over-the-counter (OTC) short-acting bronchodilators are available. The OTC drugs generally contain lesser amounts of the active agent than prescription forms and are effective for a shorter period. They may be useful, however, as temporary treatment for mild asthma attacks. Ready availability in drugstores makes the OTC products potentially helpful as a"stopgap" for patients who do not have their prescription medication at hand when an asthma attack occurs. However, patients who use OTC inhalers should still seek advice from a health professional about the long-term treatment of their asthma.

The key to effective, long-term treatment of asthma is finding the drugs and dosage plan most effective in dealing with or preventing acute episodes. But effective treatment depends as well on the patient and the caregiver knowing what the various anti-asthma drugs do, when and in what amount each drug should be used, when a change in symptoms or in the response to a particular drug requires a call or visit to the physician, and when to get emergency help. Physicians who specialize in treating asthmatics go over these points in detail as part of an overall treatment plan designed and, as necessary, adjusted to meet needs of each individual patient.

A cure for asthma is judged by experts to be still a far-off possibility. But the majority of asthma sufferers can lead essentially normal, symptom-free lives by understanding and sticking to a well-planned strategy to keep clear of asthma triggers and to use the right drugs in the right way. It isn't easy, but it works.

— by Ken Flieger

Ken Flieger is a writer in Washington, D.C.

Chapter 2

Practical and Effective Asthma Care

Asthma Care in the United States Can Be Improved

Undertreatment and inappropriate therapy are major contributors to asthma morbidity and mortality in the United States. A few examples of data that support this assertion are presented below.

* Hospitalizations due to asthma are preventable or avoidable when patients receive appropriate primary care.[2]

    1. Asthma is the third leading cause of preventable hospitalizations in the United States.[2]

    2. There are about 470,000 hospitalizations and more than 5,000 deaths a year from asthma.

* Studies from two metropolitan areas of children with asthma who used the emergency department[3] and adults hospitalized with asthma[4] found that:

    1. Less than half of these patients were receiving anti-inflammatory therapy as recommended in the EPR-2.[1]

Excerpted from "Practical and Effective Asthma Care," in *Practical Guide for the Diagnosis and Management of Asthma,* based on the *Expert Panel Report 2: Guidelines for the Diagnosis and Management of Asthma.* Produced by U.S. Department of Health and Human Services, National Heart, Lung, and Blood Institute (NHLBI), NIH Publication No. 97-4053, October 1997. For complete contact information, please refer to Chapter 68, "Resources."

2. Only 28 percent of the adult patients hospitalized for asthma had written action plans that told how to manage their asthma and control an exacerbation.[4]

Airway Inflammation Plays a Central Role in Asthma and Its Management

The management of asthma needs to be responsive to the characteristics that define asthma.

- **Asthma is a chronic inflammatory disorder of the airways.** Many cells and cellular elements play a role, in particular, mast cells, eosinophils, T-lymphocytes, macrophages, neutrophils, and epithelial cells.

- **Environmental and other factors "cause" or provoke the airway inflammation in people with asthma.** Examples of these factors include inhaled allergens to which the patient is sensitive, some irritants, and viruses. This inflammation is always present to some degree, regardless of the level of asthma severity.

- **Airway inflammation causes recurrent episodes** in asthma patients of wheezing, breathlessness, chest tightness, and coughing, particularly at night and in the early morning.

- These episodes of asthma symptoms are usually associated with widespread but **variable airflow obstruction that is often reversible** either spontaneously or with treatment. Airflow obstruction is caused by a variety of changes in the airway, including bronchoconstriction, airway edema, chronic mucus plug formation, and airway remodeling.

- **Inflammation causes an associated increase in the existing airway hyperresponsiveness** to a variety of stimuli, such as allergens, irritants, cold air, and viruses. These stimuli or **precipitants result in airflow obstruction** and asthma symptoms in the patient with asthma.

Asthma Changes over Time, Requiring Active Management

The condition of a patient's asthma will change depending on the environment, patient activities, management practices, and other factors (see Figure 2.1.). Thus, even when patients have their asthma under control, monitoring and treatment are needed to maintain control.

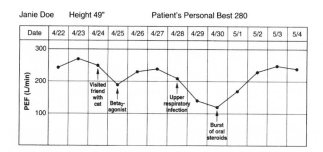

Figure 2.1. *Asthma Changes over Time: Patient Monitoring and Followup Required*

Four Key Components for Long-Term Control of Asthma

The four components of asthma therapy respond to the basic nature of asthma described previously. The four components are listed below.

- Assessment and monitoring
- Pharmacologic therapy
- Control of factors contributing to asthma severity
- Patient education for a partnership

Major Recommendations from the Expert Panel Report 2: Guidelines for the Diagnosis and Management of Asthma[1]

Diagnose asthma and initiate partnership with patient.

- **Diagnose asthma by establishing:**
  1. A history of recurrent symptoms,
  2. Reversible airflow obstruction using spirometry, and

3. The exclusion of alternative diagnoses.

- **Establish patient-clinician partnership.**

    1. Address patient's concerns.

    2. Agree upon the goals of asthma therapy.

    3. Agree upon a written action plan for patient self-management.

Reduce inflammation, symptoms, and exacerbations.

- **Prescribe anti-inflammatory medications to patients with mild, moderate, or severe persistent asthma** (i.e., inhaled steroids, cromolyn, or nedocromil).

- **Reduce exposures to precipitants of asthma symptoms.**

    1. Assess patient's exposure and sensitivity to individual precipitants (e.g., allergens, irritants).

    2. Provide written and verbal instructions on how to avoid or reduce factors that make the patient's asthma worse.

Monitor and manage asthma over time.

- **Train all patients to monitor their asthma.**

    1. All patients should monitor symptoms.

    2. Patients with moderate-to-severe persistent asthma should also monitor their peak flow.

- **See patients at least every 1 to 6 months**

    1. Assess attainment of goals of asthma therapy and patient's concerns,

    2. Adjust treatment, if needed,

    3. Review the action plan with patient, and

    4. Check patient's inhaler and peak flow technique.

Treat asthma episodes promptly.

- **Prompt use of short-acting inhaled beta 2-agonists and, if episode is moderate to severe, a 3- to 10-day course of oral steroids.**

- **Prompt communication and followup with clinician.**

References

1. National Heart, Lung, and Blood Institute, National Asthma Education and Prevention Program. *Expert Panel Report 2: Guidelines for the Diagnosis and Management of Asthma.* National Institutes of Health pub no 97-4051. Bethesda, MD, 1997.

2. Pappas G, Hadden WC, Kozak LJ, Fisher GF. Potentially avoidable hospitalizations: inequalities in rates between US socioeconomic groups. *Am J Public Health* 1997;87:811-16.

3. Friday GA Jr, Khine H, Lin MS, Caliguiri LA. Profile of children requiring emergency treatment for asthma. *Ann Allergy Asthma Immunol* 1997;78:221-224.

4. Hartert TV, Windom HH, Peebles RS Jr, Freidhoff LR, Togias A. Inadequate outpatient medical therapy for patients with asthma admitted to two urban hospitals. *Am J Med* 1996;100:386-394.

Chapter 3

Exercise-Induced Asthma

Exercise-induced asthma (EIA) can affect any susceptible person who exercises, whether he or she is a school child, recreational athlete, or elite athlete. The importance of making the proper diagnosis should not be underrated, since patients who have undiagnosed EIA may not be able to participate in athletic activities. Typical symptoms are coughing, wheezing, chest tightness, and shortness of breath during or after exercise[1,2].

Some patients with EIA have no specific symptoms of asthma but have atypical symptoms such as stomach cramps, chest pain or discomfort, nausea, headache, or feeling out of shape. In addition to those who have asthma symptoms only with exercise, most patients who have chronic asthma have increased symptoms with exertion.

The Sports Medicine Division of the U.S. Olympic Committee convened the Olympic Exercise Asthma Summit Conference in Colorado Springs in December 1994 to discuss the issues surrounding EIA (see "Participants in the Olympic Exercise Asthma Summit Conference" at the end of this article). The scientific findings and treatment recommendations from the conference are summarized below.

Excerpted from "Update on Exercise-Induced Asthma: A Report of the Olympic Exercise Asthma Summit Conference," by William W. Storms, M.D., and David M. Joyner, M.D., in *The Physician and Sportsmedicine,* Vol. 25, No.3 [Online] March 1997. Available: http://www.physsportsmed.com/issues.1997/03mar/storms.htm. © 1997 by McGraw-Hill Companies, Inc., c/o *The Physician and Sportsmedicine,* 4530 W. 77th St., Minneapolis, MN 55435. All rights reserved. Reprinted with permission.

Pathophysiology of EIA

There are two main theories on the pathophysiology of EIA. The water-loss theory[3] holds that loss of water through the bronchial mucosa into the exhaled air during exercise results in local events in the lungs that cause bronchospasm. Heat and water are transferred from the respiratory mucosa into the air in the airways when large volumes of air are moved in and out of the lungs. This leads to changes in the osmolarity, pH, and temperature of the airway epithelium, which may trigger EIA.

The thermal expenditure theory[4] states that EIA is a direct result of heat transfer from the pulmonary vascular bed into the air during and after exercise. Respiratory heat loss occurs during exercise, with heat moving to the exhaled air. This transfer of thermal energy is followed by rewarming after exercise ends, with associated dilation and hyperemia of the bronchiolar vessels. The hyperemia then leads to EIA.

Other theories for EIA have also been proposed[1,2]. One theory is that cold air leads directly to bronchoconstriction; another states that vigorous physical exertion leads to mechanical stimulation of the bronchi and surrounding tissues, leading to EIA. The osmolar theory holds that the hyperpnea of exercise causes changes in the bronchial mucosa, which lead to hyperosmolarity of the cells of the mucosa and submucosa and subsequently to EIA.

Prevalence and Aggravating Factors

The exact prevalence of EIA is unclear, but it appears to affect 15% to 20% of the general population[5-7]. Olympic-caliber athletes were found to have a prevalence of up to 11%[5]. A 1993 study[6] of a healthy military population found respiratory symptoms compatible with EIA in 31% of subjects. Rupp, et al.,[7] reported that 29% of middle school and high school athletes had reductions in FEV1 compatible with EIA, but that not all were symptomatic.

The Sports Medicine Committee of the American Academy of Allergy, Asthma and Immunology has been collecting data on a questionnaire to predict EIA[8]. These questions were put to individuals undergoing exercise challenges for a potential diagnosis of EIA. Affirmative answers to three questions independently contributed to predict a positive exercise challenge indicative of EIA: (1) Have you ever missed school or work because of chest tightness, coughing, wheezing, or prolonged shortness of breath? (2) Do you ever have chest tightness? (3) When you exercise, do you often have wheezing?

These are important questions to ask all school children and rec-reational and competitive athletes to make the diagnosis of EIA. How-ever, questionnaires are not totally predictive of EIA because some individuals have negative answers on the questionnaire but a posi-tive exercise challenge.

Many factors can influence the severity of EIA (Table 3.1.). First, the type of exercise is important, with free running being more asth-mogenic than treadmill exercise, stationary cycling, or swimming. Workload—the work itself and the rate at which it is performed—is important. Environmental factors play a significant role; for example, cold, dry air can be a potent stimulus. Other environmental factors include air pollution, particulates, smoke, and allergens.

Table 3.1. Factors That Affect the Severity of Exercise-Induced Asthma

Difficulty and Duration of Exercise
E.g., free running, treadmill, cycle ergometer

Environmental Factors
Ambient temperature and humidity
Cold air
Rapid rewarming
Air pollutants: SO_2 [sulphur dioxide], NO_2 [nitrogen dioxide], particu-lates, ozone, tobacco smoke, wood smoke, etc.
Airborne allergens

Patient's Health and Habits
Respiratory infections: Sinusitis, bronchitis
Lack of warm-up

These potential aggravating factors for EIA are important for the athlete and the physician to know, since preventive therapy may re-duce the severity of EIA. It may be best for recreational athletes or those in training to exercise indoors on very cold days and, if they have an allergy to pollen, to avoid outdoor exercise when pollen counts are high. Competitive athletes do not have a choice of when or where they compete, but they should be aware of the potential aggravating factors and adjust their medication appropriately to control these factors.

Diagnosis of EIA

The diagnosis of EIA is often made on the basis of a history alone, but the patient may not spontaneously seek medical attention for this condition. Reports of symptoms, therefore, may need to be elicited by questioning during school physicals or routine physical examinations.

If a patient reports possible symptoms but the history leaves the diagnosis in doubt, pulmonary function tests (PFTs) at rest should be performed. Abnormal PFTs indicate that the patient needs daily asthma therapy and preexercise treatment. Normal PFTs, however, dictate that the patient should be treated for EIA. If the diagnosis is in doubt, hand-held peak flow meters are useful for testing because they are portable and easy to use in the field.

If the diagnosis is in doubt after peak flow testing, or if pretreatment with an inhaled beta-agonist before exercise does not help, spirometry with flow-volume curves should be performed before and after exercise on different days with and without pretreatment with an inhaled beta-agonist. The pulmonary function measurement should be performed before exercise and at 1, 5, 10, and 25 minutes after exercise. If no symptoms occur with the exercise challenge, the patient should be tested with exercise in his or her own sport.

Asthma or EIA? An important distinction must be made: Does the patient have solitary EIA or mild, chronic, persistent asthma with exercise-induced exacerbations? This distinction is critical in regard to treatment, because nearly all EIA patients require only preexercise treatment, whereas those with persistent asthma require daily anti-inflammatory therapy plus preexercise treatment.

The distinction between solitary EIA and persistent asthma is best made by pulmonary function testing at rest. In the patient with solitary EIA, the results will be normal; in the patient with chronic persistent asthma, pulmonary function will be lower than normal. This testing can easily be done in the physician's office or clinic using a small computerized spirometer.

Nonpharmacologic Treatment

Extended warm-ups before exercise may help reduce the severity of EIA, but they do not replace pharmacologic therapy. Physicians can suggest that patients perform "subthreshold exercise" before their regular workout, carefully explaining that patients need to warm up vigorously at a level just below their maximum exercise level. For the recreational athlete who is jogging, for instance, this would mean stretching and walking, then starting slowly for the first 8 to 10 minutes. The term "subthreshold exercise" rather than "warm-up" is suggested when dealing with active patients because a warm-up can mean anything from stretching to sprinting for different people.

For patients who have a choice, exercising in a warm, humid environment is better than a cold, dry environment. Also, short-burst activities like tennis will tend to exacerbate EIA less than will prolonged, steady exercise like running.

Drug Therapy

A variety of medications are available for treating EIA (Table 3.2.), by either the inhaled or oral routes; it is important for the physician to know which are first-line drugs, second-line drugs, etc. (see below)[9]. It is particularly important to tailor drug therapy to the individual patient and his or her athletic event. For example, a wrestler participating in a 5-hour meet may have his EIA controlled best by salmeterol before the meet rather than repeated doses of albuterol. Not only are the correct medications important, but follow-up visits are crucial to ensure that the treatment is controlling the problem and to assess whether adjustments are needed.

The first drug usually chosen for control of EIA is a short-acting beta-agonist such as albuterol, metaproterenol sulfate, pirbuterol acetate, or terbutaline sulfate. The beta-agonist is administered via a metered-dose inhaler or dry powder inhaler about 15 to 30 minutes before exercise. The potential side effects are tremor and palpitations. An alternative is long-acting salmeterol[10], which can be given 30 to 60 minutes before exercise and may control EIA as long as 12 hours. Salmeterol is quite useful in school children, since it may be taken before school and should protect the patient for the entire day.

Cromolyn sodium or nedocromil sodium can also be given before exercise either alone or in combination with a beta-agonist[11]. Some physicians use cromolyn or nedocromil as first-line therapy, and it can be effective in many patients. As a general rule, either cromolyn or nedocromil or a beta-agonist is the drug of first choice, and then a drug from the other class is added in combination if the initial single-dose therapy is not adequate.

Some athletes may require a higher dose of cromolyn or nedocromil to block EIA; the dose of either of these can be increased to four puffs immediately before exercise. If these measures are not adequate to control the EIA, workshop participants suggested that ipratropium bromide can be used on a trial basis as an additional preexercise treatment.

If the patient does not obtain control of EIA with the above therapy, then daily inhaled corticosteroids should be considered. At this point, however, the patient's asthma should be re-evaluated to see if the individual is suffering from chronic persistent asthma with exercise-induced exacerbation. If this is the case, then daily anti-inflammatory inhalers (cromolyn, nedocromil, inhaled steroids) should be used for maintenance management and an inhaled beta-agonist, cromolyn, or nedocromil before exercise.

If inhaled steroids are used, the dosage is 8 to 16 puffs per day of beclomethasone dipropionate or triamcinolone acetonide, or four puffs a day of flunisolide or equivalent doses of fluticasone propionate. For cromolyn or nedocromil, the dosage is two puffs four times a day. Daily oral theophylline (5 to 10 mg/kg/day in divided doses) might also be considered.

Table 3.2. Pharmacotherapy for Exercise-Induced Asthma*

Medication	Dose	Time Taken Before Exercise	Duration of Effect	Potential Side Effects
Short-acting beta-agonists	2-4 puffs by MDI	15-30 min	2 hr	Tremor, palpitations
Salmeterol	2 puffs by MDI (not to exceed 2 puffs every 12 hr; not to be used as rescue)	30-60 min	12 hr	Tremor, palpitations
Cromolyn sodium or nedocromil sodium	2-4 puffs by MDI	10-20 min	2 hr	None
Inhaled cortico-steroids	8-16 puffs/day	Weeks**	Weeks**	Dose related
Ipratropium bromide	2-4 puffs by MDI	1 hr	2-3 hr	None
Oral theophylline	5-10 mg/kg/day in divided doses	Days**	Hours**	Nausea, tremor

MDI = metered dose inhaler

For lists of allowed, banned, and restricted substances and methods, refer to the rules and regulations or the sponsoring or governing organization for the relevant sport or contest.

**Ongoing therapy*

With either a recreational or an elite athlete, a specialist consultation should be considered if symptoms are not controlled with treatment. Other conditions can masquerade as EIA.

Recognizing the Underrecognized

Exercise-induced asthma is underrecognized and underdiagnosed, so physicians need to look for it in all patients, including school children. Appropriate treatment should prevent EIA in most patients, and those with asthma or EIA can participate in athletics, even at an elite level. For competitive athletes, the applicable sports governing organization should be consulted for its list of allowed and banned substances and pertinent regulations.

Participants in the Olympic Exercise Asthma Summit Conference*

William W. Storms, M.D., Colorado Springs (cochair)

David M. Joyner, M.D., Colorado Springs (cochair)

Paris Amani, Colorado Springs

Tom W. Bartsokas, M.D., Franklin, Tennessee

Bob Beeten, A.T.C., Colorado Springs

Peter Creticos, M.D., Baltimore

M. Craig Ferrell, M.D., Franklin, Tennessee

Clifton T. Furukawa, M.D., Seattle

Kenneth Knight, Ph.D., Terre Haute, Indiana

Roger M. Katz, M.D., Los Angeles

Roger Kruse, M.D., Maumee, Ohio

George L. Landry, M.D., Madison, Wisconsin

John L. Lehtinen, M.D., Marquette, Michigan

Reuben Lomax, Colorado Springs

Jean Lopez, Colorado Springs

David Montaluo, Colorado Springs

E. R. McFadden, Jr., M.D., Cleveland

Harold S. Nelson, M.D., Denver

Sean O'Donnell, M.D., Colorado Springs

Margaret Peter, A.T.C., Colorado Springs

Lt. Colonel John Reasoner, Jr., M.D., Fort Carson, Colorado

Troy V. Reese, Pharm.D., Colorado Springs

Denise Richardson, P.T., A.T.C., Huntington Beach, California

William S. Silvers, M.D., Englewood, Colorado

Jenny Stone, A.T.C., Colorado Springs

David Tinkelman, M.D., Augusta, Georgia

John M. Weiler, M.D., Iowa City, Iowa

*The conference, held in December 1994 in Colorado Springs, was supported by an unrestricted grant from Glaxo Wellcome.

References

1. Kumar A, Busse WW: Recognizing and controlling exercise-induced asthma. *J Respir Dis* 1995;16(12):1087-1096

2. McFadden ER Jr, Gilbert IA: Exercise-induced asthma. *N Engl J Med* 1994;330(19):1362-1367

3. Anderson SD, Daviskas E: An evaluation of the airway cooling and rewarming hypothesis as the mechanism for exercise-induced asthma, in Holgate ST (ed): *Asthma, Physiology, Immunopharmacology, and Treatment: Fourth International Symposium*. London, Academic Press, 1993

4. McFadden ER, Gilbert IA: Vascular responses and thermally induced asthma, in Holgate ST (ed): *Asthma, Physiology, Immunopharmacology and Treatment: Fourth International Symposium*. London, Academic Press, 1993

5. Voy RO: The U.S. Olympic Committee experience with exercise-induced bronchospasm, 1984. *Med Sports Exerc* 1986;18(3):328-330

6. O'Donnell AE, Fling J: Exercise-induced airflow obstruction in a healthy military population. *Chest* 1993;103(3):742-744

7. Rupp NT, Guill MF, Brudno DS: Unrecognized exercise-induced bronchospasm in adolescent athletes. *Am J Dis Child* 1992;146(8):941-944

8. Weiler JM: Use of questionnaires to predict exercise-induced asthma. Read before the Olympic Asthma Summit Conference, Colorado Springs, December 1994

9. Bierman CW: Management of exercise-induced asthma, editorial. *Ann Allergy* 1992;68(2):119-122

10. Kemp J, Bukstein D, Busse W, et al., Effect of salmeterol, albuterol, and placebo in the prevention of exercise-induced bronchospasm. *Chest* 1993;104(2 suppl):10S

11. Morton AR, Ogle SL, Fitch KD: Effects of nedocromil sodium, cromolyn sodium, and a placebo in exercise-induced asthma. *Ann Allergy* 1992;68(2):143-148

— by William W. Storms, M.D., and David M. Joyner, M.D.

Dr. Storms is an allergist in private practice in Colorado Springs and was cochair of the Olympic Exercise Asthma Summit Conference. Dr. Joyner is an orthopedic surgeon in private practice in Harrisburg, Pennsylvania, is the chair of the U.S. Olympic Sports Medicine Committee, and was cochair of the Olympic Exercise Asthma Summit Conference. Address correspondence to William W. Storms, M.D., Asthma and Allergy Associates, PC, 2709 N. Tejon St., Colorado Springs, CO 80907; e-mail to sneezedoc@aol.com.

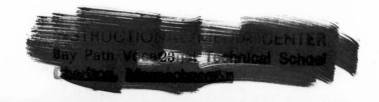

Chapter 4

Sinusitis

Sinuses are a part of the upper respiratory system. The sinuses function to lighten the skull and improve the quality of the voice. Adults and older children have four groups of sinus cavities located within the bones surrounding the nose. Very young children, however, have small sinus passages rather than fully formed sinuses. To work properly, the sinuses need adequate mucus drainage and a functioning immune system to fight off infections.

What Is Sinusitis?

Sinusitis is an inflammation of the mucous membranes that line the sinus cavities. This inflammation causes the mucous glands in the sinuses to secrete more mucus. A significant amount of inflammation and mucus can lead to obstruction of the sinuses, preventing drainage.

The common cold, allergic rhinitis or hay fever, chronic rhinitis, deviated septum, and nasal polyps can cause swelling of the nasal and sinus passages and lead to sinusitis. Also, smoking or the breathing in of second-hand smoke interferes with normal functioning of the sinuses, leading to sinusitis. Diseases such as cystic fibrosis, bronchiectasis, immune deficiencies, and immotile cilia syndrome can also

From "Med Facts: Sinusitis," [Online] Undated. Available: http://www.njc. org/MFhtml/SIN_MF.html. © 1993 by the National Jewish Medical and Research Center, 1400 Jackson St., Denver, Colorado 80206. Reprinted with permission. For complete contact information, please refer to Chapter 68, "Resources."

cause sinusitis. Very young children may be prone to developing sinusitis because their smaller sinus passages become obstructed more easily than those of adults.

What Are the Symptoms?

Sinusitis can either be acute or chronic. Acute sinusitis is usually caused by a secondary bacterial infection. It may be characterized by short term episodes with headache or pain in the area of the affected sinus, nasal obstruction, postnasal drip, cough, sore throat, and thick, yellow to green nasal drainage. If you have chronic sinusitis, which is often not associated with an infection, you may experience recurrent episodes or continuing symptoms that do not respond to treatment. These symptoms are more subtle and generally do not include headache or fever. In fact, some persons with X-ray evidence of chronic sinusitis have no symptoms.

How Is It Diagnosed?

A clinician diagnoses sinusitis after obtaining a complete medical history and physical examination. Many clinicians will obtain an X-ray of your sinuses, which can show thickening of the membrane lining and clouding by accumulation of fluid in the sinuses. As noted earlier, many people with no symptoms of sinusitis have these abnormal findings on their X-rays. This is especially true for people with asthma.

What Is the Treatment?

In treating sinusitis, the goal is to decrease the swelling and inflammation in the nose and sinus opening to improve sinus drainage. Your clinician will treat an infection, if present, and try to reduce the symptoms of a runny or stuffy nose.

Clinicians at National Jewish often recommend the following treatments:

- **Nasal Wash**—A saltwater, or saline nasal wash helps remove mucus and bacteria from the nose and sinuses. This can temporarily reduce symptoms of nasal obstruction and postnasal drip. We recommend doing a nasal wash prior to using a corticosteroid nasal spray. After performing a nasal wash, wait ten to fifteen minutes until the draining stops; then use your nasal spray as prescribed by your clinician.

- **Antibiotics**—In many cases of sinusitis, a bacteria infects the sinuses. Such an infection can be difficult to treat because the bacteria thrive in the warm, moist, and dark areas of the sinus cavities. These infections usually respond slowly to antibiotic treatment; therefore, you may need to continue medication for two to three weeks or longer. The choice of antibiotic depends on several factors such as: drug allergies, past use of antibiotics, and your particular symptoms.

- **Corticosteroid nasal spray**—A prescription corticosteroid nasal spray can decrease nasal inflammation and mucus production. This will lessen symptoms of nasal obstruction and help promote normal sinus drainage. A corticosteroid nasal spray does not provide immediate relief of symptoms however, and can require several weeks of routine use to be effective. If you have chronic sinusitis, you may benefit from continued daily use of this medication. If you have occasional sinusitis episodes, you may only require periodic use. Clinicians at National Jewish have had success in treating many cases of sinusitis with a combination of the nasal wash followed by a corticosteroid nasal spray. Several corticosteroid nasal sprays are available and include beclomethasone (Beconase®, Beconase AQ®, Vancenase®, Vancenase AQ®), triamcinolone (Nasacort®), and flunisolide (Nasalide®). Because there is little absorption of the medication into the bloodstream, the risk of systemic steroid side effects is extremely low. Local side effects that may occur are sensations of nasal burning or irritation and mild nosebleeds.

- **Decongestants**—These medications, available as tablet, syrup, or nasal spray, help unblock the openings of the sinuses and temporarily reduce symptoms of nasal obstruction. Although you can buy most decongestants without a prescription, follow your clinician's guidelines. We do not recommend prolonged use of a decongestant nasal spray because it can cause rebound congestion with increased symptoms. Commonly used decongestants include pseudoephedrine and phenylpropanolamine. Side effects can include shaking, restlessness, and urinary retention.

- **Antihistamines**—Antihistamines in tablet or syrup form help reduce mucus production. They can also reduce sneezing and itching associated with allergic rhinitis (hay fever). Many over-the-counter preparations are available and include chlorpheniramine and brompheniramine. Antihistamine side effects may include drowsiness, dry mouth, and urinary retention. A newer class of prescription antihistamines does not cause drowsiness; they include terfenadine (Seldane®), astemizole (Hismanal®), and loratadine (Claritin®).

- **Pain Relievers**—A medication to relieve pain and lessen fever may help in sinusitis, especially for acute episodes. Your clinician may recommend a medication such as acetaminophen (Tylenol®), ibuprofen or aspirin, or prescribe a stronger medication. Because some persons with asthma are sensitive to aspirin or ibuprofen, check with your clinician before taking this medication.

- **Surgery**—Occasionally, stubborn sinus infections that don't respond to aggressive medical treatment require surgery to remove the diseased tissue and restore sinus drainage. There are several surgical procedures available and your clinician can provide more information on these options. Surgery for children with chronic sinusitis is rarely indicated.

What Is the Role of National Jewish?

Clinicians at National Jewish have been evaluating, treating, and researching sinusitis for many years. Current studies include weighing the role of sinusitis as a trigger of asthma. Center scientists continue to evaluate medical and surgical methods of treatment while investigating new therapies that are more effective and less costly.

Chapter 5

Rhinitis Update: A Guide to Diagnosis and Treatment

Rhinitis is sometimes viewed—erroneously—as a trivial condition. But congestion and rhinorrhea—as well as fatigue, headache, cognitive impairment, and other systemic symptoms—can seriously diminish a patient's quality of life. Rhinitis is a significant cause of student absenteeism; it is responsible for more than 2 million lost school days in the United States annually. Direct treatment costs and indirect costs related to lost workplace productivity were estimated at $2.7 billion in 1995.

Here I present highlights of the recently published guidelines for the differential diagnosis and assessment of rhinitis developed by the Joint Task Force on Practice Parameters in Allergy, Asthma, and Immunology.[1] In [the second half of this chapter], I will recap the Task Force guidelines on therapy.

Differential Diagnosis

Rhinitis—an inflammation of the membranes lining the nose—is characterized by nasal congestion, rhinorrhea, sneezing, pruritus, and/or postnasal drainage; it may be caused by allergic, nonallergic, infectious, hormonal, occupational, or other factors. Allergic rhinitis is the most common form; it affects 10% to 30% of adults and up to

40% of children—but other causes often go unrecognized. The result is suboptimal control.

Allergic rhinitis. The severity of this condition ranges from mild to seriously debilitating. Symptoms can be classified as follows:

- Seasonal. Symptoms are caused by an IgE-mediated reaction to aeroallergens (such as pollens and molds).
- Perennial symptoms without seasonal exacerbation.
- Perennial with seasonal exacerbation. Symptoms are caused by an IgE-mediated reaction to perennial and seasonal environmental aeroallergens (such as dust mites, molds, pollen, and animal and occupational allergens).
- Sporadic. Symptoms erupt after specific exposures.

The amount of allergen required to induce an immediate response decreases each time an allergic patient is exposed to an allergen. Moreover, exposure to one allergen may promote a more exaggerated later response to another. This phenomenon reinforces the need to initiate effective anti-inflammatory therapies before pollen seasons.

Nonallergic rhinitis. These forms of rhinitis are characterized by sporadic or persistent perennial symptoms that are not IgE-mediated. When inflammatory cells are present in the mucosa, nonallergic rhinitis can be classified by inflammatory cell type:

- Infectious (acute or chronic). Symptoms of acute viral rhinitis include rhinorrhea, nasal obstruction, sneezing, and fever. A common complication is a secondary bacterial infection with sinus involvement and lingering symptoms of mucopurulent nasal discharge, facial pain and pressure, olfactory disturbances, and postnasal drainage and cough.
- Nonallergic without eosinophilia (vasomotor). Patients with vasomotor rhinitis have chronic nasal symptoms that are not immunologic or infectious and usually not associated with nasal eosinophilia. Symptoms develop in response to environmental conditions, such as cold air, high humidity, strong odors, and inhaled irritants.
- Nonallergic rhinitis with eosinophilia syndrome (NARES). This syndrome is marked by perennial sneezing, watery rhinorrhea,

nasal pruritus, and occasionally loss of sense of smell. Persons with NARES do not test positive for allergy—or there is no correlation between environmental exposures and allergens to which they may test positive—but they do have eosinophilia.

- Occupational. Symptoms of occupational rhinitis, like those of occupational asthma, are a response to airborne substances in the workplace (such as laboratory animal antigen, grain wood dusts, and chemicals) that may be mediated by allergic or nonallergic factors. This type of rhinitis often coexists with occupational asthma.

- Hormonal. Pregnancy, puberty, and hypothyroidism can provoke rhinitis symptoms. During pregnancy, symptoms may erupt from the second month to term but usually disappear after delivery.

- Drug-induced. Antihypertensive medications are the most frequently cited culprits. Angiotensin-converting enzyme inhibitors, reserpine, guanethidine, phentolamine, methyldopa, prazosin, beta blockers, chlorpromazine, aspirin and other antiinflammatory drugs, and oral contraceptives can all cause rhinitis. Repetitive use of topical alpha adrenergic nasal decongestant sprays (e.g., oxymetazoline or phenylephrine) for more than 5 to 7 days may induce rebound nasal congestion on withdrawal. Prolonged use of these nasally inhaled vasoconstrictor agents can produce a hypertrophy of the nasal mucosa known as rhinitis medicamentosa. The nasal mucosa is often beefy-red, appears inflamed, and shows areas of punctate bleeding and scant mucus. Cocaine also may produce rhinitis when used repeatedly.

- Food-related. Rhinitis following ingestion of certain foods or alcoholic products may result from vagally mediated mechanisms, nasal vasodilation, food allergy, or other causes. Rhinitis from food allergy rarely occurs without concomitant gastrointestinal, dermatologic, or systemic manifestations.

Conditions that mimic rhinitis. Nasal septal deviation, tumors, adenoidal hypertrophy, and hypertrophy of the nasal turbinates may mimic the signs and symptoms of rhinitis.

Nasal polyps. Always consider nasal polyps in the differential diagnosis of patients with invariant nasal congestion. Between 10% and 15% of patients with allergic rhinitis also have nasal polyps.

However, nasal polyps may occur in conjunction with chronic rhinitis or sinusitis of any cause and may contribute significantly to the patient's symptoms. When nasal polyps appear in children, consider the possibility of cystic fibrosis. In adults, nasal polyps may be associated with aspirin sensitivity and asthma.

Evaluation

Factors that increase the risk of allergic rhinitis include:

- A family history of atopy.
- Higher socioeconomic class.
- Exposure to indoor allergens.
- A positive allergy skin prick test

History. The complete history usually determines whether a diagnosis of rhinitis is appropriate.

- Symptoms. Do they occur daily, episodically, seasonally, or perennially? If seasonal, when and where do they occur? Do symptoms emerge after exposure to specific allergens in the workplace, or in response to weather? How long do symptoms last? Are they severe? Has severity increased, decreased, or remained the same? Does obstruction occur consistently on the same side (suggesting a polyp, foreign body, structural problem, or [rarely] tumor)? How is quality of life affected?

- Medication. Has the patient responded favorably in the past to antihistamines or intranasal corticosteroids? Is the patient taking a drug that can cause rhinitis?

- Medical history. Is there a history of other allergic conditions, such as asthma, conjunctivitis, or eczema? Is there a history of nasal trauma? Is the family history significant?

Physical examination. All patients with rhinitis should have an examination of the nose that includes assessment of the nasal passageways, secretions, turbinates, and septum and a search for nasal polyps. The nasopharynx can be examined using indirect mirror visualization or fiberoptic endoscopy.

- General. Do you observe facial pallor, mouth breathing, nasal crease, "allergic shiners," or evidence of systemic disease (such as nail clubbing)? What about eczema, skin dryness, and dermographism?

- Eyes. Is there evidence of conjunctivitis or Dennie-Morgan lines (accentuated lines or folds below the margin of the inferior eyelid)?

- Nose. Is the nose externally deformed? Can you see nasal mucosal swelling, polyps, deviated septum, septal perforation, discharge, or blood?

- Ears. Are there abnormalities of the tympanic membranes, including retraction, air-fluid levels, bubbles behind the tympanic membranes, or abnormal mobility patterns revealed by pneumatic otoscopy?

- Mouth. Is there tonsillar hypertrophy, lymphoid "streaking" in the oropharynx, pharyngeal postnasal discharge, or halitosis? Is there pain when the mouth closes (suggesting temporomandibular joint syndrome)? In children, can you detect malocclusion or high-arched palate associated with chronic mouth breathing?

- Neck. Does examination show lymphadenopathy or enlargement of the thyroid gland?

Testing for specific IgE. Skin testing for allergens is useful to provide evidence of allergy, to confirm suspected causes of the patient's symptoms, or to assess sensitivity to a specific allergen.

Special diagnostic techniques. Special techniques may be useful in certain cases. These include:

- Upper airway endoscopy. This technique provides a clear view of the nasal cavity and is the most useful diagnostic procedure when evaluating anatomic factors causing upper airway symptoms.

- Imaging techniques. Standard radiography, CT, and MRI establish the presence and extent of anatomic disease and provide an accurate reproduction of the anatomy.

- Rhinomanometry. This measures functional obstruction to airflow in the upper airway.

- Nasal cytology. There is no consensus about whether nasal cytology should be used routinely, but it is considered helpful in differentiating allergic rhinitis and NARES from other forms of rhinitis (such as vasomotor or infectious rhinitis).

33

Treatment

Fundamental to the management of rhinitis is the identification and avoidance of provoking factors, which include a wide range of allergic, nonallergic, and infectious triggers. Effective treatment is also greatly facilitated by appropriate use of pharmacologic agents.

In [the first half of this chapter], I reviewed the assessment of rhinitis in accordance with guidelines recently developed by the Joint Task Force on Practice Parameters in Allergy, Asthma, and Immunology published in the *Annals of Allergy, Asthma, and Immunology*. Here I follow up with management recommendations.

Environmental Control Measures

Effective treatment of rhinitis includes identification of triggers— such as allergens, irritants, and medications—and the implementation of effective avoidance measures. Whenever possible, enlist family cooperation.

The major classes of allergic rhinitis triggers include the following:

- Pollens. Tolerance of unavoidable triggers (such as airborne pollen) may be improved by avoidance of other allergens. Tell patients to keep doors and windows closed and to keep air-conditioning vents closed when air-conditioning is used. Remind them that indoor pollen levels are increased by window or attic fans, and that a shower or bath after outdoor activity removes pollen from the hair and skin.

- Molds. Make sure patients understand that exposure to outdoor molds is increased by walking in uncut fields and that activities such as mowing and threshing may result in very high levels of exposure. Indoor molds proliferate in damp homes, basements, cold outside walls, sinks, shower stalls, carpeting, bedding, and upholstered furniture. Mold-sensitive patients should avoid console humidifiers and cool-mist vaporizers, which are reservoirs for mold unless kept scrupulously clean. Chemical and physical measures to control indoor mold usually fail unless relative humidity and condensation are reduced.

- House dust mites. Encourage patients to avoid having carpets and upholstered furniture in their homes, to wash bedclothes in hot water (above 54.4° C [130° F]), and to decrease indoor humidity to reduce levels of dust mite allergen. They should cover mattresses, box springs, and pillows in zippered, allergen-proof casings.

- Animal allergens. The key to preventing exposure to cat or dog allergen is to remove the animal from the home. A trial removal is usually deceptive because it takes 20 weeks or longer for the allergen to dissipate. If the patient or patient's family is not willing to part with the animal, the next option is to confine the animal to an uncarpeted room—but not the patient's bedroom.

- Insect allergens. Cockroaches are a significant cause of respiratory allergy. When ordinary sanitation methods and "roach traps" fail, recommend extermination. Changing homes may be a necessary last resort.

Pharmacologic Therapy

It is important to establish the correct diagnosis before beginning therapy. Initial treatment of mild rhinitis may include avoidance measures and single-agent or combination pharmacologic therapy. Compliance with treatment is enhanced when:

- The patient has written instructions.
- Fewer daily doses are required.
- The patient schedules when doses are to be taken.
- There is a good physician-patient relationship.

When the onset of symptoms can be anticipated (as in the case of seasonal rhinitis), consider prophylactic use of medications to lessen the impact of exposure.

Antihistamines. Second-generation antihistamines are now preferred to first-generation antihistamines in most cases. Sedation and performance impairment—side effects associated with first-generation antihistamines—have been shown to cause problems ranging from learning difficulties to occupational and traffic accidents. Even when administered at bedtime, these agents can cause significant daytime sedation; decrease alertness; and impair performance in reaction time, visual-motor coordination, memory, learning, and driving. Alcohol, sedatives, hypnotics, and antidepressants may potentiate these effects.

However, there are some circumstances in which the use of first-generation antihistamines may be appropriate. When small children are agitated from the discomfort of rhinitis, mild sedation may be beneficial. The anticholinergic side effects of first-generation antihistamines are sometimes desirable because they may help reduce nasal secretions, but dry mouth and urinary retention may result.

The second-generation antihistamines—astemizole, cetirizine, fexofenadine, and loratadine—decrease sneezing, itching, nasal discharge, and the ocular symptoms of allergic conjunctivitis (Table 5.1.). Although they are probably no more effective than the first-generation agents, they do not have the same sedating effects.

Astemizole (and terfenadine, which was withdrawn from the U.S. market in 1998) may produce undesirable side effects at higher than recommended doses or if taken concurrently with azole antifungals (such as fluconazole, itraconazole, and miconazole), some macrolides (such as erythromycin and clarithromycin), or ciprofloxacin. Instruct patients to take antihistamines 2 to 5 hours before allergen exposure. Although effective on an "as-needed" basis, they work best when taken regularly. Nasal congestion is not relieved by oral antihistamines.

Intranasal antihistamines are appropriate first-line treatment for the symptoms of allergic rhinitis or in combination with intranasal corticosteroids or oral antihistamines. Unlike oral antihistamines, they may help reduce nasal congestion. However, patients may find their taste bitter, and they may cause sedation.

Table 5.1. Guidelines for the Use of Second-Generation Oral Antihistamines

Agent	Usual adult dosage	Available with decongestant?	Reduce dosage with liver disease?	Reduce dosage with renal impairment?
Astemizole	10 mg/d	No	Avoid	No
Cetirizine	5 or 10 mg/d	No	5 mg/d	5 mg/d
Fexofenadine	60 mg twice daily	Yes	No	60 mg/d
Loratadine	10 mg/d	Yes	Start at 10 mg every other day	Start at 10 mg every other day

Adapted from Dykewicz MS et al. *Ann Allergy Asthma Immunol.* 1998.[1]

Azelastine is the first intranasal antihistamine preparation approved for use in the United States. Recommended dosing is 2 sprays in each nostril twice daily for patients 12 years or older.

Oral and intranasal decongestants. An oral decongestant, such as pseudoephedrine, phenylephrine, or phenylpropanolamine, may be needed to manage nasal congestion. Prescribe these agents with caution for patients with arrhythmias, coronary heart disease, hypertension, hyperthyroidism, glaucoma, diabetes, or urinary dysfunction. Side effects may include elevated blood pressure, palpitations, loss of appetite, tremor, and sleep disturbance. The disadvantage of antihistamine-decongestant formulations is that the dose of each ingredient cannot be adjusted.

Intranasal decongestants can be useful for short-term (2 to 3 days) control of nasal congestion associated with rhinitis. These agents are not usually associated with systemic sympathomimetic reactions.

Intranasal corticosteroids. These agents most effectively control the symptoms of allergic rhinitis (Table 5.2.). Intranasal corticosteroids are particularly useful for treating more severe allergic rhinitis and—except for intranasal dexamethasone—generally are not associated with significant systemic side effects in adults. Compared with first- and second-generation antihistamines, intranasal corticosteroids provide less relief of ocular symptoms but more effectively improve allergic rhinitis symptoms.

Although local side effects are minimal if the patient is instructed in the proper use of these agents, nasal irritation and bleeding may occur. Tell patients to direct the spray away from the nasal septum to prevent repetitive direct application. Examine the nasal septum periodically to ensure that mucosal erosions do not develop; in rare instances, these may lead to nasal septal perforation.

Oral and parenteral corticosteroids. Although systemic corticosteroids are not appropriate for treating chronic rhinitis, short oral courses (3 to 7 days) may help manage very severe or intractable nasal symptoms or significant nasal polyposis. Adrenal suppression in adults is avoided with short courses at dosages equivalent to 40 mg/d of prednisone. The use of parenteral corticosteroids (particularly if administered recurrently) is discouraged because of greater potential for long-term corticosteroid side effects. Before initiating treatment with systemic corticosteroids, consider the use of intranasal corticosteroids.

Table 5.2. Recommended Dosages of Intranasal Corticosteroids

Agent	Dose per inhalation (µg)	Initial adult dosage
Beclomethasone	42	1 or 2 sprays per nostril twice daily
Budesonide	32	2 sprays per nostril twice daily or 4 sprays per nostril daily
Flunisolide	25	2 sprays per nostril twice daily
Fluticasone	50	2 sprays per nostril daily or 1 spray per nostril twice daily
Mometasone	50	2 sprays per nostril daily
Triamcinolone acetonide	55	2 sprays per nostril daily
Dexamethasone sodium phosphate	84	2 sprays per nostril 2 or 3 times daily

Adapted from Dykewicz MS et al. *Ann Allergy Asthma Immunol.* 1998.[1]

Intranasal cromolyn. Pretreatment with this agent before an anticipated allergen exposure will result in considerable diminution or ablation of the nasal allergic response. If the patient has a seasonal allergy, be sure to use cromolyn as early in the allergy season as possible. Cromolyn is also effective when used regularly during the period of exposure normally associated with allergic symptoms. The starting dosage is 1 spray in each nostril every 4 hours (during waking hours), until relief is evident. Usually, benefit is noted within 4 to 7 days, but severe cases may require several weeks of treatment for maximum effect. Maintenance treatment usually requires dosing three or four times daily.

Cromolyn is generally less effective than intranasal corticosteroids,[2] but because of its good safety profile, it is appropriate for very young children and for pregnant women. Intranasal cromolyn and intranasal antihistamines provide comparable control of allergic rhinitis.

Intranasal anticholinergics. These agents may effectively reduce rhinorrhea, but they have no effect on other nasal symptoms. Although side effects are minimal, dryness of the nasal membranes may occur. Ipratropium is the most extensively studied intranasal anticholinergic. The recommended regimen is 2 sprays in each nostril two or three times a day.

Oral antileukotriene agents. The role of these agents in the treatment of allergic rhinitis remains to be determined.

Allergen Immunotherapy

Immunotherapy may be appropriate for persons with yearly recurrent seasonal symptoms, perennial symptoms due to allergic factors, and/or significant progression of symptoms. It is generally unnecessary for persons with sensitivity to only one seasonal allergen when seasonal exposure is short.

With rare exceptions, immunotherapy is inappropriate for preschool children and elderly persons. Severe pulmonary and cardiovascular disease and the concurrent use of beta blockers are also contraindications.

Immunotherapy is best administered only by professionals familiar with the procedure who are prepared to manage anaphylaxis. Treatment should not be indefinite; generally, a 3- to 5-year period is appropriate.

Concomitant Asthma

Clinical evidence has shown that treatment of rhinitis can improve the status of coexisting asthma. For example, an intranasal corticosteroid can prevent a seasonal increase in bronchial hyperresponsiveness in patients with allergic rhinitis and asthma. In placebo-controlled trials, conventional dosages of cetirizine, fexofenadine, loratadine, and oral decongestants improved asthma symptoms and pulmonary function in patients with concomitant allergic rhinitis.

Persons with concomitant asthma may be candidates for immunotherapy, but their asthma should be well controlled when this therapy is administered. Referral to an allergist-immunologist is appropriate for these patients.

Special Groups of Patients

Special diagnostic and therapeutic considerations are warranted for children, the elderly, pregnant women, athletes, and those with rhinitis medicamentosa.

Children. When treating a child with allergic rhinitis, initiate preventive nonpharmacologic measures whenever possible. Oral antihistamines and intranasal cromolyn remain the first-line choices for childhood allergic rhinitis. As in adults, second-generation antihistamines provide a greater benefit-to-risk ratio, but not all of these agents have been approved for use in young children.

39

Intranasal corticosteroids are the most effective agents for rhinitis in children as well as in adults. However, because some intranasal corticosteroids may have a temporary adverse effect on growth in children, use these agents at the lowest possible effective dosage, monitor height routinely, and combine therapeutic approaches to minimize the dosage.

The elderly. Allergic rhinitis is an uncommon cause of perennial rhinitis in persons older than 65 years. More commonly, rhinitis in the elderly is attributable to cholinergic hyperreactivity (which may be worse after eating), congestion associated with antihypertensive drug therapy, or sinusitis. Discontinuation of an antihypertensive medication responsible for nasal congestion should be considered but may not always be feasible.

Second-generation antihistamines, such as fexofenadine and loratadine, which are not associated with significant anticholinergic effects, sedation, performance impairment, or adverse cardiac effects, are better choices than sedating antihistamines.

Pregnant women. The most common causes of nasal symptoms during pregnancy are allergic rhinitis, sinusitis, rhinitis medicamentosa, and vasomotor rhinitis. Chlorpheniramine and tripelennamine have been the preferred antihistamines for use during pregnancy, and pseudoephedrine is the preferred decongestant. However, advise patients that it is probably best to avoid oral decongestants in the first trimester; studies have linked first-trimester use with infant gastroschisis.

Nasal cromolyn is useful for allergic rhinitis and may merit first consideration because it is topically applied and has an excellent safety profile. Vasomotor rhinitis is often adequately controlled by intranasal saline instillation, appropriate exercise, and pseudoephedrine.

Athletes. Athletes and their physicians should be aware that all oral decongestants and oral or parenteral corticosteroids are banned by the U.S. Olympic Committee (USOC). Oral antihistamines are allowed by the USOC but may be banned by the international federations of certain sports. If intranasal corticosteroids are administered to olympic-class athletes, physicians must send written notification of the indication for use to the USOC.

Rhinitis medicamentosa. Use intranasal corticosteroids for patients with this syndrome, and advise them to discontinue topical decongestants as soon as symptoms abate. Occasionally, a short course of oral corticosteroids may be necessary in adults to allow for discontinuation of the topical decongestants.

When to Refer to an Allergist-Immunologist

- Medications are ineffective or produce adverse reactions.
- There is a co-morbid condition (such as asthma or chronic sinusitis).
- Symptoms interfere with the patient's ability to function or decrease quality of life.
- Symptoms have persisted for more than 3 months.
- There are complications of rhinitis (such as otitis media, sinusitis, or nasal polyposis).
- Further definition of allergic/environmental triggers of the patient's rhinitis symptoms is indicated, or patient requires more intense education.
- Allergen immunotherapy is a consideration.

References

1. Dykewicz MS, Fineman S, Skoner DP, et al. Diagnosis and management of rhinitis: parameter documents of the Joint Task Force on Practice Parameters in Allergy, Asthma, and Immunology. *Ann Allergy Asthma Immunol*. 1998;81:463-518.

2. Welsh PW, Stricker WE, Chu-Pin C, et al. Efficacy of beclomethasone nasal solution of ragweed allergy. *Mayo Clin Proc*. 1989;62:125-134.

— by Mark S. Dykewicz

Dr. Dykewicz is associate professor of internal medicine and director of the training program in allergy and immunology at Saint Louis University School of Medicine, St. Louis. He was an editor of the rhinitis parameter documents of the Joint Task Force on Practice Parameters in Allergy, Asthma, and Immunology.

Chapter 6

Cardiac Asthma and Emphysema

In the practice of medicine, physicians encounter many great imposters—in the form of diseases that exhibit symptoms very similar to other conditions.

Symptoms that appear to be asthma can actually be the work of an imposter. When asthma symptoms develop in later years it is important to make certain that an accurate diagnosis has been established. While it is entirely possible that the condition is asthma (it can develop at any age), there are other conditions which mimic asthma that must be ruled out before treatment can begin.

Cardiac asthma is the term used to describe asthma-like symptoms due to heart failure. This condition tends to occur in elderly patients. Often the patients have no history of asthma and these symptoms are a completely new problem. Patients with cardiac asthma do wheeze, but the wheezing occurs as a result of a build-up of fluid in the lungs due to the failure of the heart to pump blood effectively. In addition to a chest examination, there are several clues that doctors look for if they suspect that a patient is in heart failure, such as enlargement of the heart and liver, distension of the veins of the neck, and swelling of the ankles. In some patients, heart failure is diagnosed when a chest x-ray reveals that the heart is enlarged and there is fluid in

From "Asthma and the Elderly," [Online] 1998. Available: http://www.allergyasthma.com/archives/asthma13.html. © 1998 by Louise H. Bethea, M.D., P.A., Board Certified Allergist/Immunologist, 17070 Red Oak Dr., Ste. 107, Houston, TX 77090. Reprinted with permission. For complete contact information, please refer to Chapter 68, "Resources."

the lungs. At times, however, there are no clues and the diagnosis is more difficult to make.

The correct diagnosis is important because the therapeutic approach for cardiac asthma is different from routine asthma treatment. Diuretics are often used to reduce the fluid that has built up in the lungs. If this treatment is successful, the wheezing problem is solved.

Emphysema may also be a cause of symptoms that are suggestive of asthma. In fact, asthma and emphysema occur together. Smoking is the primary cause of emphysema. Unlike asthma, which is a reversible obstructive airway disease, the damage to the air sacs caused by emphysema is irreversible. (Yet another compelling reason to quit smoking now!)

The walls between the air sacs are permanently broken down in emphysema and as a result, there is less surface for the exchange of oxygen and carbon dioxide to occur. Less oxygen passes into the circulation, causing a build-up in the bloodstream of the body's waste product, carbon dioxide. Patients with emphysema are often short of breath and unable to exert themselves.

Dr. Bethea points out the clues that she would look for in diagnosing emphysema:

- Routine shortness of breath with moderate physical exertion (such as walking briskly or climbing stairs),

- Long history of cigarette smoking,

- Physical examination which reveals findings such as faint breath sounds when listening to the chest,

- Laboratory studies such as a chest x-ray, breathing tests including spirometry and a diffusion capacity of the lung for carbon monoxide study, and a study to determine the amount of oxygen in the arterial blood artery exercise.

If cardiac asthma and emphysema can be ruled out and a diagnosis of asthma confirmed, then treatment is basically the same as for any asthma patient. Special care is required to establish a management program which is compatible with any other chronic conditions, and age is, of course, an important consideration in determining the amount and type of medication which is prescribed.

—by Louise H. Bethea, M.D., P.A.

Chapter 7

Chronic Obstructive Pulmonary Disease

What Is COPD?

Chronic Obstructive Pulmonary Disease or COPD for short, is a progressive lung disease that affects millions of people each year. COPD is a general term used to describe specific diseases such as emphysema and chronic bronchitis. Emphysema involves destruction of the walls of the air sacs (alveoli) in the lungs. This results in a smaller number of larger air sacs that have poor gas exchange capabilities. Chronic bronchitis is characterized by a chronic cough and chronic mucus production without another known cause. A person with COPD may have either emphysema or chronic bronchitis, but most have both. Some people with COPD may also have an "asthma-like" or reactive component to their pulmonary disease.

What Are the Goals of Treatment?

At National Jewish, health care professionals believe people with COPD can lead active and full lives. By diagnosing the disease early, treating symptoms, reducing the risk of complications, and educating

From "Management of Chronic Obstructive Pulmonary Disease," "Recognizing Signs and Symptoms of Chronic Obstructive Pulmonary Disease," and "Resources for Chronic Obstructive Pulmonary Disease (Emphysema, Chronic Bronchitis)," [Online] 1994. Available: http://www.njc.org/MFhtml/. © 1994 by the National Jewish Medical and Research Center, 1400 Jackson St., Denver, Colorado 80206. Reprinted with permission. For complete contact information, please refer to Chapter 68, "Resources."

patients and families about COPD, doctors and nurses hope to improve the patients' quality of life. Our goal is to help people with COPD take charge of their breathing and regain or maintain control of their lives.

How is COPD managed?

People with COPD must become actively involved in the management of their disease. Participating in the treatment plan will help people with COPD and their families achieve the best possible results.

Exercise and Healthy Lifestyle

An exercise or conditioning program is one of the most important aspects of managing COPD. Regular exercise can enable you to improve your overall strength and endurance. By improving general fitness, respiratory muscles are strengthened. This improves your ability to perform activities despite shortness of breath. Many people with COPD enjoy walking, water aerobics and riding a stationary bike. Another important step in managing COPD is quitting smoking. If you smoke, this action is the single most important thing you can do to help stabilize your disease and prevent further damage to your lungs. Quitting smoking is a difficult task; ask your health care provider about smoking cessation programs and services that may be helpful. In addition, avoid exposure to tobacco smoke, whenever possible. This will help decrease irritation to your lungs.

Because poor nutrition is common for people with COPD, it is very important to eat a well-balanced diet and maintain a healthy weight. Shortness of breath and fatigue can interfere with your ability to eat a balanced diet. If you have special dietary needs, discuss this with a health care professional.

Avoid Infection

Because people with COPD have an increased risk of respiratory infection, vaccines are generally recommended. You can receive the influenza vaccine and pneumonia vaccine to help prevent infection. Good hand washing can also help prevent the spread of germs and infections.

Medication Therapy

Your health care professional may prescribe medications to control the symptoms of COPD. Bronchodilators help open the airways in the lungs and decrease shortness of breath. Inhaled or oral steroids may help decrease inflammation in the airways in some people. Antibiotics are often used to treat infections. For some people, expectorants can help clear mucus from the airways.

Bronchial Hygiene

In addition to medications, practicing good bronchial hygiene can help you get rid of mucus in your airways. Some people may benefit from chest physiotherapy. Treating the patient in certain positions and clapping on their chest and back can help some patients cough up thick mucus.

Breathing Retraining

Learning new breathing techniques will help you move more air in and out with less effort. This helps decrease shortness of breath. Diaphragmatic breathing, pursed lips breathing and pacing your activities can be easily learned.

Oxygen Therapy

Some people with COPD may benefit from supplemental oxygen. Supplemental oxygen is necessary when there is not enough oxygen in the blood. Some people with COPD need oxygen only with activity or while sleeping. Many people with COPD need oxygen continuously, twenty-four hours a day. To achieve the maximum benefit, use your supplemental oxygen exactly as prescribed.

Pulmonary Rehabilitation

A comprehensive pulmonary rehabilitation program includes medical and nursing management, education, physical conditioning, nutrition counseling, and consideration of psychological and social needs. A successful pulmonary rehabilitation program (such as the program offered by National Jewish) addresses the needs of each person and tailors the treatment to meet those needs.

Because of the many aspects and complexities involved in the care and management of patients with COPD, National Jewish has established a COPD rehabilitation clinic. In addition to ongoing state-of-the-art clinical care, doctors are also conducting studies in advancing the care of people with COPD.

Recognizing Signs and Symptoms of COPD

Recognizing changes in signs and symptoms of Chronic Obstructive Pulmonary Disease is an important part of managing your illness. Knowing when symptoms are changing is helpful so that treatment and other interventions can begin promptly. Early treatment is most effective. If severe symptoms are present, it is vital to begin the appropriate treatment immediately. Accurate and timely assessment of your symptoms can help you and your health care provider decide if treatment should begin in the home, at your health care provider's office, or in the emergency room.

Early symptoms or warning signs are unique to each person. These warning signs may be the same, similar, or entirely different with each episode. Usually you will be the best person to know if you are having difficulty breathing. However, some changes are more likely to be noticed by other persons, so it is important to share this information sheet with your family and those close to you.

A change or increase in the symptoms you usually experience may be the only early warning sign. You may notice one or more of the following:

- an increase or decrease in the amount of sputum produced
- an increase in the thickness or stickiness of sputum
- a change in sputum color to yellow or green or the presence of blood in the sputum
- an increase in the severity of shortness of breath, cough, and/or wheezing
- a general feeling of ill health
- ankle swelling
- forgetfulness, confusion, slurring of speech and sleepiness
- difficulty sleeping
- using more pillows or sleeping in a chair instead of a bed to avoid shortness of breath
- an unexplained increase or decrease in weight
- increased feeling of fatigue and lack of energy that continues
- a lack of sexual drive
- increasing morning headaches, dizzy spells, restlessness

Symptoms do not go away when they are ignored. Therefore, knowing when to call your health care provider is very important in managing your chronic lung disease. It is very important for you to work with your health care provider to determine the appropriate treatment for signs and symptoms of COPD.

When to Call the Doctor

- Call immediately if disorientation, confusion, slurring of speech, or sleepiness occurs during an acute respiratory infection.

- Call within 6-8 hours if shortness of breath or wheezing does not stop or decrease with inhaled bronchodilator treatments one hour apart.

- Call within 24 hours if you notice one or more of the following severe respiratory symptoms:

  1. change in color, thickness, odor, or amount of sputum persists

  2. ankle swelling lasts even after a night of sleeping with your feet up

  3. you awaken short of breath more than once a night

  4. fatigue lasts more than one day

Severe respiratory symptoms are a life-threatening emergency. Have an action plan for getting emergency care quickly in the event of severe symptoms. Inform family members and those who are close to you of this emergency action plan.

It is very important to work with your health care provider to determine the appropriate treatment steps for signs and symptoms of respiratory difficulty. These are guidelines and your specific treatment plan should be determined by you and your health care provider.

While there are many effective measures you can do at home to treat signs and symptoms, there are also actions that should be avoided. If you do any of the following, it can make your condition worse:

- Do not take any extra doses of theophylline

- Do not take codeine or any other cough suppressant

- Do not use over-the-counter nasal sprays for more than 3 days

- Do not increase the liter flow of prescribed oxygen

- Do not smoke

- Do not wait any longer than 24 hours to contact your doctor if symptoms continue

Resources for Chronic Obstructive Pulmonary Diseases

LUNG LINE® and the HealthInfo Center have compiled this list of books on COPD. [Some are available through book stores. Others marked *OP are out of print. If your local library does not have a copy your librarian may be able to help you find one through inter-library loan.] These books will provide good general information for you. Some materials may contain information that is the opinion of the author and not necessarily that of your physician, or the physicians and programs at National Jewish. Please consult your physician on specific medical questions.

Publications

Ambulatory Oxygen, by Thomas L. Petty. New York: Thieme-Stratton, 1983. 113 p. ISBN: 0-86577-113-8. *OP

The Chronic Bronchitis and Emphysema Handbook, Rev. Ed., by Francois Haas and Sheila Sperber Haas. New York: Wiley, 2000. ISBN: 0-471-23995-X.

Enjoying Life with Emphysema, by Thomas L. Petty and Louise M. Nett. 2nd ed. Philadelphia: Lea & Febiger, 1987. 178 p. ISBN: 0-8121-1102-8. *OP

Living Well with Chronic Asthma, Bronchitis, and Emphysema, by Myra B. Shayevitz and Berton R. Shayevitz. Also editors of Consumer Reports Books ed. Yonkers, NY: Consumer Reports Books, 1991. 210 p. ISBN: 0-89043-416-6. *OP

Of Life and Breath, by Jackie Dewey. New York: Warner Books, 1986. 276 p. ISBN: 0-446-30077-2. *OP

Shortness of Breath: A Guide to Better Living and Breathing, by Andrew Ries, 5th ed. St. Louis: Mosby, Inc., 1995. 210 p. ISBN: 0-8151-7339-3.

Traveling with Oxygen, published by the American Association for Respiratory Care, 1992. Call to order: (214) 243-2272. *OP

Other Resources

American Lung Association, Ph: 1-800-LUNG USA (For Nearest Chapter); National Headquarters: 1740 Broadway, New York, NY 10019; Ph: (212)315-8700

American Association For Respiratory Care, 11030 Ables Lane, Dallas, TX 75229; Ph: (972)243-2272

LUNG LINE®, National Jewish Medical and Research Center, Ph: 1-800-222-LUNG; or in Denver, CO, Ph: (303) 355-LUNG; 1400 Jackson St., Denver, CO 80206

Lung Facts®, National Jewish Medical and Research Center. To listen to taped health information 24 hours a day/7 days a week, Ph: 1-800-552-LUNG

National Heart, Lung, and Blood Institute Information Center, National Institutes of Health, P.O. Box 30105, Bethesda, MD 20824-0105; Ph: (301)592-8573

Chapter 8

Gastroesophageal Reflux: A Common Factor in Adult Asthma

Asthma and gastroesophageal reflux (GER) are distinct but inter-related diagnoses. Learning about their relationship and implementing the knowledge into clinical practice is beneficial for adult asthmatic patients. It is estimated that between 45% and 65% of adult asthmatics have GER[1,2]. In a study of difficult-to-control asthma patients, GER was identified as the single most common factor in making asthma management difficult[3]. Recent studies of direct health care costs for asthma range from $3.6 billion to $8.7 billion annually[4].

According to the National Asthma Education Panel Expert Report, asthma is "a lung disease with the following characteristics: (1) Airway obstruction (or airway narrowing) that is reversible (but not completely so in some patients) either spontaneously or with treatment. (2) Airway inflammation. (3) Airway hyperresponsiveness to a variety of stimuli[5]." Asthma management goals should focus on preventing exacerbations, controlling symptoms, and maintaining normal lung function while factoring in quality of life issues[6]. Identifying GER in the asthmatic patient and instituting appropriate reflux treatment measures may favorably impact the respiratory component and aid in asthma management efforts.

Excerpted from "Gastroesophageal Reflux: A Common Exacerbating Factor in Adult Asthma," by Carrie A. Sullivan and Wayne M. Samuelson, in *The Nurse Practitioner,* Vol. 21, No. 11, November 1996, pp. 82-6. © 1996 by Springhouse Corporation, 1111 Bethlehem Pike, Springhouse, PA 19477. Reprinted with permission. All rights reserved.

Pathophysiology

Gastroesophageal reflux has a multifactorial etiology with the key event being the retrograde movement of acid and other noxious substances from the stomach into the esophagus. All persons will demonstrate at least brief intervals of reflux under appropriate conditions. "Normal" reflux is common in the upright position and after meals. Those subjects in whom reflux results in clinically significant symptoms tend to experience more nocturnal episodes and also more prolonged reflux intervals.

Normally, reflux is prevented by an intact anti-reflux barrier consisting of the lower esophageal sphincter (LES), the crural diaphragm, and phrenoesophageal ligament[7]. The LES is a specialized bundle of circular muscle at the lower end of the esophagus with physical and pharmacologic characteristics that differ from the surrounding esophageal musculature. LES dysfunction, relaxation of the LES without swallowing or in the absence of distension of the esophagus, is the most common occurrence in GER[8].

Thus, either lax or nonexistent basal sphincter tone or inappropriate relaxation of the LES can result in reflux. Contributing factors are increased intra-abdominal pressure (e.g., obesity and straining), delayed gastric emptying causing distension, and decreased intrapleural pressure with concomitant increased intragastric pressure (as seen with bouts of coughing or during an asthma attack)[9]. Mean LES pressure is generally significantly lower in subjects with GER when compared to normal patients, but unless it is very low, LES pressure alone is of lesser utility in predicting the presence or absence of GER.

Peristalsis induced by swallowing or by esophageal distension is important in clearing the lower esophageal region. Even in subjects with comparable LES pressures (as measured by manometry), those with GER do not clear instilled acid from the lower esophagus as well as do "normals"[10,11].

The composition of the refluxed material may also influence the development of symptomatic GER. Gastric acid and pepsin both seem important in the development of symptoms. Bile salts and pancreatic enzymes may play a role in those patients in whom acid is absent. The combination of bile salts and acid is more injurious to the esophagus than is either agent alone[12].

The role of esophageal mucus, composition of swallowed saliva, and relative resistance of the esophageal mucosa to digestion are less well understood, but may also be important. LES dysfunction, composition of refluxed material, saliva, and esophageal mucus may work in concert to produce clinically significant GER. Untreated GER has been associated with strictures, Barrett's esophagus, and esophageal cancer.

The presence or absence of a hiatal hernia is of minimal concern when exploring the GER/asthma connection. Patients may have GER and not have a hiatal hernia. Patients may have a hiatal hernia and not reflux. Those with reflux and a hernia may be predisposed to worsening esophageal mucosal damage secondary to the prolonged acid exposure that occurs with repeated reflux of gastric contents in the distal esophagus.

GER and Asthma: Relationship Theories

It is generally accepted that GER and asthma are connected, but the exact nature of the relationship has yet to be determined. Asthma may promote GER and GER may provoke asthma. During an asthma attack, high negative intrapleural pressure may unfavorably alter the pressure gradient between intragastric and intraesophageal pressures allowing reflux to occur. Some asthma medications may reduce LES tone, further complicating the picture. Conversely, a patient with GER may experience pulmonary disease as a response to the esophageal acid exposure.

Three theories on the relationship between asthma and GER currently prevail. The first theory is that microaspirate, a small amount of refluxed material, is inhaled into the lungs. The microaspirate causes pulmonary inflammation and bronchial hyperresponsiveness[13]. The second theory focuses on a vagally mediated reflex pathway that occurs when acid is present in the esophagus. The hyperreactive asthmatic airways may exhibit an exaggerated response to the reflex[14]. The third theory combines the first two theories, GER-induced bronchoconstriction and the reflex pathway, to promote volatilized acid stimulation of the upper airway receptors with subsequent direct inhalation into the lungs[15].

Suspecting GER

GER may not be obvious to the clinician when obtaining a patient history, especially in an asthma patient with confounding respiratory symptoms. GER may present in patients with atypical symptoms[16] (see Table 8.1.).

Interestingly, Wiener, et al.[17], found that the severity of GER in patients with chronic hoarseness was not proportional to the incidence of traditional symptoms (heartburn, chest pain) or signs (esophagitis)

Table 8.1. Gastroesophageal Reflux Symptoms

Typical	Atypical
heartburn	odynophagia
regurgitation	chest pain
dysphagia	water brash
bloating	globus
early satiety	hoarseness
belching	pulmonary aspiration
nausea	asthma
	chronic cough

of GER. In the population studied, traditional tests for GER were usually negative. In the asthmatic patient it is crucial to assess for GER when worsening asthma is refractory to conventional therapy, especially in a patient with an atypical presentation of reflux such as nocturnal asthma symptoms[1]. GER may be precipitated in the asthmatic patient by the following factors: smoking, obesity, high-fat diet, spicy foods, caffeine, carminatives, alcohol, eating just before bed, and eating large meals[8]. Indications of worsening asthma that could be GER-related include decreasing Peak Expiratory Flow Rate measurements, increasing inhaler use, symptoms that correlate with being supine, and postprandial symptoms.

Diagnostic Evaluation of GER

The degree to which a diagnosis of GER is pursued in the asthmatic is directly related to the presence of GER symptoms and the severity of refractory respiratory symptoms. A patient that is experiencing difficult-to-control asthma even in the absence of classic GER symptoms warrants a more extensive evaluation.

Several diagnostic tests are available to the clinician to confirm the diagnosis of GER. Prolonged esophageal pH monitoring is currently considered the best clinical tool available for diagnosing pathologic GER in the asthmatic patient[18]. The use of an ambulatory esophageal 24-hour pH monitor is done on an outpatient basis. The esophageal probe tip is passed transnasally and placed just above the LES. The probe is attached to a monitor that continuously records the acid levels in the distal esophagus. The patient records mealtimes, activities, symptoms of GER, or respiratory symptoms as they occur. During the monitoring period, the patient should refrain from all drugs (especially those affecting gastric motility and gastric acid) and smoking. The patient is allowed unrestricted ambulation and a normal diet except carbonated beverages and food with a pH <5. Milk, coffee, and tea consumption should be limited to mealtimes only. The test is indicative of reflux every time there is a drop in pH to less than 4 (occurring more than 15 minutes after the end of a meal). It records the total number of single reflux episodes (both in the upright and supine positions) and prolonged reflux episodes (longer than 5 minutes)[19].

Other diagnostic tests for GER are the barium esophogram, esophageal manometry, and endoscopy[20]. The esophogram is useful in patients with dysphagia suggestive of a narrowed esophageal lumen. It assesses esophageal motility and detects a hiatal hernia. Esophageal manometry is useful prior to a surgical referral to identify patients with impaired peristaltic activity and pathologically low LES pressure. Insufficient motility identified during manometry is a contraindication for a surgical referral. Although endoscopy is useful for diagnosing esophagitis with documentation of mucosal damage severity, it is not required for the diagnosis of GER. The severity of the erosive process can be predictive of the tendency toward chronicity and relapse and would therefore influence therapeutic decisions[21].

Treatment of GER

Treatment of GER includes three types of interventions that are introduced in a stepwise approach:

- Conservative anti-reflux measures
- Medication
- Surgery

Conservative Anti-Reflux Measures

Implementing conservative anti-reflux measures (CARM) with appropriate patient education can improve the clinical course of GER by minimizing the mechanical influences that favor reflux (see Table 8.2.). Conservative therapy has been somewhat ignored in favor of the many available pharmacologic agents, yet these measures were carefully formulated based on the physiologic determinants of reflux[22].

Table 8.2. Conservative Anti-Reflux Measures

The patient should be instructed in the following measures to decrease the breaching of the anti-reflux barrier.
- Stop smoking
- Avoid alcohol
- Eliminate caffeine from diet
- Monitor/reduce fat content in diet
- Limit amount of spice used in seasoning foods
- Avoid large meals
- Avoid eating for 2 to 3 hours before bedtime
- Elevate the head of the bed 6 to 8 inches
- Maintain ideal body weight

Medical Management

The major thrust of medical management of GER is pharmacotherapy. Several different classes of medications are used to treat GER. A trial period of 4 to 6 weeks may be required before the patient responds to prescribed medication. Initially, instruct the patient on CARM if there is any suspicion of GER complicating the management of asthma. Oftentimes, additionally initiating an empiric trial of an acid suppressive agent, generally a proton pump inhibitor, is helpful to control GER. After 4 to 6 weeks the patient is reevaluated and potentially referred to a gastroenterologist for a confirmatory 24-hour ambulatory pH monitor. The patient is considered for a surgical referral if GER is documented and there is adequate esophageal motility, and if the severity of symptoms (either classic GER or asthma-related) warrant it.

One class of medication commonly prescribed to manage GER is the Histamine$_2$-Receptor Antagonists (H$_2$-RAs). These drugs [cimetidine (Tagemet), famotidine (Pepcid), nizatidine (Axid), ranitidine (Zantac)] inhibit gastric acid secretion by competitively blocking the Hz-receptors on the parietal cells. Some patients experience symptom relief with standard dosing. Others may require a high-dose regimen. Long-term treatment of GER with H$_2$-RAs is costly and about 50% of patients with GER fail to respond to high-dose therapy[2].

A newer class of medications that have proven efficacy in the treatment of GER is the proton pump inhibitors (PPIs) [lansoprazole (Prevacid), omeprazole (Prilosec)]. They decrease the episodes of GER by inhibiting the secretory ability of the parietal cell for the life of the cell, approximately 2 to 3 days. Initially there were some safety concerns about use of PPIs as a long-term therapy. Klinkenberg-Knol, et al.[24], found that omeprazole was safe and efficacious for at least 5 years in patients with GER that was resistant to treatment with H_2-RAs. The manufacturer lists omeprazole for the maintenance of healing of erosive esophagitis with the length of treatment to be determined by the individual healthcare practitioner.

Hillman, et al.[25], found in a 7-month trial that omeprazole reduced both symptoms and overall cost when compared to ranitidine. When considering the economics of treatment the clinician should note that while the daily cost of the PPIs is higher, overall the cost is lower when factoring in the high propensity for relapse with other treatments and the resultant increased number of clinic visits.

A third class of drugs that may be used in the treatment of GER is the prokinetic agents [bethanechol (Urecholine), cisapride (Propulsid), metoclopramide (Reglan)]. They enhance the LES pressure and accelerate gastric emptying. Metoclopramide hydrochloride was no more successful than the H_2-RAs in treating GER. With regular use its side effects (including drowsiness, irritability, and extrapyramidal effects) occur frequently in patients receiving 10 mg four times daily[25]. Cisapride, a newer prokinetic agent, may be as effective as some H_2-RAs in providing symptomatic relief. Cisapride does not act in the inhibitory fashion of the H_2-RAs. It raises LES pressure and stimulates the physiological process of peristalsis and gastric emptying[26].

OTC antacids or the newly available OTC-strength H_2-RAs are ineffective in healing reflux esophagitis. Even standard doses of H_2-RAs are inadequate for the management of GER. Simpson[18] reviewed several clinical trials of standard-dose H_2-RAs for treatment of GER and identified in each of the study conclusions an improvement in asthma symptoms and a decrease in medication requirements of asthmatics. While standard-dose therapy may improve respiratory symptoms, it does not adequately treat esophagitis or reduce the likelihood of relapse.

One last medication consideration is the action of the bronchodilators, theophylline, beta adrenergic agents, and anticholinergic agents. They can cause relaxation of the esophageal sphincter[8]. Judicious use of these medications should minimize LES relaxation and diminish the potential aggravation of GER while adequately managing asthma symptoms.

Surgical Intervention

Surgery may be deemed the treatment of choice for the patient with GER that remains symptomatic despite the use of mechanical anti-reflux measures and pharmacotherapy. The Nissen fundoplication (NF) is one surgical procedure used to treat GER in asthmatics. Surgical correction is achieved by improving the anti-reflux barrier and provides a lasting solution. The surgical correction of GER results in decreased pulmonary symptoms associated with asthma[27]. A study of GER patients by DeMeester, et al.[28], showed the NF was an effective, durable procedure controlling reflux symptoms for greater than 10 years in 91% of the patients followed.

With the advent of laparoscopic procedures, the NF may be used with increasing frequency in the management of GER. The laparoscopic approach, by avoiding an open abdominal procedure, has several distinct advantages. The laparoscopic approach minimizes post-operative discomfort, decreases the length of hospital stay, decreases the overall cost of surgical intervention and shortens the length of recovery.

Conclusion

GER and asthma are clearly linked. Therefore asthma patients need to be vigilantly assessed for GER when they present with either typical or atypical symptoms. Inherent to an effective treatment plan is a thorough educational component implemented by caregivers.

Educational efforts should coincide with the stepwise approach to treat GER and manage asthma. Initial therapy for GER should focus on conservative anti-reflux measures. Reflux unresponsive to these measures should be treated with mechanical measures combined with pharmacologic therapy. Finally, surgery may be necessary for an effective treatment outcome.

References

1. Allen CJ, Newhouse MT: Gastroesophageal reflux and chronic respiratory disease. *Am Rev Respir Dis* 1984;129(4):645-47.

2. Ducolone A, Vandevenne A, Jouin H, et al: Gastroesophageal reflux in patients with asthma and chronic bronchitis. *Am Rev Respir Dis* 1987;135(2):327-32.

3. Irwin RS, Curley FJ, French CL: Difficult-to-control asthma. Contributing factors and outcome of a systematic management protocol. *Chest* 1993;103(6):1662-69.

4. National Institutes of Health, Global Initiative for Asthma. January 1995; [NIH Pub. No. 95-3659].

5. Institutes of Health, National Asthma Education Program, Expert Panel. Guidelines for the diagnosis and management of asthma. August 1991; [NIH Pub. No. 91-3042] Washington, D.C., U.S. Government Printing Office.

6. National Institutes of Health, International Consensus Report on Diagnosis and Management of Asthma. March 1992; [NIH Pub. No. 92-3091].

7. Mittal RK: Current concepts of the antireflux barrier. *Gastroenterol Clin North Am* 1990;19(3):501-16.

8. Castell DO: The lower esophageal sphincter: physiological and clinical aspects. *Ann Intern Med* 1975;83(3):390-401.

9. Holloway RH, and Dent J: Pathophysiology of gastroesophageal reflux: lower esophageal sphincter dysfunction in gastroesophageal reflux disease. *Gastroenterol Clin North Am* 1990;19(3):517-35.

10. Holloway RH, Kocyan P, Dent J: Provocation of transient lower esophageal sphincter relaxations by meals in patients with symptomatic gastroesophageal reflux. *Dig Dis and Sci* 1991;36(8):1034-39.

11. Cucchiara S, Bortolotti M, Minella R, et al: Fasting and postprandial mechanisms of gastroesophageal reflux in children with gastroesophageal reflux disease. *Dig Dis and Sci* 1993;38(1):86-92.

12. Safaie-Shirazi S, DenBesten L, Zike WL: Effect of bile salts on the ionic permeability of the esophageal mucosa and their role in the production of esophagitis. *Gastroenterol* 1975;8(4):728-33.

13. Crausaz FM, Favez G: Aspiration of solid food particles into lungs of patients with gastroesophageal reflux and chronic bronchial disease. *Chest* 1988;93(3):376-78.

14. Mansfield LE, Stein MR: Gastroesophageal reflux and asthma: a possible reflex mechanism. *Ann Allergy* 1978;41(4):224-26.

15. Mansfield LE: Gastroesophageal reflux and respiratory disorders. *Compr Ther* 1992;18(3):6-10.

16. Traube M: The spectrum of the symptoms and presentations of gastroesophageal reflux disease. *Gastroenterol Clin North Am* 1990;19(3):609-16.

17. Wiener GJ, Koufman JA, Wu WC, et al: Chronic hoarseness secondary to gastroesophageal reflux disease: documentation with 24-H ambulatory pH monitoring. *Am J Gastroenterol* 1989;84(12):1503-08.

18. Simpson WG: Gastroesophageal reflux disease and asthma: diagnosis and management. *Arch Intern Med* 1995;155(8):798-803.

19. Johnson LF, DeMeester TR: Twenty-four-hour pH monitoring of the distal esophalsus. A quantitative measure of gastroesophageal reflux. *Am J Gastroenterol* 1974;62(4):325-32.

20. DeVault KR, Castell DO: Guidelines for the diagnosis and treatment of gastroesophageal reflux disease. *Arch Intern Med* 1995;155(20):2165-73.

21. Fennerty B, Castell D, Fendrick AM, et al: The diagnosis and treatment of gastroesophageal reflux disease in a managed care environment. *Arch Intern Med* 1996;156(5):477-84.

22. Kitchin LI, Castell DO: Rationale and efficacy of conservative therapy for gastroesophageal reflux disease. *Arch Intern Med* 1991;151(3):448-54.

23. Garnett WR: Efficacy, safety, and cost issues in managing patients with gastroesophageal reflux disease. *Am J Hosp Pharm* 1993;50(Supp1):S11-S18.

24. Klinkenberg-Knol EC, Festen HPM, Jansen JBMJ, et al: Long-term treatment with omeprazole for refractory reflux esophagitis:efficacy and safety. *Ann Intern Med* 1994;121(3):161-67.

25. Hillman AL, Bloom BS, Fendrick M, et al: Cost and quality effects of alternative treatments for persistent gastroesophageal reflux disease. *Arch Intern Med* 1992;152(7):1407-72.

26. Baldi F, Porro GB, Dobrilla G, et al:Cisapride versus placebo in reflux esophagitis. *J Clin Gastroenterol* 1988;10(6):614-18.

27. Larrain A, Carrasco E, Galleguillos F, et al: Medical and surgical treatment of nonallergic asthma associated with gastroesophageal reflux. *Chest* 1991;99(6):1330-35.

28. DeMeester TR, Bonavina L, Albertucci M: Nissen fundoplication for gastroesophageal reflux disease. Evaluation of primary repair in 100 consecutive patients. *Ann Surg* 1986;204(1):9-20.

—by Carrie A. Sullivan and Wayne M. Samuelson

Carrie A. Sullivan, R.N., B.S.N., is the asthma clinic coordinator at the University of Utah Health Sciences Center in Salt Lake City, Utah.

Wayne M. Samuelson, M.D., is associate professor of medicine (clinical) at the University of Utah Health Sciences Center in Salt Lake City, Utah.

Chapter 9

Vocal Cord Dysfunction

In 1983, physicians at National Jewish reported a new condition that may mimic asthma. This condition is called Vocal Cord Dysfunction, or VCD. VCD causes asthma-like symptoms because of an abnormal closing of the vocal cords. VCD can cause difficulty breathing and even wheezing. Based on these symptoms, many people with VCD may be diagnosed with asthma and treated with asthma medications, including oral steroids. Since VCD is not asthma, the symptoms do not improve with this treatment. When VCD is not treated properly, it may lead to frequent emergency room visits and hospitalizations. To complicate the situation, some people have a combination of asthma and Vocal Cord Dysfunction.

What happens with VCD?

To understand VCD, it is helpful to know how the vocal cords function normally. When you breathe in, or inhale, the vocal cords open, allowing air to flow into your windpipe (trachea) and reach your lungs. However, with Vocal Cord Dysfunction, the vocal cords close together, or constrict, when you inhale. This leaves only a small opening for air to flow into your windpipe.

From "Vocal Cord Dysfunction," [Online] 1995. Available: http://www.njc.org/MFhtml/VCD_MF.html. © 1995 by the National Jewish Medical and Research Center, 1400 Jackson St., Denver, Colorado 80206. Reprinted with permission. For complete contact information, please refer to Chapter 68, "Resources."

How is VCD diagnosed?

Making a diagnosis of VCD can be very difficult. If your physician or health care provider suspects VCD, you will be asked many questions about your symptoms. Common symptoms include a chronic cough, shortness of breath, difficulty breathing, chest tightness, throat tightness, "difficulty getting air in," hoarseness, and wheezing. Breathing tests may be normal and not show signs of asthma. A specific breathing test called a flow volume loop, can be helpful in showing VCD, especially on the "breathing in" or inspiratory part of the loop. This is only helpful if it is done while you are having symptoms.

A procedure called a laryngoscopy is the most important test in making the diagnosis of VCD. This procedure is performed by a specialized physician. Using a flexible tube, the physician can see how your vocal cords open and close. A laryngoscopy should be done when you are having symptoms because abnormal vocal cord movements do not occur all the time. Other tests may be done to trigger symptoms so that your physician can observe your vocal cords when you are having symptoms. It is important to know that people with Vocal Cord Dysfunction cannot produce symptoms voluntarily.

What can trigger VCD symptoms?

Possible triggers of VCD are often similar to asthma triggers. Triggers may include upper respiratory infections, fumes, odors, cigarette smoke, singing, emotional upset, post-nasal drip, and exercise. Sometimes the trigger is not known.

How is VCD treated?

Once you are diagnosed with VCD, you can begin a specific treatment program. If VCD is your only condition, your asthma medications may be stopped. If you have a combination of asthma and VCD, asthma medications may be continued, but may often be decreased.

Speech therapy is a very important part of the treatment for VCD. Special exercises increase your awareness of abdominal breathing and relax your throat muscles. This enables you to have more control over your throat. You will learn to practice these exercises while you are symptom-free in order to effectively use the exercises during VCD episodes. These exercises help overcome the abnormal vocal cord movements and improve airflow into your lungs.

Another important part of treatment is supportive counseling. Counseling can help you adjust to a new diagnosis and a new treatment program. Counseling can also help you identify and deal positively with stress which may be an underlying factor in VCD. Most people with VCD find counseling to be very beneficial.

The Role of National Jewish

Physicians and researchers at National Jewish are continuing to discover more about Vocal Cord Dysfunction, a condition that may mimic asthma. In addition, National Jewish offers a variety of programs that can help individuals with known or suspected VCD. Physicians and a team of specialists can work together to evaluate your condition and determine the best treatment program. National Jewish's long-standing intensive specialization in respiratory diseases has been instrumental in our success in treating this newly recognized medical condition.

Chapter 10

Chronic Cough

Cough is a defense mechanism for clearing secretions and inhaled and noxious substances from the tracheobronchial tree. Coughing may be voluntary but is more often the result of an involuntary reflex response to stimulation of cough receptors in the airways. The cough reflex is quite complex and as yet is not completely understood. A variety of peripheral sites are connected to the cough center in the medulla, including the nose, auditory canal, nasopharynx, larynx, trachea, intrapulmonary bronchi, and pleural surfaces. Stimulation of receptors in these sites can result in cough.[1]

Definition and Prevalence

A chronic cough may be defined as one of greater than three weeks duration.[2] In the nonsmoking population, persistent cough is reported to occur in 14 to 23 percent of adults[3,4] and is a frequent reason for visits to primary care physicians.[5] From 17 to 24 percent of adults smoke, and the incidence of chronic cough caused by smoking is directly related to the number of cigarettes smoked per day. Approximately 25 percent of those who smoke one half pack per day report a chronic cough, while over 50 percent who smoke more than two packs

From "Chronic Cough," by Elizabeth B. Philp, in *American Family Physician,* Vol. 56, No. 5, October 1, 1997, pp. 1395-1404. © 1997 by American Academy of Family Physicians, 8880 Ward Pkwy., Kansas City, MO 64114. Reprinted with permission.

per day have a chronic cough. Many smokers will not report their cough to their physicians or seek medical attention for it.

Chronic cough may be caused by multiple factors in addition to smoking (Table 10.1.).[6] In patients referred to a pulmonary clinic for chronic cough, a study[2] concluded that in 94 percent of patients, chronic cough was caused by four conditions: postnasal drip, asthma, chronic bronchitis, or gastroesophageal reflux. In 82 percent of patients, cough had a single cause, and in 18 percent of cases, multiple causes were found. Tailoring treatment to specific causes of chronic cough resulted in sustained resolution of the cough in 97 percent of patients.

Table 10.1. Differential Diagnosis of Chronic Cough

Common causes	Less common causes
Smoking and other environmental irritants	Congestive heart failure
Postnasal drip	Cancer (bronchogenic or esophageal)
Asthma	Interstitial lung disease (emphysema or sarcoidosis)
Gastroesophageal reflux	Bronchiectasis
Chronic bronchitis	Tuberculosis and other chronic lung infections (e.g., fungal)
Transient airway hyperresponsiveness (e.g., after viral upper respiratory infection)	Cystic fibrosis
Recurrent aspiration (e.g., post-stroke, frequent vomiting [bulimia], alcoholism) Medication-related (ACE inhibitors, beta blockers)	Pressure from an intrathoracic mass (e.g., thoracic aneurysm, thyromegaly, mediastinal lymphadenopathy)
	Irritation of cough receptors in ear (e.g., impacted cerumen, hair, foreign body)
	Opportunistic infections in immunosuppressed patients
	Lymphangitis carcinomatosis
	Foreign body
	Chronic inhalation of bronchial irritants (occupational)
	Psychogenic

ACE = angiotensin-converting enzyme.

70

Management of Chronic Cough

Evaluation of chronic cough should begin with a careful history focused on eliciting symptoms associated with the most common causes of chronic cough (Tables 10.1. and 10.2.). The physical examination should focus on readily accessible anatomic locations known to contain receptor sites for the cough reflex (e.g., the nose, the nasopharynx, the lungs).

By proceeding in a stepwise fashion from common causes of chronic cough to less common causes, the invasiveness and expense of the work-up can be minimized. While the history and physical examination can often identify the cause of chronic cough, empiric treatment for common etiologies is frequently necessary.

Avoid Lung 'Toxins'

Cigarette smoking. Cigarette smoking is the leading cause of chronic cough, and cessation of smoking usually leads to a dramatic decrease in cough within one month. Physicians should take every opportunity to advise their patients to stop smoking and can use target symptoms, such as chronic cough, to motivate these patients to quit smoking. Family physicians can increase their success rate in smoking cessation by providing time for patient counseling and by educating patients about the use of nicotine patches or nicotine gum to help them stop smoking.[10]

Occupational exposure. In patients who note an improvement in their cough during vacations or other time away from their workplace, an occupational exposure (e.g., dust, fumes, other irritants) may be playing a role in their chronic cough. These patients should be counseled to inquire about available engineering controls at their workplace to reduce their exposure. This may mean improving air circulation, or wearing a face mask or other protective clothing. In extreme circumstances, a change of job may be necessary.

Discontinue Medications Causing Cough

Angiotensin-converting enzyme inhibitors. Angiotensin-converting enzyme (ACE) inhibitors are useful in the treatment of hypertension or congestive heart failure because of their minimal side effects. Cough was first described as a side effect of ACE inhibitor therapy in 1985,[11] and since then numerous case reports and studies

71

Table 10.2. Checklist for Use in Determining Common Causes of Chronic Cough

Smoking
How many cigarettes a day does the patient smoke?
Is coughing worse on awakening in the morning?

Postnasal drip
Does patient note mucus drainage from the nose?
Does patient frequently "clear" the throat or swallow mucus?
Does patient have a history of allergies or sinus complaints?

Asthma
Does patient note more coughing at night?
Is coughing brought on by specific irritants (e.g., smoke, pollen, dust, fumes, chemicals)?
Is there a family history of allergies/asthma/eczema?
Does patient note wheezing/chest discomfort/difficulty breathing?
Has patient changed residences recently?

Gastroesophageal reflux
Does patient complain of heartburn or sour belches?
Are symptoms worse when patient is lying down?
Is the cough improved by use of antacids or over-the-counter H_2 blockers?

Chronic bronchitis
Is patient a smoker?
Is the cough usually productive?

Medication-related
Review medication list for use of ACE inhibitors or beta blockers, including $beta_2$-blocker eyedrops

Airway hyperresponsiveness following upper respiratory infection
Did the cough begin during an upper respiratory infection?
Is the chronic cough usually nonproductive?

Underlying malignancy or serious infection (i.e., tuberculosis)
Does patient have fever, chills, or night sweats?
Has patient coughed up any blood?
Has patient lost weight recently without trying to?

ACE = angiotensin-converting enzyme.

describing this condition have been published. A recent review[12] of the literature concludes that cough occurs in 5 to 20 percent of patients treated with an ACE inhibitor. The cough resolves rapidly when the drug is withdrawn. If the cough resolves, the patient should be given an alternate class of medication, because cough would recur with reintroduction of the same or another ACE inhibitor.

Beta blockers. Beta blockers are used in the management of hypertension, angina, cardiac arrhythmias, hyperthyroidism, prophylaxis of migraine, and glaucoma. Blockade of beta-adrenergic receptors in the bronchi and bronchioles can cause increased airway resistance resulting from unopposed parasympathetic activity, especially in patients who already have obstructive lung disease (e.g., asthma, emphysema). Cough provoked by this class of drugs will resolve when the drug is withdrawn, and a drug from a different class should be substituted for treatment of the primary disease.

Identify Post-Upper Respiratory Infection Airway Hyperresponsiveness

Acute cough is frequent in upper respiratory infections. Most patients will have total resolution of all symptoms within three weeks. However, a subgroup of patients develop airway hyperresponsiveness with a persistent cough that can last two months or so.[9,13] Studies suggest that airway epithelial damage that follows an upper respiratory infection can lead to hypersensitivity of the airway receptors to inhaled irritants. In these patients, the cough, if unresponsive to treatment with an antihistamine, should be treated with inhaled steroids.[9]

Identify Chronic Bronchitis

Chronic bronchitis is associated with excessive mucus produced in the tracheobronchial tree. Patients who have an expectorant cough for three or more months of the year for more than two consecutive years fit the clinical definition of chronic bronchitis.[14,15] Patients with longstanding disease may also have overlapping asthma or emphysema.

Although cigarette smoking is the single most important etiologic factor, the physician should also inquire about environmental and occupational exposure to dusts, fumes, and other air pollutants. Inhaled ipratropium (Atrovent), an anticholinergic bronchodilator, has theoretic advantages, including decreased mucus production and peripheral antitussive effect, and may be more effective than standard beta-agonist bronchodilator treatment.[16,17]

Patients should be evaluated with chest radiographs and a pulmonary function test. A tuberculosis skin test should be administered in high-risk patients (e.g., patients with human immunodeficiency virus [HIV] infection, intravenous drug users, prison inmates, homeless persons, immigrants from endemic areas).

Management must start with discontinuation of smoking and avoidance of environmental irritants and toxins. An exercise program will increase exercise tolerance and provide an improved sense of well-being. Immunizations with pneumococcal vaccine, as well as annual influenza vaccinations, are important preventive health measures. Treatment of community-acquired respiratory infections with an appropriate antibiotic for seven to 10 days should be promptly instituted. Optimum bronchodilator therapy, postural drainage, and hydration are the basics of good management. Patients who fail to improve with these measures may require the addition of oral steroid therapy.[18] In some cases, correction of malnutrition is an important adjunctive therapy because of the higher incidence of poor nutritional status in patients with chronic lung disease.

Identify Weight Loss or Other Symptoms of Serious Disease

Patients with serious underlying disease seldom present with only one symptom, such as chronic cough. Inquiry should be made about such symptoms as fever, chills, or night sweats (suggesting pulmonary tuberculosis), hemoptysis or recent weight loss (suggesting lung cancer), and dyspnea, orthopnea, or pedal edema (suggesting congestive heart failure). If any of these symptoms are acknowledged, appropriate diagnostic evaluation should be undertaken.

In patients with chronic cough as the only presenting symptom, and having excluded the etiologies already discussed, the physician can move to step one in the algorithm for management of chronic cough.

An Empiric Treatment Algorithm

Step one. For one week, give all patients empiric treatment for postnasal drip using an older-generation antihistamine-decongestant combination.[19] Evidence indicates that the newer generation histamine$_1$

antagonists are inferior in treating cough caused by postnasal drip,[17] and their use should be avoided unless sedation is a major side effect with the older agents. If the cough improves, the antihistamine-decongestant combination should be continued until the cough is resolved or until there is no further improvement. Nasal steroids should be added in patients whose cough is not controlled by antihistamine-decongestant medications.

If symptoms persist after one to two weeks of nasal steroid use, a computed tomographic (CT) examination of the sinuses should be performed. If chronic sinusitis is identified, the patient should be treated with an empiric trial of antibiotics such as amoxicillin-clavulanate potassium (Augmentin) or trimethoprim-sulfamethoxazole (Bactrim, Septra), or a second- or third-generation oral cephalosporin. In addition, some data indicate that patients may benefit from a short (three-day) course of treatment with an over-the-counter nasal oxymetazoline decongestant spray (Afrin, Allerest, Dristan) plus an oral antihistamine-decongestant combination drug. When all of these measures fail, the patient may require aspiration or irrigation of the sinuses and may benefit from a consultation with an ear, nose, and throat specialist.

Step two. Patients who continue to cough despite the treatments in step one should be evaluated for asthma. Asthma is a disease characterized by reversible airflow obstruction caused by airway inflammation, edema, mucus production, and smooth muscle constriction.[14] Clinically, asthma presents as acute, recurrent episodes of dyspnea, coughing, or wheezing. Physicians should bear in mind that patients with asthma may present with only a chronic, usually nonproductive cough. This is often termed "cough-variant asthma." Physical examination of asthma patients outside periods of acute symptoms is essentially normal. In one study[20] of nonsmoking patients with chronic cough, asthma was found to be the cause of cough in 24 percent of patients, and more than one fourth of these patients had so-called cough-variant asthma.

The expert panel of the National Asthma Education Program[21] has suggested a sequence for assessing a patient suspected of having asthma, and an algorithm for diagnosing asthma has been developed. The algorithm suggests that airflow obstruction should be objectively evaluated by spirometry.[22-24] A reduced peak expiratory flow rate and a reduced ratio of forced expiratory volume in one second (FEV_1) to forced vital capacity (FVC) is diagnostic of obstructive lung disease. Following bronchodilator therapy, an increase of at least 15 percent in the FEV_1 may be expected in the patient with asthma.

When the results of spirometry are equivocal, a bronchoprovocation test using methacholine (Provocholine) may be helpful in evaluating airway hyperresponsiveness.[25,26] Patients diagnosed with asthma should be counseled about avoidance of allergens, treated prophylactically with intranasal and inhaled cromolyn (Intal, Nasalcrom), and with beta-agonist and/or steroid inhalers and oral corticosteroids, as required.

Step three. Chest and sinus radiographs should be obtained at this point, if they are not already available. Any clinically significant abnormality should be evaluated and treated.

Step four. Patients in whom a diagnosis has not been reached by this time and who remain symptomatic should be given an empiric gastric-acid suppression test, along with antireflux measures for treatment of possible GERD.

Patients with GERD usually complain of heartburn or chest discomfort. However, some patients may have chronic cough as their only presenting symptom.[27] Mild degrees of GERD, involving only the distal esophagus, can still irritate the nerve fibers that initiate the cough reflex. Actual aspiration of gastric contents causing cough is uncommon.

GERD can be ruled out in most patients if symptoms do not improve during a limited period of gastric-acid suppression therapy. High doses of proton-pump inhibitors (e.g., omeprazole, in a dosage of 80 mg per day) are used to ensure complete suppression. This test has a sensitivity of 83 to 90 percent.[28,29] Discontinuing certain medications that can exacerbate GERD (e.g., anticholinergic drugs, calcium channel blockers, theophylline, other smooth muscle relaxants) may be necessary. A protective agent, such as sucralfate (Carafate), in a dosage of 1 g taken one hour before meals, may be helpful, as may the addition of a prokinetic agent, such as metoclopramide (Reglan) or cisapride (Propulsid), before meals and at bedtime.

Nonresponding patients should be further evaluated using 24-hour esophageal pH monitoring, which is the most sensitive and specific test for the diagnosis of GERD.[30,31] Patients with abnormal results should receive aggressive therapy with a proton-pump inhibitor for at least eight weeks.

Step five. Patients who still continue to cough at this stage should receive bronchoscopic examination. If this procedure does not produce a diagnosis, a repeat course of antiasthmatic therapy with a beta agonist and steroids should be tried.

76

Final Comment

In following this protocol, patients whose cough improves with one therapy but does not resolve completely should continue with the initial therapy and proceed to the next step in the management algorithm, because in some patients, two or three diseases may be contributing to their cough.[3,7]

If cough still persists, the physician should institute a careful search for less common causes (Table 10.1.). Less than 6 percent of patients with chronic cough have one of these less common diagnoses, and it would be unusual for cough to be the only presenting symptom in patients with serious underlying disease. Patients with lung cancer, interstitial lung disease, chronic lung infections, or aneurysm could be expected to be identified by chest radiographs and/or bronchoscopy. A CT scan of the chest would be appropriate in these patients, and lymph-node biopsy may be necessary in diagnosing sarcoidosis or bronchogenic carcinoma. In the absence of clinical signs of congestive heart failure, two-dimensional echocardiography may aid in diagnosis.

Any child who coughs and has a history of recurrent pneumonia and/or failure to thrive should have a sweat chloride test for cystic fibrosis. Finally, an evaluation for immunosuppression caused by HIV infection or IgA deficiency may be indicated. If all of this evaluation and treatment fails, a careful history should be repeated, with emphasis on occupational or home exposure to an airway irritant.

If no pathology can be found, psychogenic cough must be considered.[8,32] A careful psychosocial history may elicit the abnormal family dynamics that led to this attention-seeking symptom. A harmless subset of this group of patients includes those whose cough is a nervous tic, occurring when they become upset or nervous.

References

1. Braunwald E. Cough and hemoptysis. In: *Harrison's Principles of internal medicine*. 13th ed. New York: McGraw-Hill, 1994:171-8.

2. Irwin RS, Corrao WM, Pratter MR. Chronic persistent cough in the adult: the spectrum and frequency of causes and successful outcome of specific therapy. *Am Rev Respir Dis* 1981;123(4 Pt 1):413-7.

3. Di Pede C, Viegi G, Quackenboss JJ, Boyer-Pfersdorf P, Lebowitz MD. Respiratory symptoms and risk factors in an

Arizona population sample of Anglo and Mexican-American whites. *Chest* 1991;99:916-22.

4. Wynder EL, Lemon FR, Mantel N. Epidemiology of persistent cough. *Am Rev Respir Dis* 1965;91:679-700.

5. Braman SS, Corrao WM. Chronic cough. Diagnosis and treatment. *Prim Care* 1985;12:217-25.

6. Braman SS, Corrao WM. Cough: differential diagnosis and treatment. *Clin Chest Med* 1987;8:177-88.

7. Pratter MR, Bartter T, Akers S, DuBois J. An algorithmic approach to chronic cough. *Ann Intern Med* 1993;119:977-83.

8. Bucca C, Rolla G, Brussino L, De Rose V, Bugiani M. Are asthma-like symptoms due to bronchial or extrathoracic airway dysfunction? *Lancet* 1995;346:791-5.

9. Poe RH, Harder RV, Israel RH, Kallay MC. Chronic persistent cough. Experience in diagnosis and outcome using an anatomic diagnostic protocol. *Chest* 1989;95(4):723-8.

10. Danis PG, Seaton TL. Helping your patients to quit smoking. *Am Fam Physician* 1997;55:1207-14, 1217-8.

11. Sesoko K, Kaneko Y. Cough associated with the use of captopril. *Arch Intern Med* 1985;145:1524.

12. Israili ZH, Hall WD. Cough and angioneurotic edema associated with angiotensin-converting enzyme inhibitor therapy. A review of the literature and pathophysiology. *Ann Intern Med* 1992;117:234-42.

13. Empey DW, Laitinen LA, Jacobs L, Gold WM, Nadel JA. Mechanisms of bronchial hyperreactivity in normal subjects after upper respiratory tract infection. *Am Rev Respir Dis* 1976;113:131-9.

14. Standards for the diagnosis and care of patients with chronic obstructive pulmonary disease (COPD) and asthma. This official statement of the American Thoracic Society was adopted by the ATS Board of Directors, November 1986. *Am Rev Respir Dis* 1987;136:225-44.

15. Definition and classification of chronic bronchitis for clinical and epidemiological purposes. A report to the Medical Research

Council by their Committee on the Aetiology of Chronic Bronchitis. *Lancet* 1965;1(389):775-8.

16. Irwin RS, Curley FJ. The treatment of cough. A comprehensive review. *Chest* 1991;99:1477-84.

17. Irwin RS, Curley FJ, Bennett FM. Appropriate use of antitussives and protussives. A practical review. *Drugs* 1993;46:80-91.

18. Ingram RH. Chronic bronchitis, emphysema and airways obstruction. In: *Harrison's Principles of internal medicine*. 13th ed. New York: McGraw-Hill, 1994:1197-205.

19. Irwin RS, Pratter MR, Holland PS, Corwin RW, Hughes JR. Postnasal drip causes cough and is associated with reversible upper airway obstruction. *Chest* 1984;85(3):346-52.

20. Irwin RS, Curley FJ, French CL. Chronic cough. The spectrum and frequency of causes, key components of the diagnostic evaluation, and outcome of specific therapy. *Am Rev Respir Dis* 1990;141:640-7.

21. Guidelines for the diagnosis and management of asthma. Bethesda, Md.: National Asthma Education Program, National Heart, Lung, and Blood Institute, Department of Health and Human Services, 1991; DHHS publication no. 91-3042.

22. Morris JF, Koski A, Johnson LC. Spirometric standards for healthy nonsmoking adults. *Am Rev Respir Dis* 1971;103:57-67.

23. Dickman ML, Schmidt CD, Gardner RM. Spirometric standards for normal children and adolescents (ages 5 years through 18 years). *Am Rev Respir Dis* 1971;104:680-7.

24. Morris JF, Temple WP, Koski A. Normal values for the ratio of one-second forced expiratory volume to forced vital capacity. *Am Rev Respir Dis* 1973;108:1000-3.

25. Townley RG, Bewtra AK, Nair NM, Brodkey FD, Watt GD, Burke KM. Methacholine inhalation challenge studies. *J Allergy Clin Immunol* 1979;64(6 Pt 2):569-74.

26. Pratter MR, Irwin RS. The clinical value of pharmacologic bronchoprovocation challenge. *Chest* 1984;85:260-5.

27. Irwin RS, French CL, Curley FJ, et al. Chronic cough due to gastroesophageal reflux. *Chest* 1993;104(5):1511-7.

28. Young MF, Sanowski RA, Talbert GA, Harrison ME, Walker BE. Omeprazole administration as a test for gastroesophageal reflux [Abstract]. *Gastroenterology* 1992;102(4 Pt 2):A192.

29. Schindlbeck NE, Klauser AG, Voderholzer WA, Muller-Lissner SA. Empiric therapy for gastroesophageal reflux disease. *Arch Intern Med* 1995;155:1808-12.

30. Schindlbeck NE, Heinrich C, Konig A, Dendorfer A, Pace F, Muller-Lissner SA. Optimal thresholds, sensitivity, and specificity of long-term pH-metry for the detection of gastroesophageal reflux disease. *Gastroenterology* 1987;93:85-90.

31. Schindlbeck NE, Ippisch H, Klauser AG, Muller-Lissner SA. Which pH threshold is best in esophageal pH monitoring? *Am J Gastroenterol* 1991;86:1138-41.

32. Corrao WM, Braman SS, Irwin RS. Chronic cough as the sole presenting manifestation of bronchial asthma. *N Engl J Med* 1979;300:633-7.

— by Elizabeth B. Philp, M.B., Ch.B.

Elizabeth B. Philp, is associate professor of family medicine at the University of Alabama School of Medicine, Tuscaloosa, where she is also the chairperson of the Objective Structured Clinical Examination and Standardized Patient Program. Dr. Philp is a graduate of Edinburgh University Medical School, Scotland.

Part Two

Asthma Statistics

Chapter 11

Asthma Surveillance and Intervention Programs

An increasingly organized and privatized health care system, dominated by large managed care organizations, obscures the role of state public health agencies in preventing clinically important diseases. What makes a disease a matter of public health importance and therefore of concern to health departments?

A disease first becomes a public health issue when an unexpected number of cases are found. After a decade of decline, both the morbidity and mortality associated with asthma are increasing in the United States; more than 14 million people are affected today.[1] At the national level, this has led to an increased awareness of asthma as a public health concern.

Public health agencies traditionally conduct surveillance in response to the unexpected—to learn whether an apparent increase in disease is real and to find the causes. In the case of asthma, are the states aware of the extent of the problem? Have they undertaken surveillance activities?

When a disease has an environmental cause, public health agencies have a second important role: to control or eliminate causal environmental exposures. Asthma is triggered by a variety of environmental allergens and irritants; thus state health agencies have an important role to play in the detection and prevention of asthma.

Excerpted from "Asthma: The States' Challenge," by Clive M. Brown, Henry A. Anderson, and Ruth A. Etzel, in *Public Health Reports,* Vol. 112, No.3, May-June 1997, pp.198-205. © 1997 by U.S. Department of Health and Human Services. Reprinted with permission.

In 1996, the Council of State and Territorial Epidemiologists (CSTE), in conjunction with the Centers for Disease Control and Prevention (CDC), conducted a survey of asthma surveillance and control efforts. We found that most states and territories lack coordinated asthma programs and few have implemented programs to achieve the health goals related to asthma in Healthy People 2000,[2] [See "Healthy People 2000 Asthma Goals" at end of article] which, among other things, called for the establishment of 35 state-based asthma surveillance programs. These programs would allow states to identify high risk communities for targeted intervention and allow them to monitor progress in reducing the burden of disease.[3]

Who Gets Asthma?

Asthma is a chronic inflammatory disorder of the airways characterized by intermittent, recurrent episodes of wheezing, breathlessness, chest tightness, and cough, particularly at night or in the early morning or both.[4] In the United States, asthma is the most common chronic disease of childhood,[5] affecting almost five million children below the age of 18, and has become the fourth leading cause of disability among children less than 18 years old.[6] Inner-city children have the highest prevalence of asthma and the highest asthma-associated hospitalization rates.[7,8] Studies have shown that asthma mortality is higher among inner-city children than other children,[7,8] higher among poor children than other children,[9] and higher among African Americans than other groups.[5,10] A recent CDC analysis of mortality data from its multiple-cause-of-death files found that between 1980 and 1993 African Americans ages 15 to 24 years consistently had the highest asthma-associated death rates.[1]

The association between poverty and adverse asthma outcomes seen among children in the United States is not evident in Great Britain or Canada.[11] This may be due at least in part to differences in health care systems.[11] Lack of access to care and reliance on emergency departments for primary care are associated with poor health outcomes in rural and inner-city poverty areas.[9,12] Maternal smoking during pregnancy[13] and exposure to dust mites[14] and cockroaches[14] are associated with asthma in inner-city children. Exposure to indoor allergens appears to be more common in these populations.[15]

Why Is Asthma on the Increase?

Many scientists are puzzled by the recent apparent increase in asthma morbidity and mortality. Bronchial airway hyper-reactivity in asthma is the respiratory manifestation of sensitization to allergens and irritants in the environment. The major role of genetics in predisposition to airway hyper-reactivity in people with asthma is supported by twin and genetic linkage studies. However, since changes in the genetic make-up of individuals occurs over generations, the rapid increase in the prevalence of asthma during the past decade suggests that changes at the genetic level are unlikely to be the cause.

Some of this increase in the prevalence of asthma may be due to increased recognition and diagnosis of the disease given greater awareness on the part of physicians of the pathophysiology of asthma and the clinical signs and symptoms associated with the disease and given the recent publication of asthma management guidelines by, for example, the National Heart, Lung, and Blood Institute.[4] However, these factors are also unlikely to account for all of the increase in prevalence.

Monitoring of environmental exposures related to asthma is usually restricted to epidemiologic or clinical studies, including the investigation of acute clusters of asthma symptoms or occupational exposures. There are few biomarkers to indicate exposure (especially acute exposure) to environmental factors. We are therefore unable to determine whether the increase in asthma is due to an increase in airborne levels of indoor or outdoor allergens and irritants.

One theory is that urbanization has increased our exposure to environmental allergens and irritants. By building more energy-efficient homes and by using more carpeting, it may be that we are providing the opportunity to collect more dust and to concentrate pollutants in the dust. Psychosocial factors that cause us to spend more time indoors and overcrowding in certain neighborhoods and in the home may lead to increased exposure to indoor pollutants. Overcrowding may also predispose to increases in the number of pests such as cockroaches and rodents. Socioeconomic factors related to lack of access to health care and to specialist services may also be related to an increase in asthma attacks.

Although there has been an overall decline in the proportion of people that are exposed to environmental tobacco smoke, the rate of smoking has increased in some populations, including young women. If these women are exposing their children to environmental tobacco smoke, especially during the perinatal period, this could be associated with an increase in the prevalence of asthma.

In summary, the increased prevalence of asthma seems to be related to a variety of factors, including increased diagnosis of the disease, increased exposure to environmental allergens and irritants, increased exposure of children to mothers' tobacco smoke, and psychosocial and socioeconomic factors.

Treatment and Prevention

Asthma is generally treated in ambulatory settings. Between 1965 and 1992 the estimated annual number of visits to physicians by people with asthma in this country approximately doubled, rising to an estimated annual average of 15 million visits.[16] Today, fewer visits for asthma are made to general practitioners and more to specialists.[16] While the total number of prescriptions filled annually in the United States rose by approximately 23% between 1988 and 1994, the number of asthma prescriptions filled during the same period increased by 48%, due primarily to increased use of anti-inflammatory drugs—inhaled corticosteroids and inhaled [beta.sub.2]-agonists. At the same time, the number of prescriptions for bronchodilators—xanthines—decreased significantly.[17] The use of anti-inflammatory drugs reflects the current view of asthma as a chronic inflammatory disorder of the airways. Yet despite an improved understanding of the pathophysiology of the disorder and advances in treatment, the prevalence of asthma and asthma-related morbidity and mortality continue to rise.

Education of patients and parents can play an important role in reducing the prevalence and severity of asthma. While the exact etiology of asthma is unknown, we know that a variety of environmental allergens and irritants trigger the bronchial hyper-responsiveness and airway obstruction that characterize the disease. These exposures can be avoided or reduced. Indoor air pollutants show the strongest association with exacerbations of asthma symptoms. Exposure to allergens from house dust mites[18] and cockroaches[14,15,19] and environmental tobacco smoke[20] usually contribute more than outdoor air pollutants.[21,22] Studies have shown that the environmental control of allergens,[23,24] including avoidance of environmental tobacco smoke, is effective in preventing attacks. Increasing parental knowledge of the effects of "secondhand smoke"[25] and patient and provider education programs[26,27] also reduce the severity of the disease and frequency of hospitalizations.

The management of the person with asthma should ideally incorporate both clinical treatment and preventive approaches that mobilize the family and the community to learn about asthma management. State and local health departments are essential to an effective effort; they have important roles to play in measuring the burden of disease in their areas and in identifying high risk populations and the pollutants associated with asthma. These departments should lead the development of targeted interventions to reduce the burden of disease. Unfortunately, the CSTE/CDC survey found that most states lacked the necessary funding and personnel.

State-Based Asthma Activities

We surveyed asthma surveillance and intervention programs in public health departments in the United States and asked about barriers to establishing such programs. CSTE/CDC sent questionnaires to 50 state and four territorial epidemiologists affiliated with CSTE, asking that the person most knowledgeable about asthma prevention and control programs in the state complete the questionnaire. Responses were received from 48 states and three territories.

State-level asthma control programs. In responding to the survey, only eight of the health departments reported that they had implemented any type of asthma control project within the previous 10 years. The two most important reasons given for not having an asthma control program were lack of funds and shortage of staff; however, 10 of the responding health departments indicated that they did not regard asthma as a public health priority.

Availability of data. In order for state health departments to understand the scope of [the] problem, they need to evaluate local data. All state health departments have access to mortality data; 82% (42) of the respondents reported that hospital discharge data were available, and 31% (16) reported that data on emergency department visits were available. Only 20% (10) reported being able to evaluate the use of public or private health care services for asthma care, with 8% (4) being able to identify first-time users of such services. Four responding health departments (8%) reported having data on the quality of life of people with asthma.

Use of data. Simply having data available does not mean that those data are used. For example, although 82% of respondents reported having access to hospital discharge data, only 34% of the respondents having those data had used them. In addition to legal constraints and technological barriers, states reported that ownership and cost issues made it difficult to obtain information, especially from private sources such as firms conducting health care analyses under contract with providers.

Most of the 10 health departments reporting that asthma was not a priority had not evaluated the asthma data for their jurisdictions.

None of the 10 had ever done a survey to determine the prevalence of asthma, and although hospital discharge data were available to nine of the 10, only three used them to study asthma. None of the 10 health departments had data available to them on emergency department visits, the use of public or private ambulatory care services for asthma, or the quality of life of people with asthma. None had a surveillance system in place to monitor trends in asthma.

Using national data sources. In written comments, survey respondents suggested additional sources of data on asthma—for example, adding state- and territory-specific questions about asthma to the Behavioral Risk Factor Survey (BRFSS), a monthly telephone survey of adults, which uses standard protocols and standard interviewing methods to inquire about behavioral risk factors. Our survey respondents also recognized the utility of using Medicaid data and of making diagnosis of asthma a performance measure in the Health Plan and Employer Data, an information set produced and used by the nation's managed care plans.

We agree that exploring the use of such national data sources could be beneficial and result in savings of both time and money. BRFSS data could be used to estimate the prevalence of asthma and its effects, and HEDIS or Medicaid data monitored over time could form the basis of a surveillance system by providing estimates of services used by asthmatics. Our findings suggest that state public health officials need to explore ways of removing barriers to the use of existing data in order to develop asthma surveillance systems and novel intervention programs.

State-based surveys and surveillance. A survey to determine the local burden of asthma and the environmental exposures related to asthma in specific geographic areas is a good first step toward an asthma program. An ongoing surveillance system is needed to monitor trends in the disease and the effectiveness of interventions. Only 20% of respondents (10) reported that they had ever done a survey to determine the prevalence of asthma. Prevalence data would allow a department to target intervention at populations with the greatest need. Only one health department reported having a surveillance system in place to monitor trends in asthma.

Intervention programs. About half of the responding health departments reported involvement in intervention programs to control asthma in communities within their jurisdiction at some point during the previous 10 years. In addition to state-level programs sponsored by the health departments, these included activities initiated or sponsored by other agencies or groups.

Twenty-six health departments indicated that they had implemented or helped implement limited asthma intervention programs in communities within their jurisdictions. Only three health departments told us they were currently involved in an intervention program. Unfortunately, only one state has an ongoing asthma surveillance system that would allow it to monitor the impact of these interventions.

Of the 25 asthma intervention programs reported by the health departments surveyed, 56% (14) involved public education, 56% (14) involved patient education, 48% (12) involved the education of health care providers, and 20% (5) involved legislation. Only 8 of the 22 environmental control programs included active intervention measures such as efforts to reduce dust and allergens in dust or financial incentives to enroll in smoking cessation programs. The remaining 14 were passive programs, which provided people with information but did not offer concrete support.

Plans for future programs. Of 48 responding departments not involved in an asthma intervention or control program at the time of the survey, seven indicated that they planned to develop a program in the near future. Of the remaining 41 states and territories, 34 said they would be interested in starting a program. Of the seven states not interested in starting an asthma control program, five reported that asthma was not considered a public health priority.

We asked respondents to tell us where an asthma intervention or control program might be located within their organizations. About half (23/43) of the health departments that had not been involved with an asthma control program in the last 10 years indicated that a future asthma control program would probably be located within existing chronic disease programs, while 26% (11/43) suggested the program would probably be shared among two or more program areas. Asthma programs at the CDC are in the Center for Environmental Health, which focuses on the environmental exposures; thus to attack clinical and health education issues, CDC will need to draw on resources from other centers and coordinate efforts.

Implementing New Asthma Surveillance and Control Programs

Starting and maintaining asthma programs may seem costly, yet asthma itself—measured in terms of both direct and indirect costs—

represents a large economic burden. The estimated medical costs associated with asthma were nearly 1% of total U.S. health care costs in 1985, increasing from $4.5 billion to $6.2 billion between 1985 and 1990.[28] Programs to limit the exposure for people with asthma to allergens and irritants and thus reduce exacerbations of symptoms could potentially result in great savings to society.

We asked for estimates of the start-up cost of an asthma surveillance system. Thirty-eight percent (17/45) of those answering the question indicated a cost between $100,000 and $250,000, and 44% (20/45) between $50,000 and $100,000. For an asthma intervention program, 54% (22/41) of those answering the question estimated start-up costs at between $100,000 and $250,000, and 29% (12/41) between $50,000 and $100,000.

Using the upper bounds of these estimates, we calculate the total start-up cost for state-based asthma surveillance systems across the United States at approximately $9 million and the cost of starting asthma intervention programs at approximately $10 million. Because costs would differ depending on the nature and scope of the program, the size of the population, and the prevalence of asthma, it might be prudent to start with demonstration intervention and surveillance programs in a few states. Evaluating the prevention effectiveness ("the systematic assessment of the impact of public health policies, programs, and practices on health outcomes"[29] of these demonstration projects would produce an estimate of the direct and indirect medical costs saved. These demonstration projects could serve as models for other states and territories.

Clinical guidelines. The National Asthma Education Program of the National Heart, Lung, and Blood Institute (NHLBI) has developed guidelines for the diagnosis and management of asthma.[4,30] Of the health departments in our survey, 57% knew about the NHLBI guidelines. Seventy-eight percent reported being unsure if their public health clinics used the guidelines, while 12% stated that their clinics did not use the NHLBI guidelines. (It should be kept in mind that not all health departments offer clinical services.) Cooperation between CDC, NHLBI, and state and territorial health departments could assure distribution of the guidelines to providers serving populations with the greatest need for clinical services.

Recommendations

In addition to a responsibility for the health of the whole population, public health agencies have traditionally provided clinical services to medically underserved populations.[31] For asthma, these jobs come together because the populations that have often relied on the health department for medical care are also the groups with a high prevalence of asthma. Thus we recommend that with regard to asthma, state and territorial public health departments should be able to:

- Access and interpret existing asthma-related data on hospital discharges and emergency department visits;

- Access and interpret existing asthma-related data from nontraditional sources such as Medicaid and HEDIS;

- Conduct surveys to assess the prevalence of asthma and the prevalence of environmental exposures associated with asthma;

- Implement targeted intervention programs for high risk populations based on local data; and

- Develop novel asthma surveillance systems to monitor local trends in the disease.

We believe that collaboration is essential to the design and implementation of comprehensive community-based asthma prevention programs. Providers, payers, and patient representatives as well as academic centers and community and citizen groups must work with state and local health departments, which in turn must work with CDC and other Federal agencies. Surveillance systems are needed from the start to help us understand asthma, to direct interventions, and for accurate evaluation of our progress against the disease.

A national strategy is needed too, to assure that every person with asthma has access to state-of-the-art case management and appropriate care and to assure that every state and local public health department and the programs they coordinate can abate the air pollutants that put people with asthma at risk. With a coordinated approach we anticipate decreasing the burden of asthma on people with the condition, on their families, and on the health care system.

Healthy People 2000 Asthma Goals

Health goals related to asthma in Healthy People 2000: National Health Promotion and Disease Prevention Objectives (11.1, 17.4, 17.14b, 11.16).[2]

- Reduce hospitalizations from 188 per 100,000 to 160 per 100,000.

- Reduce from 19% to 10% the proportion of people with asthma whose activities are limited by the disease.

- Increase the proportion of people with asthma who get formal patient education from 9% to 50%.

- Establish and monitor 35 state-based plans to define and track sentinel respiratory diseases triggered by environmental factors.

References

1. Centers for Disease Control and Prevention (U.S.). Asthma mortality and hospitalization among children and young adults—United States, 1980-1993. *MMWR Morbid Mortal Wkly Rep* 1996;45:350-3.

2. Public Health Service (U.S.). Healthy People 2000: national health promotion and disease prevention objectives. Washington: Department of Health and Human Services; 1991. Pub. No. (PHS) 91-50212.

3. Centers for Disease Control and Prevention (U.S.). Asthma surveillance programs in public health departments—United States. *MMWR Morbid Mortal Wkly Rep* 1996;45:802-4.

4. National Heart, Lung, and Blood Institute, National Institutes of Health (U.S.). Global initiative for asthma: global strategy for asthma management and prevention. Bethesda (MD): The Institute; 1995. Pub. No. 95-3659.

5. Adams PF, Marano MA. Current estimates from the National Health Interview Survey, 1994. Vital and Health Statistics Vol. 10, No. 94. Hyattsville (MD): National Center for Health Statistics (US); 1995.

6. Centers for Disease Control and Prevention (U.S.). Disabilities among children aged less than or equal to 17 years—United States, 1991-1992. *MMWR Morbid Mortal Wkly Rep* 1995;44:609-13.

7. Centers for Disease Control and Prevention (U.S.). Asthma—United States, 1982-1992. *MMWR Morbid Mortal Wkly Rep* 1995;43: 952-5.

8. Weiss KB, Gergen PJ, Crain EF. Inner-city asthma: the epidemiology of an emerging U.S. public health concern. *Chest* 1993;101: 362S-367S.

9. Malveaux F, Houlihan D, Diamond EL. Characteristics of asthma mortality and morbidity in African-Americans. *J Asthma* 1993;30: 431-7.

10. Weitzman M, Gortmaker SL, Sobol AM, Perrin JM. Recent trends in the prevalence and severity of asthma. *JAMA* 1992;268:2673-7.

11. Gergen P. Social class and asthma—distinguishing between the disease and the diagnosis [editorial]. *Am J Public Health* 1996;68: 1361-2.

12. St. Peter RF, Newacheck PW, Halfon N. Access to care for poor children. *JAMA* 1992;267:2760-4.

13. Oliveti JF, Kercsmar CM, Redline C. Pre- and perinatal risk factors for asthma in inner-city African American children. *Am J Epidemiol* 1996;143:570-7.

14. Call RS, Smith TF, Morris E, Chapman MD, Platts-Mills T. Risk factors for asthma in inner-city children. *J Pediatr* 1992;121:862-6.

15. Kang BC, Johnson J, Veres-Thosner C. Atopic profile of inner-city children with a comparative analysis of the cockroach-sensitive and ragweed-sensitive subgroups. *J Allergy Clin Immunol* 1993;92: 802-11.

16. Fitzgerald ST, Huss K, Huss RW. The diagnosis and management of asthma: an update. *AAOHN J* 1996;44:94-102.

17. Terr AI, Bloch D. Trends in asthma therapy in the United States: 1965-1992. *Ann Allergy Asthma Immunol* 1996;76:273-81.

18. Sporik R, Holgate ST, Platts-Mills TA, Cogswell JJ. Exposure to house-dust mite allergen (*Der p I*) and the development of asthma in childhood: a prospective study. *N Engl J Med* 1990;323:502-7.

19. Kang B, Vellody D, Hombarger H, Yuninger JW. Cockroach: cause of allergic asthma. *J Allergy Clin Immunol* 1979;63:80-6.

20. Martinez FD, Cline M, Burrows B. Increased incidence of asthma in children of smoking mothers. *Pediatrics* 1992;89:21-6.

21. Ostro BD, Braxton-Owens H, White MC. Air pollution and asthma: exacerbations among African-American children in Los Angeles. 1995;7:711-22.

22. White MC, Etzel RA, Wilcox WD, Lloyd C. Exacerbations of childhood asthma and ozone pollution in Atlanta. *Envir Res* 1994;65: 56-68.

23. Ehnert B, Lau-Schadendorf S, Weber A, Buettner P, Schou C, Wahn U. Reducing domestic exposure to dust mite allergen reduces bronchial hyperactivity in sensitive children with asthma. *J Allergy Clin Immunol* 1992;90:135-8.

24. DeBlay F, Chapman MD, Platts-Mills TA. Airborne cat allergen (*Fel d I*): environmental control with the cat in-situ. *Am Rev Respir Dis* 1991;143:1334-5.

25. Murray AB, Morrison BJ. The decrease in severity of asthma in children of parents who smoke since the parents have been exposing them to less cigarette smoke. *J Allergy Clin Immunol* 1993;91:102-110.

26. Huss K, Rand CS, Butz AM, Eggleston PA, Murigande C, Thompson LC, et al. Home environmental risk factors in urban minority asthmatic children. *Ann Allergy* 1994;72:173-7.

27. Carswell F, Robinson EJ, Hek G, Shenton T. A Bristol experience: benefits and cost of an "asthma nurse" visiting homes of asthmatic children. *Bristol Medico-Chirurgical J* 1989;104:11-2.

28. Weiss KB, Gergen PJ, Hodgson TA. An economic evaluation of asthma in the United States. *N Eng J Med* 1992;326:862-6.

29. Teutsch SM. A framework for assessing the effectiveness of disease and injury prevention. *MMWR Morbid Mortal Wkly Rep* 1992;41(RR-3):i-iv, 1-12.

30. National Heart, Lung, and Blood Institute, National Institutes of Health (U.S.). Guidelines for the diagnosis and management of asthma. Bethesda (MD): The Institute; 1991. NIH Pub. No. 91-3042.

31. Starfield B. Public health and primary care: a framework for proposed linkages [editorial]. *Am J Public Health* 1996;68:1365-9.

— *by Clive M. Brown, Henry A. Anderson, and Ruth A. Etzel*

Dr. Brown and Dr. Etzel are with the Division of Environmental Hazards and Health Effects, National Center for Environmental Health, Centers for Disease Control and Prevention, Atlanta, GA. Dr. Brown is a Medical Epidemiologist with the Air Pollution and Respiratory Health Branch. At the time of this study, Dr. Etzel was Chief of the Air Pollution and Respiratory Health Branch; she currently is Assistant Director for Special Projects for the Division. Dr. Anderson is an Environmental Epidemiologist Consultant with the Council of State and Territorial Epidemiologists, Atlanta, GA.

Address correspondence to Dr. Brown, Air Pollution and Respiratory Health Branch, Division of Environmental Hazards and Health Effects, National Center for Environmental Health, CDC, 4770 Buford Highway, MS-F39, Chamblee, GA 30341; tel. 770-488-7697; fax 770-488-3507; e-mail <cmb8@cdc.gov.

Chapter 12

Asthma by Race, Sex, Age, and State

Introduction

Asthma is a chronic inflammatory disorder of the airways characterized by variable airflow obstruction and airway hyperresponsiveness in which prominent clinical manifestations include wheezing and shortness of breath[1]. It is a multifactorial disease that has been associated with familial, infectious, allergenic, socioeconomic, psychosocial, and environmental factors[2,3]. Asthma morbidity and mortality are largely preventable with improved patient education regarding the factors associated with asthma and medical management[1,4]. Surveillance information on asthma, with the exception of mortality data, are not available at the state or local level. Such information is needed to identify high-risk populations and to design and evaluate interventions aimed at preventing the development or exacerbation of this disease. This report summarizes and reviews national data for self-reported asthma prevalence (1980-1994), asthma office visits (1975-1995), asthma emergency room visits (1992-1995), asthma hospitalizations

Excerpted from "Surveillance for Asthma—United States, 1960-1995," by David M. Mannino, M.D., David M. Homa, Ph.D., Carol A. Pertowski, M.D., Annette Ashizawa, Ph.D., Leah L. Nixon, M.P.H., Carol A. Johnson, M.P.H., Lauren B. Ball, D.O., M.P.H., Elizabeth Jack, and David S. Kang, in *Morbidity and Mortality Weekly Review (MMWR)*, Surveillance Summaries, Vol. 47, SS-1, April 24, 1998, pp. 1-28 [Online] October 5, 1998. Available: http://www.cdc.gov/epo/mmwr/preview/mmwrhtml/00052262.htm. Produced by the Centers for Disease Control and Prevention (CDC). For complete contact information, please refer to Chapter 68, "Resources."

(1979-1994), and asthma deaths (1960-1995). In addition, this report describes several asthma surveillance programs at the state and local levels that may be useful to other states that are developing asthma surveillance systems.

Methods

We used existing databases to evaluate self-reported asthma prevalence, asthma office visits, asthma emergency room visits, asthma hospitalizations, and asthma mortality. At the state level, only asthma mortality data are reported; the other endpoints are available only at regional and national levels. The four regions represent standardized geographical divisions defined by the U.S. Bureau of the Census. We used data from the 1960, 1970, 1980, and 1990 censuses and the 1996 intercensal estimate to calculate denominators for office visit rates, emergency room visit rates, hospitalization rates, and death rates. We stratified each censal dataset by region, sex, race (white, black, and other), and age group (i.e., 0-4 years, 5-14 years, 15-34 years, 35-64 years, and greater than or equal to 65 years). The 1960 census reported only whites and nonwhites; therefore, we used the 1970 region-, sex-, and age-specific proportions between black and other nonwhite populations and applied this proportion to the 1960 region-, sex-, and age-specific population of nonwhites. We used linear interpolation to estimate the population for years in which there was neither census data nor the intercensal estimate. We used the civilian, noninstitutionalized population of the United States as our denominator for prevalence rates.

The diagnosis of asthma is less reliable among persons aged less than 5 years and those aged greater than 35 years[5] compared with persons aged 5-34 years. Persons in these same age groups, however, are the ones most likely to be adversely affected by asthma[6,7]. The figures in this summary depict the asthma endpoints, by region, both among the overall population and among persons aged 5-34 years.

For most datasets, we grouped the data into 3-year groups. We also race-, sex-, and age-adjusted our estimates to the 1970 U.S. population, using the five age groups (i.e., 0-4 years, 5-14 years, 15-34 years, 35-64 years, and greater than or equal to 65 years). We used 1970 as a reference population because we had complete race, sex, and age data available from the 1970 census. All analyses were done using SAS (SAS Institute, Cary, NC) and SUDAAN (RTI, Research Triangle Park, NC). We used the procedure REG in SAS to determine whether the trends over time in asthma prevalence rates, asthma office visit rates, asthma emergency room visit rates, asthma hospitalization rates, and asthma death rates were significant. We used two-tailed t tests to compare asthma hospitalization rates and asthma emergency room visit rates between regions, racial groups, age groups, and males and females in a single year or group of years. Using the Bonferroni adjustment for multiple comparisons in up to five groups, we considered a p value of 0.05 as significant.

Self-Reported Prevalence

The National Health Interview Survey (NHIS) is conducted annually among a probability sample of the civilian, noninstitutionalized population of the United States by the National Center for Health Statistics (NCHS)[8]. The NHIS questionnaire asks participants about their own present health status and that of other persons in their families, including whether they have had any recent illnesses. Each year, one sixth of the sample (approximately 20,000 of 120,000 persons) are asked whether they have had any one of 17 chronic respiratory diseases, including asthma, during the preceding 12 months. We used this subset of NHIS to determine the prevalence of self-reported asthma, using NHIS weights to determine national estimates of the population affected. Information on chronic conditions is collected on NHIS core questionnaires in which questions are asked about all family members. Although all members of the family are invited to participate in the interview, in many cases, a single respondent provides information for other family members. Thus, for adults, information on asthma may not have been reported by subjects themselves; for children, all information would have been provided by an adult responding for the family. We used SUDAAN to determine the relative standard errors (RSEs) of the estimates and to indicate which estimates were reliable (i.e., RSE less than 30%, which is equivalent to a relative confidence interval less than 59%).

Office Visits

Ambulatory medical care is the predominant means of providing health care services in the United States. Since 1975, NCHS has administered the National Ambulatory Medical Care Survey (NAMCS), collecting information on ambulatory patient visits to physicians' offices[9]. Of the 3,507 physicians included in the 1975 NAMCS sample, 2,081 actually participated in the survey. Approximately 2,000 physicians participated in the survey in subsequent years that the survey was administered (i.e., 1980, 1981, 1985, and 1989-1995). For each year, 30,000-60,000 patient encounters were included in the database. We identified visits for which asthma (International Classification of Diseases, Ninth Revision, Clinical Modification {ICD-9-CM}, code 493) was the first-listed diagnosis. Sample weights were used to obtain national estimates of annual office visits for asthma. We used the RSEs, which are listed with the database documentation, to indicate which estimates were reliable (i.e., RSE less than 30%).

Emergency Room Visits

Since 1992, information on visits to hospital emergency and outpatient departments has been collected annually by NCHS in the National Hospital Ambulatory Medical Care Survey (NHAMCS)[10]. For this analysis, we included only the emergency room database. For each year, records from 25,000 to 45,000 emergency room visits were included in the survey. We identified emergency room records for which asthma (ICD-9-CM-493) was listed as the first diagnosis. We used the survey weights to obtain national estimates of emergency room visits for asthma. We used the RSEs to indicate which estimates were reliable (i.e., RSE less than 30%).

Hospitalizations

To investigate national trends in hospitalizations attributable to asthma in the United States during 1979-1994, we analyzed hospitalization data from the National Hospital Discharge Survey (NHDS)[11], which is conducted annually by NCHS. These data were obtained from a sample of inpatient records from a national sample of non-federal general and short-stay specialty hospitals in the United States. Hospitalizations considered attributable to asthma were those with ICD-9-CM-493 listed as the primary discharge diagnosis. Data on race were missing for 5%-20% of the sample in any given year[12]; we excluded these subjects from the race-specific rate calculations but included them in all of the other rate calculations. Thus, the race-specific, age-adjusted rates underestimate the true hospitalization rates. We used the RSEs to indicate which estimates were reliable (i.e., RSE less than 30%). The survey was redesigned in 1988; our trend analysis was done on data during 1988-1994[13].

Mortality

We reviewed the Underlying Cause of Death dataset from NCHS[14] for 1960 through 1995 to identify all deaths in which asthma was selected as the underlying cause of death. During this period, three different ICD classifications were used to indicate a diagnosis of asthma: ICD-7 (code 241, 1960-1967), International Classification of Diseases, Eighth Revision (Adapted) (ICDA-8) (code 493, 1968-1978), and ICD-9 (code 493, 1979-1995). The comparability ratio for asthma (ICD-9/ICDA-8) is 1.35, indicating that approximately 35% more deaths would be attributed to asthma as the underlying cause of death under ICD-9 as compared with ICDA-8[15]. Part of this change was related to classifying "asthmatic bronchitis" as "bronchitis" in ICDA-8 but as "asthma" in ICD-9[16]. The comparability ratio for asthma (ICDA-8/ICD-7) is 0.70, indicating that approximately 30% fewer deaths would have been assigned to asthma under ICDA-8 compared with ICD-7[17]. For 1960 and 1961 mortality data, race was classified as white and nonwhite. For these years, we estimated the number of blacks and persons of other races within the nonwhite stratum (by state, race, and age) by using the proportion of blacks and persons of other races in that same stratum during 1962-1963. We used a similar technique to estimate the number of deaths among blacks and whites in New Jersey for 1962 and 1963, as no race data were available for that state for those years. In addition to the regional analysis, we did a state-by-state analysis of death rates among blacks and whites within 6-year periods. Among blacks, we restricted our analysis to states in which two or more asthma deaths occurred annually over the 6-year period, corresponding to an RSE of less than 30%. Our trend analysis was limited to data during 1979-1995.

Results

During the preceding 15 years, prevalence and death rates for asthma have increased both nationally and regionally. Regional differences were apparent for some endpoints (e.g., hospitalization rates and emergency room visit rates) but not for others (e.g., prevalence rates).

Self-Reported Prevalence

The self-reported prevalence rate for asthma increased 75% from 1980 to 1994; by 1993-1994, an estimated 13.7 million persons reported asthma during the preceding 12 months (Table 12.1.). This increasing trend in rates was evident among all race strata, both sexes, and all age groups (p less than 0.05 for all). The most substantial increase occurred among children aged 0-4 years (160%, from 22.2

per 1,000 to 57.8 per 1,000; p less than 0.05) and persons aged 5-14 years (74%, from 42.8 per 1,000 to 74.4 per 1,000; p less than 0.05) (Table 12.2.). During 1993-1994 the self-reported prevalence rate for asthma was slightly higher among persons aged less than or equal to 14 years than among persons aged greater than or equal to 15 years. The increasing trend in asthma prevalence rates during 1980-1994 was evident and significant (p less than 0.05) in every region of the United States, with the prevalence patterns in the overall population similar to those among persons aged 5-34 years. During 1993-1994, asthma prevalence rates were similar in all four regions of the country.

Office Visits

From 1975 to 1993-1995, the estimated annual number of office visits for asthma more than doubled, from 4.6 million to 10.4 million (Table 12.3.). Repeat visits could not be separated out in the data; therefore, the number of persons affected cannot be determined. Increasing rates were evident among all race strata, both sexes, and all age groups (Table 12.4.). Estimated regional rates for asthma office visits also increased, but not uniformly. During 1993-1995, the rate for office visits for asthma was lowest among persons aged 15-34 years (p less than 0.05) (Table 12.4.). We did not report on hospital outpatient visits for asthma, which comprise less than 10% of total visits for asthma[18], and for which data were only available for 1992-1995.

Emergency Room Visits

Data for emergency room visits are available for 1992-1995. Over this period, the national rate of emergency room visits for asthma did not change significantly (p less than 0.05). In 1995, there were an estimated greater than 1.8 million emergency room visits for asthma (Table 12.5.). Blacks had consistently higher rates for emergency room visits than whites (p less than 0.05), and rates decreased as age strata increased (Table 12.6.). In 1995, the Northeast had higher rates than the South and West, both among the entire population and among persons aged 5-34 years (p less than 0.05). For each year, the rate for emergency room visits for asthma decreased with increasing age (Table 12.6.).

Hospitalizations

Between 1979-1980 and 1993-1994, the estimated national number of asthma-related hospitalizations increased from 386,000 to

466,000 (Table 12.7.), whereas the national asthma hospitalization rate was not significantly changed (p greater than 0.05; Table 12.8.). During this period, hospitalization rates for asthma were consistently higher among blacks than they were among whites (p less than 0.05; Table 12.8.). During 1988-1994, asthma hospitalization rates increased in the Northeast but decreased in the Midwest and West (p less than 0.05). By 1993-1994, age-adjusted asthma hospitalization rates were higher among persons residing in the Northeast than they were among those residing in the West (p less than 0.05). A similar pattern was exhibited in the rates among persons aged 5-34 years. In every grouping of years, asthma hospitalization rates were highest among persons aged 0-4 years, lowest among persons aged 15-34 years, and intermediate among persons aged greater than or equal to 35 years (Table 12.8.).

Mortality

Overall rates of death with asthma as the underlying cause decreased from 1960-1962 through 1975-1977, and gradually increased again in all race, sex, and age strata (Table 12.9. and Table 12.10.). Blacks had consistently higher death rates than whites. Death rates were consistently higher in older age strata. In most race-, sex-, and age-strata, death rates were lower during 1968-1978, when the ICDA-8 coding system was being used, than in other years. Changes in ICD codes also may have affected death rates by region. We found a difference in the regional death rates for the entire population when compared with the death rates among persons aged 5-34 years; the West had the highest death rates in the overall population, whereas the Northeast and Midwest had the highest rates among persons aged 5-34 years. Death rates also varied among states within regions among both whites (Table 12.11.) and among blacks (Table 12.12.).

Table 12.1. Estimated Average Annual Number of Persons with Self-Reported Asthma during the Preceding 12 Months, by Race, Sex, and Age Group—United States, National Health Interview Survey, 1980-1994*

Category	1980	1981-1983	1984-1986	1987-1989	1990-1992	1993-1994
Race						
White	5,790,000	6,560,000	7,430,000	8,270,000	9,110,000	10,700,000
Black	880,000	1,020,000	1,030,000	1,510,000	1,590,000	1,880,000
Other	100,000+	180,000+	320,000+	280,000+	380,000	540,000
Sex						
Male	3,350,000	3,730,000	4,080,000	4,910,000	5,260,000	6,150,000
Female	3,410,000	4,110,000	4,680,000	5,290,000	6,060,000	7,400,000
Age group (yrs)						
0-4	360,000	550,000	600,000	620,000	870,000	1,280,000
5-14	1,520,000	1,560,000	1,790,000	2,130,000	2,360,000	2,790,000
15-34	2,160,000	2,410,000	2,810,000	3,210,000	3,320,000	4,050,000
35-64	1,960,000	2,410,000	2,460,000	2,980,000	3,630,000	4,090,000
≥65	770,000	920,000	1,100,000	1,260,000	1,150,000	1,480,000
Total§	6,770,000	7,850,000	8,760,000	10,200,000	11,330,000	13,690,000

*All relative standard errors are <30% (i.e., relative confidence interval <59%) unless otherwise indicated. +Relative standard error of the estimate is 30%-50%; the estimate is unreliable. §Numbers for each variable may not add up to total because of rounding error.

Table 12.2. Estimated Average Annual Rate* of Self-Reported Asthma during the Preceding 12 Months, by Race, Sex, and Age Group—United States, National Health Interview Survey, 1980-1994+

Category	1980	1981-1983	1984-1986	1987-1989	1990-1992	1993-1994
Race§						
White	30.4	33.9	37.7	41.1	44.7	50.8
Black	34.0	38.0	36.4	51.7	52.2	57.8
Other	22.5@	31.7@	28.2@	32.7@	39.7	48.6
Sex§						
Male	32.0	34.3	36.8	43.0	45.3	51.1
Female	29.2	34.7	38.4	42.3	47.5	56.2
Age group (yrs)						
0-4	22.2	32.6	34.3	33.9	46.1	57.8
5-14	42.8	44.7	51.1	60.7	65.9	74.4
15-34	27.7	30.2	35.1	40.1	41.7	51.8
35-64	28.	33.1	32.0	36.8	42.3	44.6
≥65	30.7	34.4	38.9	42.1	36.4	44.6
Total§	30.7	34.6	37.6	42.9	46.6	53.8

*Per 1,000 population. +All relative standard errors are <30% (i.e., relative confidence interval <59%) unless otherwise indicated. §Age-adjusted to the 1970 U.S. population. @Relative standard error of the estimate is 30%-50%; the estimate is unreliable.

Table 12.3. Estimated Average Number of Office Visits for Asthma as the First-Listed Diagnosis, by Race, Sex, and Age Group—United States, National Ambulatory Medical Care Survey, 1975-1995*

Category	1975	1980-1981	1985	1989	1990-1992	1993-1995
Race						
White	4,084,000	4,804,000	5,663,000	5,471,000	6,980,000	8,316,000
Black	463,000+	584,000+	702,000	893,000	1,196,000	1,373,000
Other	&	&	&	&	290,000	686,000
Sex						
Male	2,173,000	2,643,000	2,972,000	2,458,000	3,695,000	4,252,000
Female	2,460,000	2,830,000	3,531,000	4,364,000	4,866,000	6,122,000
Age group (yrs)						
0-4	429,000+	517,000+	556,000	626,000+	950,000	1,024,000
5-14	867,000	1,629,000	1,520,000	975,000	1,821,000	2,004,000
15-34	1,009,000	1,140,000	1,206,000	1,580,000	1,984,000	1,876,000
35-64	1,743,000	1,506,000	2,275,000	2,684,000	2,617,000	3,982,000
≥65	584,000	680,000	945,000	957,000	1,187,000	1,488,000
Total@	4,632,000	5,472,000	6,502,000	6,822,000	8,559,000	10,374,000

*All relative standard errors are <30% (i.e., relative confidence interval <59%) unless otherwise indicated. +Relative standard error of the estimate is 30%-50%; the estimate is unreliable. &Relative standard error of the estimate exceeds 50%. @Numbers for each variable may not add up to total because of rounding error and missing race for 1989 and 1990-1992.

Table 12.4. Estimated Average Rates* of Office Visits for Asthma as the First-Listed Diagnosis, by Race, Sex, and Age Group—United States, National Ambulatory Medical Care Survey, 1975-1995+

Category	1975	1980-1981	1985	1989	1990-1992	1993-1995
Race§						
White	22.2	26.2	29.3	26.2	34.6	39.6
Black	19.7@	22.4@	26.8	29.9	39.5	43.8
Other	**	**	**	**	17.3	34.1
Sex§						
Male	21.1	25.8	27.3	21.0	31.2	33.9
Female	21.5	23.7	28.3	32.7	36.7	43.6
Age group (yrs)						
0-4	25.3@	30.4@	30.7	32.7@	48.2	50.3
5-14	22.5	45.6	42.6	27.0	49.3	51.5
15-34	14.1	13.9	14.6	19.0	23.9	22.8
35-64	25.4	20.7	28.8	31.7	29.5	41.7
≥65	25.3	25.8	33.0	30.9	37.0	44.0
Total§	21.4	25.0	27.9	27.0	34.1	39.0

*Per 1,000 population. +All relative standard errors are <30% (i.e, relative confidence interval <59%) unless otherwise indicated. §Age-adjusted to the 1970 U.S. population. @Relative standard error of the estimate is 30%-50%; the estimate is unreliable. **Relative standard error of the estimate exceeds 50%.

Table 12.5. Estimated Annual Number of Emergency Room Visits for Asthma as the First-Listed Diagnosis, by Race, Sex, and Age Group—United States, National Hospital Ambulatory Medical Care Survey, 1992-1995*

Category	1992	1993	1994	1995
Race				
White	925,000	1,000,000	927,000	1,018,000
Black	488,000	642,000	635,000	775,000
Other	54,000+	43,000+	45,000+	73,000+
Sex				
Male	667,000	766,000	735,000	725,000
Female	800,000	920,000	872,000	1,140,000
Age group (yrs)				
0-4	288,000	334,000	298,000	248,000
5-14	291,000	317,000	313,000	322,000
15-34	438,000	488,000	517,000	566,000
35-64	361,000	473,000	400,000	630,000
≥65	89,000	74,000	79,000	101,000
Total&	1,467,000	1,686,000	1,607,000	1,867,000

*All relative standard errors are <30% (i.e., relative confidence interval <59%) unless otherwise indicated. +Relative standard error of the estimate is 30%-50%; the estimate is unreliable. &Numbers for each variable may not add up to total because of rounding error.

Table 12.6. Estimated Annual Rate* of Emergency Room Visits for Asthma as the First-Listed Diagnosis, by Race, Sex, and Age Group—United States, National Hospital Ambulatory Medical Care Survey, 1992-1995[+]

Category	1992	1993	1994	1995
Race[&]				
White	46.8	50.3	46.1	48.8
Black	151.9	197.4	191.2	228.9
Other	28.6[@]	23.7[@]	21.9[@]	33.1[@]
Sex[&]				
Male	55.5	62.6	53.4	57.8
Female	61.4	69.7	65.9	82.3
Age group (yrs)				
0-4	143.5	164.3	145.5	120.7
5-14	77.1	82.8	80.3	81.3
15-34	52.9	59.0	62.8	69.2
35-64	39.6	50.7	41.8	64.4
≥65	27.7	22.6	23.5	29.5
Total[&]	58.8	66.6	62.9	70.7

*Per 10,000 population. [+]All relative standard errors are <30% (i.e., relative confidence interval <59%) unless otherwise indicated. [&]Age-adjusted to the 1970 U.S. population. [@]Relative standard error of the estimate is 30%-50%; the estimate is unreliable.

109

Table 12.7. Estimated Average Number of Hospitalizations for Asthma as the First-Listed Diagnosis, by Race, Sex, and Age Group—United States, National Hospital Discharge Survey, 1979-1994*

Category	1979-1980	1981-1983	1984-1986	1987-1989	1990-1992	1993-1994
Race						
White	271,000	317,000	322,000	296,000	254,000	240,000
Black	67,000	94,000	94,000	111,000	124,000	115,000
Other	12,000	17,000	23,000	27,000	23,000	26,000
Missing†	35,000	23,000	40,000	42,000	83,000	85,000
Sex						
Male	167,000	193,000	204,000	205,000	206,000	191,000
Female	219,000	259,000	275,000	271,000	277,000	275,000
Age group (yrs)						
0-4	56,000	72,000	85,000	95,000	111,000	97,000
5-14	56,000	66,000	66,000	65,000	73,000	67,000
15-34	68,000	75,000	75,000	76,000	74,000	78,000
35-64	127,000	148,000	146,000	135,000	132,000	139,000
≥65	79,000	90,000	106,000	105,000	94,000	85,000
Total§	386,000	451,000	478,000	476,000	484,000	466,000

*All relative standard errors are <30% (i.e., relative confidence interval <59%). †Race data was not collected by some hospitals in the survey. §Numbers for each variable may not add up to total because of rounding error.

Table 12.8. Estimated Average Rates* of Hospitalizations for Asthma as the First-Listed Diagnosis, by Race, Sex, and Age Group—United States, National Hospital Discharge Survey, 1979-1994[+]

Category	1979-1980	1981-1983	1984-1986	1987-1989	1990-1992	1993-1994
Race[§]						
White	14.2	16.2	15.9	14.1	11.9	10.9
Black	26.0	34.8	33.2	38.1	40.1	35.5
Other	28.2	30.6	32.7	33.6	24.4	23.0
Sex[§]						
Male	16.3	18.4	18.7	18.3	18.0	15.9
Female	18.7	21.4	21.8	21.0	20.8	20.0
Age group (yrs)						
0-4	34.3	42.8	48.5	52.2	58.3	49.7
5-14	15.9	19.2	18.9	18.7	20.6	18.0
15-34	8.7	9.5	9.5	9.5	9.3	10.0
35-64	18.2	20.3	19.0	16.7	15.4	15.2
≥65	31.5	33.6	37.5	35.2	29.7	25.6
Total[§]	17.6	20.0	20.5	19.8	19.7	18.1

*Per 10,000 population. [+]All relative standard errors are <30% (i.e., relative confidence interval <59%). [§]Age-adjusted to the 1970 U.S. population.

Table 12.9a. (continued in Table 12.9b.) Average Number of Deaths with Asthma as the Underlying Cause of Death Diagnosis, by Race, Sex, and Age Group—United States, Underlying Cause of Death Dataset, 1960-1995*

Category	1960-1962[+]	1963-1965	1966-1967	1968-1971[+]	1972-1974	1975-1978
Race						
White	4,342	3,928	3,499	1,786	1,588	1,466
Black	682	701	688	560	428	377
Other	43	44	45	36	22	28
Sex						
Male	3,226	2,806	2,392	1,052	879	782
Female	1,841	1,867	1,839	1,330	1,159	1,089
Age group (yrs)						
0-4	86	77	62	52	32	22
5-14	77	89	100	76	50	39
15-34	272	272	274	256	197	176
35-64	2,239	2,102	1,947	1,130	920	745
≥65	2,393	2,134	1,848	868	840	888
Total[§]	5,067	4,674	4,231	2,382	2,039	1,870

*All relative standard errors are <30%, (i.e., relative confidence interval <59%). [+]International Classification of Diseases (ICD), Seventh Revision: 1960-1967; ICD, Eighth Revision (Adapted): 1968-1978; and ICD, Ninth Revision: 1979-1995. [§]Numbers for each variable may not add up to total because of rounding error.

Table 12.9b. (continued from Table 12.9a.) Average Number of Deaths with Asthma as the Underlying Cause of Death Diagnosis, by Race, Sex, and Age Group—United States, Underlying Cause of Death Dataset, 1960-1995*

Category	1979-1980[+]	1981-1983	1984-1986	1987-1989	1990-1992	1993-1995
Race						
White	2,193	2,542	2,947	3,520	3,800	4,084
Black	514	652	769	972	1,022	1,182
Other	38	62	84	116	141	165
Sex						
Male	1,213	1,352	1,534	1,800	1,894	2,036
Female	1,532	1,904	2,266	2,809	3,069	3,394
Age group (yrs)						
0-4	27	27	28	28	40	34
5-14	53	76	91	103	108	136
15-34	223	309	331	392	420	489
35-64	962	1,164	1,305	1,541	1,588	1,798
≥65	1,481	1,679	2,045	2,545	2,807	2,972
Total[§]	2,745	3,255	3,800	4,609	4,963	5,429

*All relative standard errors are <30%, (i.e., relative confidence interval <59%). [+]International Classification of Diseases (ICD), Seventh Revision: 1960-1967; ICD, Eighth Revision (Adapted): 1968-1978; and ICD, Ninth Revision: 1979-1995. [§]Numbers for each variable may not add up to total because of rounding error.

Table 12.10a. (continued in Table 12.10b.) Rates* of Death with Asthma as the Underlying Cause of Death Diagnosis, by Race, Sex, and Age Group—United States, Underlying Cause of Death Dataset, 1960-1995[+]

Category	1960-1962[&]	1963-1965	1966-1967	1968-1971[&]	1972-1974	1975-1978
Race[@]						
White	26.6	23.1	20.0	9.8	8.3	7.2
Black	42.0	40.8	38.0	28.4	20.7	17.3
Other	25.7	23.0	22.3	15.3	8.1	8.4
Sex[@]						
Male	38.6	32.6	27.0	11.4	9.1	7.7
Female	19.5	18.7	17.7	12.3	10.0	8.8
Age group (yrs)						
0-4	4.3	4.0	3.4	3.0	1.9	1.3
5-14	2.1	2.4	2.6	1.8	1.3	1.1
15-34	5.6	5.2	4.9	4.3	3.0	2.4
35-64	36.9	33.9	30.8	17.5	13.8	10.9
≥65	141.5	118.8	98.1	43.6	38.7	37.6
Total[@]	28.2	24.9	21.8	11.8	9.5	8.2

*Per 1,000,000 population. [+]All relative standard errors are <30% (i.e., relative confidence interval <59%). [&]International Classification of Diseases (ICD), Seventh Revision: 1960-1967; ICD, Eighth Revision (Adapted): 1968-1978; ICD, Ninth Revision: 1979-1995. [@]Age-adjusted to the 1970 U.S. population.

Table 12.10b. (continued from Table 12.10a.) Rates* of Death with Asthma as the Underlying Cause of Death Diagnosis, by Race, Sex, and Age Group—United States, Underlying Cause of Death Dataset, 1960-1995+

Category	1979-1980&	1981-1983	1984-1986	1987-1989	1990-1992	1993-1995
Race@						
White	10.2	11.4	12.5	14.2	14.6	15.1
Black	22.2	26.7	30.0	36.1	35.6	38.5
Other	10.3	13.6	15.3	17.6	18.7	17.7
Sex@						
Male	11.5	12.2	13.2	14.7	14.8	15.1
Female	11.6	13.8	15.5	18.2	18.9	20.0
Age group (yrs)						
0-4	1.6	1.6	1.6	1.5	2.1	1.8
5-14	1.5	2.2	2.6	2.9	3.0	3.7
15-34	2.8	3.9	4.1	4.9	5.3	6.3
35-64	13.8	16.0	17.0	19.0	18.5	19.6
≥65	58.6	63.0	72.3	85.0	89.0	89.8
Total@	11.5	13.1	14.4	16.6	17.1	17.9

*Per 1,000,000 population. +All relative standard errors are <30% (i.e., relative confidence interval <59%). &International Classification of Diseases (ICD), Seventh Revision: 1960-1967; ICD, Eighth Revision (Adapted): 1968-1978; ICD, Ninth Revision: 1979-1995. @Age-adjusted to the 1970 U.S. population.

Discussion

This report describes several trends, raises questions, and highlights the need for improved surveillance of asthma and other chronic respiratory diseases. The overall picture of asthma is changing. National statistics indicate that asthma prevalence and mortality have increased in recent years, despite numerous advancements in the diagnosis and treatment of asthma. The reasons for these increases are not clear[2]. The data cannot be used to differentiate between a true increase in asthma versus an increase in the diagnosis of asthma by physicians[19].

Asthma-related deaths varied substantially by age group. Although asthma prevalence was lowest for persons aged greater than or equal to 35 years, this group accounted for greater than 85% of the asthma mortality. This may reflect an overlap in diagnosis of asthma with chronic obstructive pulmonary disease (COPD), an overlap most likely to occur among older persons. Clinically, the key difference between these conditions is that decreases in airway function are reversible in asthma, but not in COPD. However, persons with longstanding asthma, especially if inadequately treated, can develop irreversible changes in lung function[20]. Conversely, many persons with COPD can improve their lung function with interventions such as smoking cessation or medication[21]. Trends in overall asthma mortality through the 1960s and 1970s may have been affected by both changes in clinical diagnosis and changes in the ICD coding system[16]. At the state level, only mortality data are available for asthma. Age-adjusted death rates for asthma during 1990-1995 varied substantially from state to state, even among states in the same region (Table 12.11. and Table 12.12.).

We have used several measures of asthma morbidity: self-reported prevalence, office visits, emergency room visits, and hospitalizations. The overall national increase in the prevalence of asthma, which has been previously reported, occurred in all regions of the United States. We observed different trends, however, in hospitalization rates. In 1979, the four regions had similar hospitalization rates, both for the overall population and for persons aged 5-34 years. By 1994, overall rates in the Northeast were more than twice the rates in the West; among persons aged 5-34 years, the difference was more than threefold. The possible reasons for these differences include differences among the regions in asthma severity[22], asthma treatment[23], physician diagnosis[22], access to health care[24,18], climatic and home heating factors[25], or exposure to air pollutants[26,27]. Caution should be exercised in interpreting trends over time, in that methods of data collection, disease coding, and disease recognition have changed over the years[13,16].

The summary differences in asthma morbidity outcomes among regions raise the question of whether rates within the regions are also heterogeneous. The previously described state-to-state differences in death rates suggest that morbidity may also differ within regions and highlight the need for asthma surveillance data at the state and local level.

A 1996 survey by the Council of State and Territorial Epidemiologists and CDC revealed an interest in establishing asthma surveillance systems among states and territories that do not have programs[28]. Of the 43 state respondents who did not have an asthma-control program, 37 (86%) were interested in establishing such programs. Respondents cited funding and manpower limitations as the main reasons for not having an asthma-control program. Forty-two states had hospital discharge data available for characterizing asthma, but only 14 (33%) had used the data to examine asthma morbidity. In some states, legislative restraints and incompatible data formats contributed to an inability to use the data[28].

Several states have used existing data or have initiated other approaches to examine asthma morbidity. Wisconsin analyzed billing data from hospital emergency rooms to develop a low-cost surveillance system for asthma. The main data source came from billing data for emergency room visits for 1990-1994 from Children's Hospital of Wisconsin in Milwaukee. Data collected included demographic information, date of visit, diagnosis, and length of stay (if the patient was hospitalized). Patients aged less than 19 years who had a diagnosis of asthma (ICD-9-CM-493), acute pharyngitis (ICD-9-CM-462), upper respiratory infections (ICD-9-CM-465), or acute bronchitis or bronchiolitis (ICD-9-CM-466) were included[29,30]. Results from this study revealed that 20% of the children in the study accounted for 50% of the total number of emergency room visits, and 8% of these children accounted for 38% of all hospital admissions. Researchers also found that asthma admissions increased when sulfur dioxide levels in ambient air increased[29,30].

The Michigan Department of Community Health has examined hospital data from the Michigan Inpatient Discharge Database for 1989-1993 for children aged less than 15 years with a primary diagnosis of asthma (ICD-9-CM-493)[31]. Results indicated that the rate for asthma hospitalizations was higher for boys than for girls (43 per 10,000 versus 25 per 10,000) and that the rate for blacks was higher than for whites (81.3 per 10,000 versus 25.6 per 10,000). The data also demonstrated local differences, with three groups of counties in the southeast, southwest, and eastern parts of Michigan having higher hospitalization rates for asthma than the rest of the state[31].

Other potential sources of asthma surveillance include billing data from Medicaid and Medicare and data from managed-care organizations. In 1995, Arizona had a higher asthma death rate than the overall U.S. population (2.8 versus 2.1 per 100,000), with particularly high rates in Maricopa County, in which the city of Phoenix is located. Billing data and managed-care data from Maricopa County demonstrated high hospital discharge rates, particularly among blacks and Hispanics[32].

The Behavioral Risk Factor Surveillance System (BRFSS) is an ongoing random-digit-dialed telephone survey in which 45 states participate. The purpose of the survey is to ascertain the prevalence of behaviors and practices related to certain risk factors (e.g., cigarette smoking) associated with the leading causes of death in the United States. The system has core questions (e.g., about diabetes and tobacco use), which all state participants are required to ask and standardized modules (e.g., about health care utilization and weight control), which are optional. States may also include additional health questions as part of the survey, although these questions are not nationally standardized. Since 1996, New Hampshire, New York, and Oregon have included additional questions about asthma, and in 1997, Washington added questions about asthma. Respondents from all four states were asked if a doctor or other health professional had told them that they had asthma. New Hampshire, New York, and Oregon had questions on medication usage. New Hampshire and Washington included questions regarding children in the household with asthma, whereas New York and Oregon included a question on emergency room and urgent-care visits.

Oregon and New Hampshire have analyzed BRFSS data on asthma-specific questions. The American Lung Association of Oregon assisted in analyzing data for Oregon. These data, which are specific to adults, indicated that 6.6% of the 1995 respondents (n=2,371) and 7.4% of the 1996 respondents (n=2,932) reported active asthma (i.e., positive responses for wheezing during the preceding year and ever being told by a health provider that they had asthma). Nine percent of the respondents who had been told that they had asthma reported receiving emergency care for asthma during the year preceding the survey[33]. Data from New Hampshire revealed that 11% of the respondents (n=1,502) reported that they had been told that they had asthma. Of those with asthma (n=166), 19.9% of the males and 44.6% of the females had used medication. Almost 10% of the respondents reported that they had a child with asthma (L. Powers, New Hampshire Department of Health and Human Services, personal communication, 1997).

Asthma surveillance data collected by states have many uses. Researchers in Wisconsin have demonstrated that asthma surveillance data can be used to investigate correlations between environmental events and asthma morbidity. States are also using data to develop prevention strategies. In Michigan, prevention strategies have been implemented in areas with elevated hospital discharge rates for asthma. In southeast Michigan, an area where hospitalization rates for asthma are high, asthma has been made a health priority in a seven-county area. One county health department has organized an advisory committee to develop strategies for prevention (K. Wilcox, Michigan Department of Health, personal communication, 1997). The experience in Arizona highlights the importance of partnerships between the public and private sectors in collecting and analyzing surveillance data. Nationwide, CDC can help states identify potential partners in collecting surveillance data and also can help promote collaborative efforts.

One component of a proposed national strategy for asthma control and surveillance is to support the development of state-based asthma surveillance systems, using existing databases. As indicated by the state systems highlighted in this report, developing state-based surveillance systems for asthma will likely require the use of several sources of data. These data sources should be easily accessible and not costly. Some surveillance data that already exist include hospital discharge data, billing and insurance data, and managed-care data[34]. Hospital discharge data and the billing and insurance data (e.g., Medicare and Medicaid) would probably be the most accessible and least costly data sources in many states. Because managed-care organizations are private entities, use of their data may require the development of specific collaborative projects[32]. Potential national activities to promote the development of state surveillance systems include providing technical assistance on the design and implementation of systems and developing standardized data elements and case definitions for use by states. National activities can also encourage states to share information on data collection and analysis and on the development and assessment of control measures.

A second component of a proposed national strategy for asthma control and surveillance is to develop new databases that can provide estimates of morbidity at the state level. One approach that may meet these criteria is the BRFSS, which, in its present form, can obtain data reliable for adults but not for children. The use of an asthma module with randomly selected households can permit researchers to estimate asthma rates among adults. Another potential new source of data is the State and Local Integrated Telephone Survey, which is being piloted by NCHS and is modeled after NHIS. It could be used to obtain data on both persons with diagnosed asthma and persons with asthma symptoms (e.g., coughing or wheezing) but no diagnosis.

This report presents data on asthma morbidity and mortality and highlights the need for better state and local surveillance of asthma outcomes. Collecting local asthma data can aid in assessing the etiology of asthma and in evaluating prevention strategies. State-specific data can help public health officials direct prevention efforts and allocate resources. Finally, asthma surveillance systems can provide an opportunity for health departments to develop partnerships with voluntary associations, managed-care organizations, and other groups to better understand, prevent, and treat a growing and expensive health problem that affects both children and adults[4].

Table 12.11. Rates* of Death with Asthma as the Underlying Cause of Death among Whites, by Year, Region, and State—United States, Underlying Cause of Death Dataset, 1960-1995 **(Continued on next page)**

Region/State	1960-1965+	1966-1971&	1972-1977+	1978-1983&	1984-1989+	1990-1995
Northeast						
Connecticut	16.4	—	6.7	—	10.9	10.2
Maine	35.0	—	10.2	—	15.7	13.0
Massachusetts	25.3	—	8.1	—	14.7	14.1
New Hampshire	35.8	—	8.9	—	13.4	12.4
New Jersey@	17.5	—	4.5	—	9.4	11.3
New York	19.8	—	8.4	—	16.7	17.0
Pennsylvania	22.5	—	6.9	—	10.0	11.6
Rhode Island	28.0	—	6.1	—	8.6	9.5
Vermont	27.1	—	9.9	—	11.9	14.7
Midwest						
Illinois	21.5	—	7.0	—	11.8	14.5
Indiana	26.9	—	6.9	—	12.3	14.4
Iowa	29.6	—	6.8	—	14.9	16.6
Kansas	26.9	—	8.7	—	13.7	14.8
Michigan	30.6	—	9.1	—	12.5	14.1
Minnesota	26.0	—	8.1	—	15.7	18.1
Missouri	27.8	—	6.9	—	9.0	12.7
Nebraska	36.2	—	9.1	—	20.6	23.0
North Dakota	33.0	—	10.7	—	19.5	20.0
Ohio	22.8	—	6.3	—	11.2	11.7
South Dakota	33.6	—	6.6	—	16.3	18.3
Wisconsin	23.3	—	7.8	—	14.0	14.9

121

Table 12.11. (continued from previous page) Rates* of Death with Asthma as the Underlying Cause of Death among Whites, by Year, Region, and State—United States, Underlying Cause of Death Dataset, 1960-1995

Region/State	1960-1965+	1966-1971&	1972-1977+	1978-1983&	1984-1989+	1990-1995
South						
Alabama	20.4	—	7.0	—	9.3	10.1
Arkansas	18.4	—	5.6	—	9.5	15.3
Delaware	22.8	—	4.2	—	7.7	12.7
District of Columbia	20.2	—	7.3	—	13.0	12.1
Florida	22.5	—	6.6	—	9.8	11.5
Georgia	21.1	—	6.9	—	11.8	13.3
Kentucky	34.6	—	11.5	—	13.9	14.1
Louisiana	22.9	—	7.3	—	12.0	15.3
Maryland	18.8	—	6.2	—	9.4	11.1
Mississippi	19.8	—	5.6	—	10.3	11.1
North Carolina	24.0	—	8.7	—	14.1	16.4
Oklahoma	31.1	—	7.3	—	13.6	16.0
South Carolina	18.6	—	7.4	—	12.6	14.1
Tennessee	24.3	—	7.5	—	10.3	14.2
Texas	21.5	—	6.9	—	11.3	15.4
Virginia	22.4	—	7.5	—	15.4	16.3
West Virginia	33.6	—	11.4	—	14.1	15.4

West

State					
Alaska	25.8	—	9.4	—	11.6	5.3
Arizona	89.4	—	15.3	—	23.5	20.4
California	24.8	—	7.8	—	15.8	17.0
Colorado	29.9	—	10.6	—	23.2	21.3
Hawaii	27.3	—	11.5	—	14.9	23.3
Idaho	34.2	—	9.7	—	19.4	16.9
Montana	34.0	—	10.1	—	21.8	22.4
Nevada	36.9	—	10.2	—	14.1	15.8
New Mexico	43.1	—	12.4	—	22.9	22.9
Oregon	31.3	—	10.0	—	20.4	21.5
Utah	23.9	—	10.3	—	18.0	18.8
Washington	28.4	—	9.7	—	16.2	18.2
Wyoming	34.5	—	7.9	—	14.3	17.2

*Per 1,000,000 population, age-adjusted to the U.S. 1970 population. +International Classification of Diseases (ICD), Seventh Revision: 1960-1967; ICD, Eighth Revision (Adapted): 1968-1978; ICD, Ninth Revision: 1979-1995. &Rates are not reported for these year groupings because they cross ICD classifications. @For 1962 and 1963, the number of deaths among whites was estimated.

Northeast = Connecticut, Maine, Massachusetts, New Hampshire, New Jersey, New York, Pennsylvania, Rhode Island, and Vermont; Midwest = Illinois, Indiana, Iowa, Kansas, Michigan, Minnesota, Missouri, Nebraska, North Dakota, Ohio, South Dakota, and Wisconsin; South = Alabama, Arkansas, Delaware, District of Columbia, Florida, Georgia, Kentucky, Louisiana, Maryland, Mississippi, North Carolina, Oklahoma, South Carolina, Tennessee, Texas, Virginia, and West Virginia; and West = Alaska, Arizona, California, Colorado, Hawaii, Idaho, Montana, Nevada, New Mexico, Oregon, Utah, Washington, and Wyoming.

Table 12.12. Rates* of Death with Asthma as the Underlying Cause of Death among Blacks, by Year, Region, and State[+]—United States, Underlying Cause of Death Dataset, 1960-1995

Region/State	1960-1965[&***]	1966-1971[@]	1972-1977[**]	1978-1983[@]	1984-1989[**]	1990-1995
Northeast						
Connecticut	39.5	—	16.1	—	26.0	30.1
Massachusetts	52.9	—	33.8	—	32.2	36.4
New Jersey[++]	34.4	—	16.1	—	29.1	36.1
New York	46.9	—	24.7	—	45.8	49.0
Pennsylvania	34.3	—	15.1	—	27.9	34.0
Midwest						
Illinois	28.0	—	21.0	—	45.4	60.8
Indiana	46.8	—	12.0	—	29.8	30.2
Kansas	56.4	—	20.9	—	42.5	23.2
Michigan	46.6	—	18.0	—	32.1	38.5
Missouri	53.7	—	20.8	—	31.3	41.1
Ohio	48.7	—	15.9	—	31.5	32.2
Wisconsin	44.6	—	17.1	—	29.5	48.5
South						
Alabama	31.1	—	19.8	—	26.0	26.5
Arkansas	33.8	—	7.9	—	30.1	45.0
Delaware	11.9	—	21.1	—	30.8	19.2
District of Columbia	51.7	—	18.8	—	34.3	44.9
Florida	58.6	—	25.5	—	28.5	30.4
Georgia	39.3	—	19.3	—	36.5	30.9
Kentucky	44.3	—	23.2	—	20.0	32.8

State						
Louisiana	47.0	—	21.0	—	32.9	35.0
Maryland	45.3	—	17.3	—	23.5	25.6
Mississippi	30.8	—	13.1	—	27.6	32.2
North Carolina	32.2	—	20.7	—	30.2	31.7
Oklahoma	61.8	—	12.4	—	26.6	29.4
South Carolina	20.6	—	14.1	—	30.7	31.0
Tennessee	49.6	—	20.2	—	29.6	32.8
Texas	39.9	—	14.8	—	25.1	32.9
Virginia	42.4	—	22.6	—	26.4	36.7
West Virginia	46.2	—	24.8	—	12.0	26.3
West						
Arizona	104.1	—	20.4	—	39.4	40.6
California	40.3	—	18.1	—	37.9	36.6
Colorado	84.7	—	17.2	—	58.8	50.6
Washington	34.6	—	13.9	—	34.0	42.0

*Per 1,000,000 population, age-adjusted to the 1970 U.S. population. +Includes only data from states in which two or more asthma deaths occurred among blacks annually. &For 1960 and 1961, the number of deaths among blacks was estimated for all states. @Rates are not reported for these year groupings because they cross ICD classifications. **International Classification of Diseases (ICD), Seventh Revision: 1960-1967; ICD, Eighth Revision (Adapted): 1968-1978; ICD, Ninth Revision: 1979-1995. ++For 1962 and 1963, the number of deaths among blacks was estimated.
Northeast = Connecticut, Maine, Massachusetts, New Hampshire, New Jersey, New York, Pennsylvania, Rhode Island, and Vermont; Midwest = Illinois, Indiana, Iowa, Kansas, Michigan, Minnesota, Missouri, Nebraska, North Dakota, Ohio, South Dakota, and Wisconsin; South = Alabama, Arkansas, Delaware, District of Columbia, Florida, Georgia, Kentucky, Louisiana, Maryland, Mississippi, North Carolina, Oklahoma, South Carolina, Tennessee, Texas, Virginia, and West Virginia; and West = Alaska, Arizona, California, Colorado, Hawaii, Idaho, Montana, Nevada, New Mexico, Oregon, Utah, Washington, and Wyoming.

References

1. Sheffer AL, Taggart VS. The National Asthma Education Program: expert panel report guidelines for the diagnosis and management of asthma. *Med Care* 1993;31(suppl):MS20-MS28.

2. Weiss KB, Gergen PJ, Wagener DK. Breathing better or wheezing worse? The changing epidemiology of asthma morbidity and mortality. *Annu Rev Public Health* 1993;14:491-513.

3. Barbee RA, Dodge R, Lebowitz ML, Burrows B. The epidemiology of asthma. *Chest* 1985; 87(suppl):21S-25S.

4. Weiss KB, Gergen PJ, Hodgson TA. An economic evaluation of asthma in the United States. *N Engl J Med* 1992;326:862-6.

5. Sears MR, Rea HH, de Boer G, et al. Accuracy of certification of deaths due to asthma: a national study. *Am J Epidemiol* 1986;124:1004-11.

6. Infante-Rivard C. Young maternal age: a risk factor for childhood asthma? *Epidemiology* 1995; 6:178-80.

7. Tilles SA, Nelson HS. New onset asthma in the elderly. *Immunology and Allergy Clinics of North America* 1997;17:575-86.

8. Massey JT, Moore TF, Parsons VL, Tadros W. Design and estimation for the National Health Interview Survey, 1985-1994. Hyattsville, MD: U.S. Department of Health and Human Services, Public Health Service, CDC, National Center for Health Statistics, 1989; DHHS publication no. (PHS)89-1384. (Vital and health statistics; series 2, no. 110).

9. Nelson C, McLemore T. The National Ambulatory Medical Care Survey: United States, 1975-81 and 1985 trends. Hyattsville, MD: U.S. Department of Health and Human Services, Public Health Service, CDC, National Center for Health Statistics, 1988; DHHS publication no. (PHS)88-1745. (Vital and health statistics; series 13, no. 93).

10. McCaig LF, McLemore T. Plan and operation of the National Hospital Ambulatory Medical Survey. Hyattsville, MD: U.S. Department of Health and Human Services, Public Health Service, CDC, National Center for Health Statistics, 1994; DHHS publication no. (PHS)94-1310. (Vital and health statistics; series 1, no. 34).

11. Simmons WR, Schnack GA. Development and design of the NCHS Hospital Discharge Survey. Rockville, MD: U.S. Department of Health, Education, and Welfare, Public Health Service, CDC, National Center for Health Statistics, 1977; DHEW publication no. (HRA)77-1199. (Vital and health statistics; series 2, no. 39).

12. Kozak LJ. Underreporting of race in the National Hospital Discharge Survey. Hyattsville, MD: U.S. Department of Health and Human Services, Public Health Service, CDC, National Center for Health Statistics, 1995. (Advance data from vital and health statistics; no. 265.) DHHS publication no. (PHS)95-1250.

13. Survey. Hyattsville, MD: U.S. Department of Health and Human Services, Public Health Service, CDC, National Center for Health Statistics, 1992; DHHS publication no. (PHS)92-1772. (Vital and health statistics; series 13, no. 111).

14. National Center for Health Statistics. Vital statistics of the United States, 1990. Vol II: Mortality, part A. Technical appendix. Washington, DC: Public Health Service, 1994; DHHS publication no. (PHS)95-1101.

15. Klebba AJ, Scott JH. Estimates of selected comparability ratios based on dual coding of 1976 death certificates by the eighth and ninth revisions of the International Classification of Diseases. Hyattsville, MD: U.S. Department of Health, Education, and Welfare, Public Health Service, CDC, 1980; DHEW publication no. (PHS)80-1120. (Vital statistics report; vol 28, no. 11, suppl).

16. Evans III R, Mullally DI, Wilson RW, et al. National trends in the morbidity and mortality of asthma in the U.S.—prevalence, hospitalization, and death from asthma over two decades: 1965-1984. *Chest* 1987;91(suppl):65S-74S.

17. National Center for Health Statistics. Provisional estimates of selected comparability ratios based on dual coding of 1966 death certificates by the seventh and eighth revisions of the International Classification of Diseases. Washington, DC: U.S. Department of Health, Education, and Welfare, Public Health Service, 1968. (Monthly vital statistics report; vol. 17, no. 8, suppl).

18. Burt CW, Knapp DE. Ambulatory care visits for asthma: United States, 1993-94. Hyattsville, MD: U.S. Department of Health and Human Services, Public Health Service, CDC, National Center for Health Statistics, 1996. (Advance data from vital and health statistics; no. 277.) DHHS publication no. (PHS)96-1250.

19. Whallett EJ, Ayres JG. Labelling shift from acute bronchitis may be contributing to the recent rise in asthma mortality in the 5-34 age group. *Respir Med* 1993;87:183-6.

20. Lebowitz MD, Holberg CJ, Martinez FD. A longitudinal study of risk factors in asthma and chronic bronchitis in childhood. *Eur J Epidemiol* 1990;6:341-7.

21. Anthonisen NR, Connett JE, Kiley JP, et al. Effects of smoking intervention and the use of an inhaled anticholinergic bronchodilator on the rate of decline of FEV_1 : the Lung Health Study. *JAMA* 1994;272:1497-505.

22. Erzen D, Roos LL, Manfreda J, Anthonisen NR. Changes in asthma severity in Manitoba. *Chest* 1995;108:16-23.

23. O'Brien KP. Managed care and the treatment of asthma. *J Asthma* 1995;32:325-34.

24. Finkelstein JA, Brown RW, Schneider LC, et al. Quality of care for preschool children with asthma: the role of social factors and practice setting. *Pediatrics* 1995;95:389-94.

25. Lintner TJ, Brame KA. The effects of season, climate, and air-conditioning on the prevalence of Dermatophagoides mite allergens in household dust. *J Allergy Clin Immunol* 1993;91:862-7.

26. Schwartz J, Slater D, Larson TV, Pierson WE, Koenig JQ. Particulate air pollution and hospital emergency room visits for asthma in Seattle. *Am Rev Respir Dis* 1993;147:826-31.

27. White MC, Etzel RA, Wilcox WD, Lloyd C. Exacerbations of childhood asthma and ozone pollution in Atlanta. *Environ Res* 1994;65:56-68.

28. CDC. Asthma surveillance programs in public health departments—United States. *MMWR* 1996;45:802-4.

29. Morris RD, Hersch M, Naumova EM. Development and implementation of asthma surveillance in Milwaukee: final report

to the Council of State and Territorial Epidemiologists. Milwaukee, WI: Medical College of Wisconsin, Center for Environmental Epidemiology, June 14, 1995.

30. Morris RD, Goldring J, Hersch M, Naumova EN, Munasinghe RL, Anderson H. Childhood asthma surveillance in Milwaukee, Wisconsin, using computerized billing records. Milwaukee, WI: Medical College of Wisconsin, June 20, 1997.

31. Wilcox KR, Hogan J. An analysis of childhood asthma hospitalization and deaths in Michigan, 1989-1993. Lansing, MI: Michigan Department of Community Health, Division of Epidemiology, 1997.

32. O'Neil R. Tackling asthma in Arizona: The Asthma Coalition. Phoenix, AZ: Arizona Public Health Association, 1997.

33. London MR. Behavioral Risk Factor Surveillance System (BRFSS) 1996 results (compared to 1995 results): Oregon asthma prevalence. Portland, OR: American Lung Association of Oregon, 1997.

34. Meriwether RA. Blueprint for a national public health surveillance system for the 21st century. Atlanta, GA: Council of State and Territorial Epidemiologists, October 15, 1995.

— by David M. Mannino, M.D.(1), David M. Homa, Ph.D.(1), Carol A. Pertowski, M.D.(1), Annette Ashizawa, Ph.D.(1,2), Leah L. Nixon, M.P.H.(1), Carol A. Johnson, M.P.H.(1), Lauren B. Ball, D.O., M.P.H.(1), Elizabeth Jack(1), and David S. Kang(1).
(1) = Division of Environmental Hazards and Health Effects National Center for Environmental Health; (2) = Council of State and Territorial Epidemiologists.

Chapter 13

Forecasted Estimates of Self-Reported Asthma Prevalence by State

Asthma is a chronic inflammatory disorder of the lungs characterized by episodic and reversible symptoms of airflow obstruction[1].
During 1993-1994, an estimated 13.7 million persons in the United
States reported having asthma, and from 1980 to 1994 the prevalence
of self-reported asthma in the United States increased 75%[2]. Despite
this increase, surveillance data are limited for asthma at the state
and local levels[3]. To estimate the 1998 prevalence rate of asthma for
each state, CDC analyzed national self-reported asthma prevalence
data from 1995. This report summarizes the results of the analyses,
which project that approximately 17 million persons in the United
States have asthma.

For this analysis, persons were considered to have asthma if they
had had asthma diagnosed by a physician at some time in their life and
had reported symptoms of asthma during the preceding 12 months. Using methods that have been applied elsewhere to forecast cancer rates[4],
state-specific asthma prevalence estimates for 1998 were calculated
using a three-step procedure: 1) race-, sex-, and age-specific asthma
prevalence rates were calculated for each of the four U.S. census regions using data from the 1995 National Health Interview Survey

From "Forecasted State-Specific Estimates of Self-Reported Asthma Prevalence—United States, 1998 ," by S. Rappaport, M.P.H., and B. Boodram, M.P.H.,
in *Morbidity and Mortality Weekly Review (MMWR)*, Vol. 47, No. 47, December
4, 1998, pp. 1022-5 [Online] December 3, 1998. Available: http://www.cdc.gov/
epo/mmwr/preview/mmwrhtml/00055803.htm. Produced by the Centers for
Disease Control and Prevention (CDC). For complete contact information,
please refer to Chapter 68, "Resources."

(NHIS); 2) each state's 1998 demographic composition as estimated by the Bureau of Census was multiplied by the corresponding regional prevalences; and 3) linear extrapolations of region-specific increases in asthma prevalence from 1980 to 1994 were applied to the 3-year period from 1995 to 1998 for each state. Confidence intervals and relative standard errors for all estimates were calculated using regression parameters provided by CDC's National Center for Health Statistics for prevalence of chronic conditions[5].

In 1998, asthma affected an estimated 17,299,000 persons in the United States. The state with the largest estimated number of persons with asthma was California (2,268,300), followed by New York (1,236,200) and Texas (1,175,100) (Table 13.1.). State-specific prevalence rates ranged from 5.8% to 7.2%. Differences in asthma prevalence rates between states were not significant. By region, 1-year period prevalence estimates ranged from 6.4% to 6.8% in the Northeast, 5.8% to 6.1% in the South, 6.6% to 6.7% in the Midwest, and 6.0% to 7.2% in the West.* The narrow range of prevalence rates within each of these regions indicates that state-specific differences in demographic composition minimally influenced estimated asthma prevalence.

Editorial Note

The findings in this report project state-specific prevalence rates of 5.8% to 7.2%. These findings are consistent with those from a study in Oregon, which estimated asthma prevalence at 6%-7%[6]. However, surveys of self-reported asthma prevalence in Bogalusa, Louisiana[7], Chicago, Illinois[8], and Bronx, New York[9,] all indicated estimates considerably higher than those in this report. State program planners can use these findings to estimate the burden of asthma within their states.

The findings in this report are subject to at least two limitations. First, the findings assume a linear growth in asthma prevalence since 1995. Although this linear assumption was selected after review of regional growth trends in asthma prevalence during the preceding 15 years[2], changes in the trends of self-reported asthma rates that may have occurred in the 3-year interval during 1995-1998 could not be captured by these linear extrapolations. Second, these results are based on the assumption that age, sex, and race-specific rates of asthma do not vary within any of the four geographic regions of the United States. Each state's estimated prevalence reflects its regional placement in the United States and its demographic composition.

These analyses do not account for differences among states in the relative presence or absence of environmental risk factors in asthma prevalence, possible differences in genetic susceptibility toward the condition, or other sociodemographic indicators (e.g., poverty status). As a result, these findings underestimate the variability in asthma prevalence between states within regions. They also do not accurately represent asthma prevalence in geographic subpopulations within states.

Asthma is the ninth leading cause of hospitalization nationally[10]. Its severity can be managed with appropriate medical treatment, education, and environmental modification[1]. However, fewer than 10 states have conducted asthma prevalence surveys. The initiation of state-based asthma control and management programs will require better state and local data on asthma prevalence to evaluate the effectiveness of these programs. State-level surveillance could incorporate existing data such as hospital discharge data and managed-care data. Questions about asthma could also be added to state and community-level surveys such as the State and Local Integrated Telephone Survey and other surveys conducted in individual states such as the Behavioral Risk Factor Surveillance System.

State-based surveys should include questions related to asthma diagnosis, severity, management techniques, and known geographic and household risk factors. These surveillance data will provide a foundation for planning and evaluating asthma-control programs, identifying high-risk and hard-to-access populations, and structuring health promotion and education initiatives.

Table 13.1. Forecasted Estimates of Self-Reported Asthma Prevalence*, by State—United States, 1998 **(continued on next page)**

Region/State	No. Cases	Estimated Prevalence	(95% CI⁺)	Standard Error
Northeast				
Connecticut	215,900	6.6%	(5.6%-7.5%)	7.2%
Maine	80,300	6.4%	(5.4%-7.4%)	7.8%
Massachusetts	401,000	6.5%	(5.6%-7.5%)	7.2%
New Hampshire	78,500	6.6%	(5.5%-7.6%)	7.8%
New Jersey	540,400	6.7%	(5.7%-7.6%)	7.2%
New York	1,236,200	6.8%	(5.8%-7.8%)	7.3%
Pennsylvania	800,900	6.6%	(5.6%-7.5%)	7.2%
Rhode Island	64,400	6.5%	(5.5%-7.4%)	7.3%
Vermont	39,500	6.5%	(5.5%-7.6%)	7.8%
Total	3,241,200	6.7%	(5.7%-7.6%)	7.3%
Midwest				
Iowa	190,100	6.6%	(5.6%-7.6%)	7.5%
Illinois	795,200	6.7%	(5.7%-7.6%)	7.5%
Indiana	398,400	6.7%	(5.7%-7.7%)	7.3%
Kansas	174,900	6.7%	(5.7%-7.6%)	7.3%
Michigan	642,300	6.7%	(5.7%-7.7%)	7.5%
Minnesota	318,600	6.7%	(5.8%-7.7%)	7.1%
Missouri	362,300	6.1%	(4.7%-7.4%)	11.3%
Nebraska	112,100	6.7%	(5.7%-7.7%)	7.4%
North Dakota	43,600	6.7%	(5.7%-7.6%)	7.3%
Ohio	748,200	6.7%	(5.7%-7.6%)	7.4%
South Dakota	51,000	6.7%	(5.8%-7.7%)	7.3%
Wisconsin	350,800	6.7%	(5.7%-7.7%)	7.2%
Total	4,187,600	6.6%	(5.6%-7.6%)	7.4%
South				
Alabama	280,500	6.0%	(4.8%-7.1%)	9.5%
Arkansas	162,600	5.9%	(4.9%-6.9%)	6.9%
District of Columbia	31,400	5.9%	(3.6%-8.2%)	19.7%
Delaware	44,300	5.9%	(4.9%-6.9%)	8.5%
Florida	863,900	5.8%	(4.9%-6.8%)	8.0%
<tbl>Georgia	458,700	6.0%	(4.9%-7.2%)	9.7%
Kentucky	232,800	5.9%	(4.9%-6.9%)	8.2%
Louisiana	265,500	6.1%	(4.8%-7.3%)	10.5%
Maryland	307,300	6.5%	(5.6%-7.5%)	7.2%
Mississippi	167,900	6.1%	(4.7%-7.4%)	11.3%
North Carolina	447,200	5.9%	(4.9%-7.0%)	8.9%
Oklahoma	191,700	5.8%	(4.8%-6.7%)	7.9%
South Carolina	228,600	6.0%	(4.8%-7.2%)	10.1%
Tennessee	328,300	5.9%	(4.9%-6.9%)	8.3%
Texas	1,175,100	6.0%	(5.0%-7.0%)	8.2%
Virginia	403,400	5.9%	(4.9%-6.9%)	8.6%
West Virginia	108,600	5.8%	(4.9%-6.8%)	8.2%
Total	5,697,800	5.9%	(4.9%-7.0%)	8.8%

Table 13.1. (continued) Forecasted Estimates of Self-Reported Asthma Prevalence*, by State—United States, 1998

Region/State	No. Cases	Estimated Prevalence	(95% CI+)	Standard Error
West				
Alaska	42,500	6.7%	(5.7%-7.7%)	7.7%
Arizona	316,200	6.9%	(6.0%-7.9%)	6.9%
California	2,268,300	7.1%	(6.1%-8.0%)	6.8%
Colorado	283,700	7.1%	(6.1%-8.0%)	6.8%
Hawaii	73,100	6.0%	(4.1%-7.8%)	15.3%
Idaho	86,100	6.7%	(5.7%-7.8%)	7.6%
Montana	61,600	6.6%	(5.7%-7.6%)	7.4%
Nevada	125,700	7.2%	(6.3%-8.1%)	6.4%
New Mexico	121,800	6.8%	(5.8%-7.8%)	7.2%
Oregon	225,900	6.9%	(5.9%-7.8%)	6.9%
Utah	141,200	6.7%	(5.6%-7.8%)	8.1%
Washington	391,900	6.9%	(5.9%-7.8%)	6.8%
Total	4,172,400	7.0%	(6.0%-8.0%)	7.0%
Total	**17,299,000**	**6.4%**	**(5.5%-7.5%)**	**7.8%**

*Persons were considered to have asthma if they had had asthma diagnosed by a physician at some time in their life and had reported symptoms of asthma during the preceding 12 months. +Confidence interval.

Northeast = Connecticut, Maine, Massachusetts, New Hampshire, New Jersey, New York, Pennsylvania, Rhode Island, and Vermont; Midwest = Illinois, Indiana, Iowa, Kansas, Michigan, Minnesota, Missouri, Nebraska, North Dakota, Ohio, South Dakota, and Wisconsin; South = Alabama, Arkansas, Delaware, District of Columbia, Florida, Georgia, Kentucky, Louisiana, Maryland, Mississippi, North Carolina, Oklahoma, South Carolina, Tennessee, Texas, Virginia, and West Virginia; West = Alaska, Arizona, California, Colorado, Hawaii, Idaho, Montana, Nevada, New Mexico, Oregon, Utah, Washington, and Wyoming.

References

1. National Institutes of Health. Practical guide for the diagnosis and management of asthma. Washington, DC: U.S. Department of Health and Human Services, National Institutes of Health. (Publication no. 97-4053).

2. CDC. Surveillance for asthma—United States, 1960-1995. *MMWR* 1998;47(no. SS-1).

3. Brown CM, Anderson HA, Etzel RA. Asthma: the states' challenge. *Public Health Reps* 1997;112:198-205.

4. Landis SH, Murray T, Bolden S, Wingo PA. Cancer statistics, 1998. *CA Cancer J Clin* 1998;48:6-9.

5. CDC. Vital and health statistics: design and estimation for the National Health Interview Survey. Washington, DC: U.S. Department of Health and Human Services, CDC, National Center for Health Statistics, 1989; DHHS publication no. (PHS) 89-1384. (Series 2, no. 110).

6. Ertle AR, London MR. Insights into asthma prevalence in Oregon. *J Asthma* 1998;35:281-9.

7. Farber HJ, Wattigney W, Berenson G. Trends in asthma prevalence: The Bogalusa Heart Study. *Ann Allergy Asthma Immunol* 1997;78:265-9.

8. Persky VW, Slezak J, Contreras A, et al. Relationships of race and socioeconomic status with prevalence, severity, and symptoms of asthma in Chicago school children. *Ann Allergy Asthma Immunol* 1998;81:266-71.

9. Crain EF, Weiss KB, Bijur PE, Hersh M, Westbrook L, Stein RE. An estimate of the prevalence of asthma and wheezing among inner-city children. *Pediatrics* 1994;94:356-62.

10. CDC. National Hospital Discharge Survey: annual summary, 1995. Washington, DC: U.S. Department of Health and Human Services, CDC; DHHS publication no. (PHS) 98-1794. (Series 13, no. 133).

—by S. Rappaport, M.P.H., and B. Boodram, M.P.H.,
Epidemiology and Statistics Unit,
American Lung Association, New York City;
Air Pollution and Respiratory Health Br., Div. of Environmental
Hazards and Health Effects, National Center for Environmental
Health; and an EIS Officer, CDC.

Chapter 14

Seasonal Variation of Hospitalizations for Asthma, Bronchitis, and Emphysema

Respiratory diseases such as asthma, chronic bronchitis, and emphysema are among the leading causes of morbidity and mortality in many countries and appear to be on the rise.[1-5] This upward trend is in contrast to sharply downward trends for heart disease, stroke, and other chronic diseases. Trends in asthma morbidity and mortality have been studied, and emergency department visits, hospitalization, and deaths have been shown to be increasing in all age groups over the past two decades in many countries.[6] These increases may be due to changes in asthma prevalence, incidence, and/or modification of the management of asthma or exposure to triggers.[7,8]

Seasonal patterns in asthma morbidity have long been recognized and may shed insight into the triggers provoking hospital-based care for asthma.[9,10] For example, such patterns have been linked to seasonal exposure to specific antigens,[11,12] periodicity of infections,[13] and periodicity in high levels of air pollutants.[14,15]

Less is known about seasonal patterns in morbidity for chronic bronchitis and emphysema. These diseases are excluded from analyses of morbidity due to asthma. Indeed, many of the studies of asthma morbidity have been limited to children and young adults to minimize diagnostic overlap of asthma with chronic bronchitis and emphysema.

Excerpted from "Periodicity of Asthma, Emphysema, and Chronic Bronchitis in a Northwest Health Maintenance Organization," by Molly L. Osborne, William M. Vollmer, and A. Sonia Buist, in *Chest,* Vol. 110, No. 6, December 1996, pp. 1458-62. © 1996 by the American College of Chest Physicians, 3300 Dundee Rd., Northbrook, IL 60062-2348. Reprinted with permission.

The aims of this study were (1) to examine seasonal variation in patterns of hospitalizations for asthma, chronic bronchitis, and emphysema among members of a large health maintenance organization, and (2) to contrast these patterns for different age-sex subgroups.

Materials and Methods

Population

The data for this analysis derive from the abstracted medical records of Kaiser Permanente (KP), Northwest region, a large health maintenance organization centered in Portland, Ore. The KP membership, which grew from 221,743 to 310,819 during the years covered by this study (1979 to 1987), is generally representative of the area population as a whole.[16,17] No evidence exists of systematic selection of healthy individuals either into or out of the system.

Data Systems

Data for the study have been derived from the abstracted inpatient medical records of the entire KP membership. Details of this database are given elsewhere.[18,19] Briefly the inpatient database includes information about each discharge from the two Portland area KP hospitals and from the contracted hospitals in Salem and Longview since 1966. Data include, but are not limited to, primary hospital discharge diagnosis and up to eight secondary discharge diagnoses, each coded according to the *International Classification of Diseases (ICD)* coding system in effect at the time of the discharge. This report uses information only from 1979 to 1987 *(ICD-9)*.

Because the diagnoses of chronic bronchitis and emphysema often overlap with asthma, we examined utilization data for asthma and for the combination of chronic bronchitis and emphysema. To determine the extent to which some of the seasonal variation in hospitalizations might be attributable to infections, we also examined secondary hospital discharge diagnoses of pneumonia and influenza *(ICD-9* codes 480-487).

Statistical Methods

We used standard nonparametric methods (Pearson[2]) for the analysis of contingency table data, and log-linear models[20] to examine the joint influence of age, sex, and season on hospitalizations. We further used two methods to quantify "season." The first was simply the month in which the utilization occurred. Although these divisions do not correspond to any natural definitions of season, variation in outcome from month to month should be indicative of seasonal variation. The second method used three-month groupings (January to March, April to June, July to September, October to December) that roughly correspond to winter, spring, summer, and fall.

Results

In all, we observed 2,060 primary hospital discharges for asthma and 1,121 primary hospital discharges for emphysema or chronic bronchitis over the 9-year period. For asthma, the 3-month moving average of hospital discharges varied significantly by age. The 0- to 14-year-old group showed a small spring peak and a larger fall peak. Although hospitalizations in this age group appear to be highest in October, this is an artifact of the 3-month moving averages. The peak actually occurs in September (15.3% of all asthma hospitalizations), following a lull in July (5.1%) and August (4.9%). The 15- to 64-year-old group showed only a spring peak, while the over-64-year-old group exhibited a single peak in the late winter/early spring months. In general, these age-related seasonal patterns were similar for male and female patients. For the 15- to 64-year-old group, however, the patterns did differ significantly by gender (p=0.005). In general, the peak was accentuated in female patients, with female patients having higher peaks in May and June and lower troughs in the fall, particularly September and October. Log-linear models indicated statistically significant interactions of both age and sex with month.

For the combination of chronic bronchitis and emphysema, the monthly patterns of hospital discharges differed from asthma and also varied significantly by age. The two younger groups each showed a single peak, although these were somewhat out of phase with each other. The 0- to 14-year-old group peaked in the fall/winter months (the actual peak was in October), while the 15- to 64-year-old group peaked in the late winter and early spring months. We found no seasonal variation in the 65+-year age group.

Generally, we found little evidence of diagnostic overlap between hospitalizations for asthma and hospitalizations for chronic bronchitis/emphysema. Of the 3,181 hospitalizations for which either asthma or chronic bronchitis/emphysema was listed as the primary hospital discharge diagnosis, only 205 (6.4%) included both diagnoses on the discharge summary (Table 14.1.). Even in the 65+-year age group, this figure was less than 10%.

139

To explore the extent to which these seasonal patterns might be explained by seasonal trends in infections, we also determined the extent to which pneumonia and influenza were listed as secondary diagnoses (comorbidities) when either asthma or chronic bronchitis/ emphysema was listed as a primary diagnosis (Table 14.2.). Overall, 4.8% of primary asthma discharges and 6.3% of chronic bronchitis/ emphysema discharges listed pneumonia or influenza as a comorbidity. In both asthma and chronic bronchitis/emphysema, pneumonia/influenza was most common from January through June. This was statistically significant only for chronic bronchitis/emphysema. Whether there was inadequate statistical power to identify the trend in both groups is unclear. Certainly the proportion of hospitalizations involving pneumonia or influenza as a secondary morbidity was relatively low and accounted for only a small minority of hospitalizations in these groups.

Discussion

We have demonstrated age-related seasonal patterns in the occurrence of hospitalizations for asthma and for chronic bronchitis/emphysema. The differences in these seasonal patterns by age are unlikely to be related to diagnostic overlap between asthma and chronic bronchitis/ emphysema, as the joint occurrence of these conditions as hospital discharge diagnoses was low. However this does not exclude misclassification that may have occurred in older patients. Indeed, following asthma in administrative databases is increasingly unreliable with increasing age because of the likelihood of misclassification of smoking-related COPD.

Table 14.1. Diagnostic Overlap for Hospitalizations, KP, Northwest Region, 1979 to 1987*

Age, yr., at discharge	No.	Asthma only, No. (%)	Chronic bronchitis/ emphysema only, No. (%)	Asthma and chronic bronchitis/ emphysema, No. (%)
0-14	786	721 (91.7)	64 (8.1)	1 (0.1)
15-64	1,130	774 (68.5)	275 (24.3)	81 (7.2)
65+	1,265	415 (32.8)	727 (57.5)	123 (9.7)
Total	**3,181**	**1,910 (60.0)**	**1,066 (33.5)**	**205 (6.4)**

χ^2 test for independence = 767.9 on 4 df, p<0.0001.

The reasons for differences in seasonal patterns between age groups in both asthma and the combination of chronic bronchitis and emphysema are unclear. In case of chronic bronchitis/emphysema, the seasonal variations in morbidity decrease with age, with the least seasonal variation seen in the 65+-year-old patients. Reviewing the *ICD-9* codes for the children aged 0 to 14 years reveals that the large majority (n=64) had *ICD-9* code 490 bronchitis, NOS (not otherwise specified). Furthermore, the seasonal variation suggests that most of the hospitalizations were in the late fall and early winter. Therefore, we think it likely that these children had either acute or chronic bronchitis. However, it is conceivable that some of the patients are misclassified, with either underlying cystic fibrosis or α_1-antitrypsin deficiency. In any event, the pathophysiologic condition is presumably inflammatory and quite different from that resulting in chronic bronchitis/emphysema in the older population, with COPD much more common in the latter population, and likely to be related to cigarette smoking.

While our data do not permit us to identify the causes of these seasonal patterns, similar patterns for hospitalization for asthma have been reported by Weiss,[9] drawing on the National Hospital Discharge Survey. Many explanations have been suggested. For example, the

Table 14.2. Proportion of Hospitalizations Involving Pneumonia or Influenza as a Secondary Morbidity, KP, Northwest Region 1979 to 1987

Primary diagnosis	Month	No. of discharges	Proportion with secondary diagnosis of influenza, %	p value*
Asthma	Jan.-Mar.	518	5.8	
	Apr.-June	552	5.2	0.48
	July-Sept.	472	3.8	
	Oct.-Dec.	518	4.4	
	Total	**2,060**	**4.8**	
Chronic	Jan.-Mar.	312	8.3	
bronchitis/	Apr.-June	279	7.9	0.018
emphysema	July-Sept.	274	2.6	
	Oct.-Dec.	256	5.9	
	Total	**1,121**	**6.3**	

*Two-sided p value based on Pearson's χ^2 statistic.

seasonal pattern in asthma morbidity has been attributed to seasonal fluctuations in the following: specific aeroallergen exposures;[11,12,21-23] "atmospheric" factors such as temperature or humidity; [24,25] infections; [21] and irritant gases such as ozone and sulfur dioxide.[26,27]

Specifically in our cohort, the spring and fall peaks for asthma that we observed in the younger cohorts appear to correlate with seasonal patterns of aeroallergens and, in the 0- to 14-year-old group, with infections associated with the start of school. However, there may be a different explanation for the fall peak in chronic bronchitis/emphysema since the peak is slightly later than that for asthma whether comparing the monthly peak or the 3-month moving average. That the peak in health-care utilization for asthma in early fall may be related to exposure to infectious agents as children return to school has been suggested elsewhere.[14] Similarly, the fall peaks in chronic bronchitis hospitalizations in the 0 to 14-year-old group (essentially all chronic bronchitis hospitalizations in this age range) suggest more of a link with infections than with aeroallergens.[28,29]

However, it is important to recognize that different mechanisms of inflammation might be additive or synergistic, that both aeroallergens and infections may contribute to the increase in fall hospitalizations. For example, Avres[30] has suggested that sensitization to aeroallergens in the summer might make patients with asthma more susceptible to effects of viral infections in the fall. Similarly, Molfino, et al.,[31] have demonstrated that exposure to low concentrations of ozone potentiates the airway allergic response in patients with asthma.

In conclusion, we have demonstrated age-related seasonal patterns for hospitalizations for asthma and for the combination of chronic bronchitis and emphysema. The patterns for asthma differ from those for the combination of chronic bronchitis and emphysema. A better understanding of the causes of the age-specific seasonal patterns in these obstructive respiratory diseases may help to reduce the morbidity that is associated with them.

References

1. Guidotti TL, Jhangri GS. Mortality from airways disorders in Alberta, 1927-1987: an expanding epidemic of COPD, but asthma shows little change. *J Asthma* 1994; 31:227-90

2. Sherrill DL, Lebowitz MD, Burrows B. Epidemiology of chronic obstructive pulmonary disease. *Clin Chest Med* 1990; 11:375-87

3. Evans III R, Mulally DI, Wilson RW, et al. National trends in the morbidity and mortality of asthma in the US. *Chest* 1987; 91(suppl):65S-73S

4. Burney PGJ. Asthma mortality in England and Wales: evidence for a further increase 1974-1984. *Lancet* 1986; 2:323-26

5. Cooreman J, Thom TJ, Higgins MW. Mortality from chronic obstructive pulmonary disease and asthma in France 1969-1983. *Chest* 1990; 97:213-19

6. Mitchell EA. International trends in hospital admission rates for asthma. *Arch Dis Child* 1985; 60:376-78

7. Dowse GK, Turner KJ, Stewart GA, et al. The association between Dermatophagoides mites and the increasing prevalence of asthma in village communities within the Papua New Guinea highlands. *J Allerg Clin Immunol* 1985; 75:75-83

8. Molfino NA, Slutsky AS. Near-fatal asthma. *Eur Respir J* 1994; 7:981-90

9. Weiss KB. Seasonal trends in US asthma hospitalizations and mortality. *JAMA* 1990; 263:2323-28

10. Khot A, Burn R, Evans N, et al. Seasonal variation and time trends in childhood asthma in England and Wales 1975-81. *BMJ* 1984; 289:235-37

11. Platts-Mills TE, Hayden ML, Chapman MD, et al. Seasonal variation in dust mite and grass-pollen allergens in dust from the houses of patients with asthma. *J Allergy Clin Immunol* 1987; 79:781-91

12. O'Hollaren MT, Yunginger JW, Offord KP, et al. Exposure to an aeroallergen as a possible precipitating factor in respiratory arrest in young patients with asthma. *N Engl J Med* 1991; 324:359-63

13. Clarke CW. Relationships of bacterial and viral infections to exacerbations of asthma. *Thorax* 1979; 34:344-47

14. Bates DV. Baker-Anderson M, Sizto R. Asthma attack periodicity: a study of hospital emergency visits in Vancouver. *Environ Res* 1990; 51:51-70

15. Schwartz J, Slater D, Larson TV, et al. Particulate air pollution and hospital emergency room visits for asthma in Seattle. *Am Rev Respir Dis* 1993; 147:826-31

16. Greenlick MR, Hurtado AV, Pope CR, et al. Determinants of medical care utilization. *Health Serv Res* 1968; 3:296-315

17. Greenlick MR, Freeborn DK, Pope CR. *Health care research in an HMO: two decades of discovery*. Baltimore: Johns Hopkins University, Press, 1988

18. Vollmer WM, Buist AS, Osborne ML. Twenty year trends in hospital discharges for asthma among members of a health maintenance organization. *J Clin Epidemiol* 1992; 45:999-1006

19. Vollmer WM Osborne ML, Buist AS. Temporal trends in hospital-based episodes of asthma care in a health maintenance organization. *Am Rev Respir Dis* 1993; 147:347-53

20. Feinberg SE. *The analysis of cross-classified categorical data*. Cambridge, Mass: MIT Press, 1977

21. Carlsen KH, Orstavik I, Leegaard J, et al. Respiratory virus infections and aeroallergens in acute bronchial asthma. *Arch Dis Child*. 1984; 59:310-15

22. Jenkins PF, Mullins J, Davies BH, et al. The possible role of aero-allergens in the epidemic of asthma deaths. *Clin Allergy* 1981; 11:611-20

23. Gelber LE, Seltzer LH, Bouzoukis JK, et al. Sensitization and exposure to indoor allergens as risk factors for asthma among patients presenting to hospital. *Am Rev Respir Dis* 1993; 147:573-78

24. Greenberg L, Fielf F, Reed JI, et al. Asthma and temperature change. *Arch Environ Health*; 1964; 8:742-47

25. O'Byrne PM, Ryan G, Morris M, et al. Asthma induced by cold air and its relation to nonspecific bronchial responsiveness to methacholine. *Am Rev Respir Dis* 1982; 125:281-85

26. Goldstein IF, Currie B. Seasonal patterns of asthma: a clue to etiology. *Environ Res* 1984; 33:201-15

27. Lebowitz MD, Collins L, Holberg CJ. Time series analyses of respiratory responses to indoor and outdoor environmental phenomena. *Environ Res* 1987; 43:332-41

28. La-Via WV, Grant SW, Stutman HR, et al. Clinical profile of pediatric patients hospitalized with respiratory syncytial virus infection. *Clin Pediatr* 1993; 32:461-62

29. Jamjoom GA, Al-Semrani AM, Board A, et al. Respiratory syncytial virus infection in young children hospitalized with respiratory illness in Riyadh. *J Trop Pediatr* 1993; 39:346-49

30. Ayres JG. Trends in asthma and hay fever in general practice in the United Kingdom 1976-83. *Thorax* 1986; 41:111-16

31. Molfino NA, Wright SC, Katz I, et al. Effect of low concentrations of ozone on inhaled allergen responses in asthmatic subjects. *Lancet* 1991; 338:199-203.

Chapter 15

Asthma by Family Income and Age

The 1995 National Health Interview Survey

The following table was excerpted from the 1995 National Health Interview Survey (NHIS) which provides detailed data on the health of the resident civilian noninstitutionalized population living at the time of the interview in the United States. The survey presents estimates on acute conditions, episodes of persons injured, restriction in activity, prevalence of chronic conditions, limitation of activity due to chronic conditions, respondent-assessed health status, and the use of medical services—including physician contacts and short-stay hospitalization.

It should be noted that the sample population described by the NHIS estimates does not include persons residing in nursing homes, members of the armed forces, institutionalized persons, or U.S. nationals living abroad.

Asthma Data

Information in Table 15.1. is based on data collected in a continuing nationwide survey by household interview. Each week a probability

Excerpted from "Current Estimates from the National Health Interview Survey, 1995," by Veronica Benson and Marie A. Marano, in *Vital and Health Statistics,* Series 10, No. 199, October 1998. Produced by the Centers for Disease Control and Prevention (CDC), National Center for Health Statistics (NCHS). For complete contact information, please refer to Chapter 68, "Resources."

147

sample of the population was interviewed by personnel of the U.S. Bureau of the Census. Information was obtained about the prevalence of chronic asthma by age and family income in each household.

Because of a federal furlough in 1995, the NHIS was fielded only for 48 of the 52 calendar weeks of 1995.This resulted in a slightly smaller sample size. The interviewed sample for 1995 consisted of 39,239 households containing 102,467 persons. The total noninterview rate was 6.2 percent: 4.4 percent was the result of respondent refusal, and the remainder was primarily the result of failure to locate an eligible respondent at home after repeated calls.

Definitions of Terms

Chronic condition—A condition is considered chronic if (a) the respondent indicates it was first noticed more than 3 months before the reference date of the interview, or (b) it is a type of condition that ordinarily has a duration of more than 3 months.

Table 15.1. Reported Chronic Asthma per 1,000 Persons, by Family Income and Age: United States, 1995

	Family Income			
	Less than $10,000	$10,000- $19,999	$20,000- $34,999	$35,000 or more
Age (yrs)	No. of cases of chronic asthma per 1,000 persons			
<45	79.2	65.9	53.6	61.9
45-64	101.7	65.9	39.9	54.1
65-74	*93.1	*49.0	*39.6	*33.3
75 and over	*36.8	*38.7	*10.9	*21.7

Data are based on household interviews of the civilian noninstitutionalized population.
*Figure does not meet standard of reliability or precision.

Age—The age recorded for each person is the age at last birthday. Age is recorded in single years and grouped in a variety of distributions depending on the purpose of the table.

Income of family—Each member of a family is classified according to the total income of the family of which he or she is a member. Within the household, all persons related to each other by blood, marriage, or adoption constitute a family. The income recorded is the total of all income received by members of the family in the 12-month period preceding the week of interview. Income from all sources—for example, wages, salaries, rents from property, pensions, government payments, and help from relatives—is included.

Chapter 16

Missing the Mark: U.S. Not Meeting Asthma Goals

Overview

[*Asthma in America*], one of the largest and most comprehensive surveys of public, patient, and professional knowledge, attitudes, and behavior toward asthma in the United States, was conducted between mid-May and mid-July 1998. The survey explored asthma prevalence, the frequency and severity of symptoms, utilization of emergency care, quality of life, and quality of care issues. Interviews were completed with a national sample of 2,509 adults with asthma or parents of children with asthma. The national sample of asthma patients was identified by systematically screening a national sample of 42,022 households in the United States. A national cross-sectional sample of 1,000 adults in the general public was also conducted for comparison to the national asthma sample. Finally, a national sample of more than 700 healthcare providers—comprising 512 doctors, 101 nurses, and 113 pharmacists—was interviewed as part of the survey.

The survey was conducted by the national public-opinion research organization, Schulman, Ronca and Bucuvalas, Inc. (SRBI). Serving as advisors to the project were Nancy Sander, President of Allergy and

Asthma Network/Mothers of Asthmatics, and Dr. Scott Weiss, an asthma expert and lead epidemiologist with Brigham and Women's Hospital, Harvard Medical School, and Harvard School of Public Health. The survey was funded by Glaxo Wellcome Inc., a research-based pharmaceutical company.

The survey yields five major conclusions about the current state of asthma in America:

- Asthma management in America is falling far short of the goals established by the National Heart, Lung, and Blood Institute (NHLBI), part of the National Institutes of Health. (*Expert Panel Report 2: Guidelines for the Diagnosis and Management of Asthma,* NHLBI, May 1997.) Indeed, it would not be an exaggeration to say that asthma is out of control for many patients.

- Poorly controlled asthma symptoms cause hospitalizations, emergency room and urgent care visits, sick days, and activity limitations that may cause asthma sufferers to accept a much lower quality of life than need be.

- Although doctors report that they are following NHLBI guidelines and patients are generally satisfied with their care, the level of care reported by patients does not meet current standards.

- Another key finding is the widespread misunderstanding by patients of the underlying condition that causes asthma symptoms, as well as confusion about appropriate treatment and other aspects of asthma management.

- People with asthma recognize the need for greater patient education—71% believe there is a strong need for more patient education about asthma.

The survey findings about asthma are particularly important because of the number of American households affected. The population prevalence of asthma found by the survey is consistent with previous government estimates that about one in twenty Americans, or nearly 15 million people, suffer from asthma. However, the survey finds that far more Americans are directly affected by asthma. Nearly half of the American public (48%) have had asthma themselves, or in their household, or in their immediate family. Another three out of ten (29%) know friends, co-workers, or someone else personally who has asthma. Hence, nearly four out of five Americans (77%) are affected.

U.S. Not Meeting Asthma Goals

Asthma in America reveals that the United States is not meeting the goals for asthma management established last year by the National Heart, Lung, and Blood Institute (NHLBI).* A point-by-point comparison:

Table 16.1. Missing the Mark

National Goals	Survey Findings
No sleep disruption	30 percent of asthma patients awakened by breathing problems at least once a week
No missed school or work	49 percent of children with asthma—and 25 percent of adults with asthma—missed school or work because of asthma in past year
No (or minimal) need for ER visits/hospitalizations	32 percent of children with asthma went to emergency room for asthma attacks in the past year
	41 percent of all people with asthma sought urgent care from the ER, clinic, or hospital last year
Maintain normal activity levels	48 percent of patients limited in sports/recreation
	36 percent limited in normal physical exertion
	25 percent limited in their social activities
Have normal or near-normal lung function	Only 35 percent of patients report having had a lung-function test in past year
	Only 28 percent have peak-flow meters to monitor their airflow; 9 percent report using one at least once a week

*According to the NHLBI's Practical Guide for the Diagnosis and Management of Asthma: "The goals of asthma therapy provide the criteria that the clinician and patient will use to evaluate the patient's response to therapy."

Chapter 17

Mortality and Markers of Risk of Asthma Death

Despite major advances in the treatment for bronchial asthma over the past decades, especially increasing use of inhaled corticosteroids, mortality rates for asthma appear to have been gradually but steadily increasing in North America and in many other Western countries.[1-3] This increase is of particular concern because it comes at a time when mortality from most other causes is on the decline. There is no general accepted definition of asthma[4] and therefore, the increase in asthma deaths might be attributed to a combination of diagnostic difficulties and inaccurate coding of the cause of death.[5] As the national mortality statistics are derived from death certificates, inaccurate coding due to lack of knowledge of the clinical history may lead to imprecise estimation of mortality rates from asthma[42,6] Compared with the number of review articles published concerning asthma mortality,[1-3,7] remarkably few studies have been published regarding mortality among asthmatics in whom the diagnosis has been objectively verified.[8-11] Reliable markers of asthma severity are of utmost importance to clinicians in their attempt to identify patients who are at increased risk of death,[12] and specific information of these markers may as well provide etiologic clues as to the mechanisms leading to asthma deaths.

From "Mortality and Markers of Risk of Asthma Death among 1,075 Outpatients with Asthma," by Charlotte Suppli Ulrik and Jens Frederiksen, in *Chest*, Vol. 108, July 1995, p. 10. © 1995 by the American College of Chest Physicians, 3300 Dundee Rd., Northbrook, IL 60062-2348. Reprinted with permission.

155

The purpose of the present study was to describe mortality among patients with asthma referred to an outpatient clinic by comparing the observed mortality with that of a matched group of nonasthmatic patients, and furthermore, to identify risk factors for subsequent death from asthma.

Materials and Methods

Patients with Asthma (Cases)

The study population consisted of subjects >15 years of age referred to the Allergy and Chest Clinic at Frederiksberg Hospital, Copenhagen, by general practitioners because of known or suspected asthma (ICD-8 code 498.0) during the years 1974 to 1990. Patients were included in the analysis only if they met at least two, unless stated otherwise, of the following criteria for asthma: (1) typical history, that is, attacks of breathlessness, wheezing, or both, chest tightness and dry cough either spontaneously or triggered by exercise, allergens, respiratory infections, or irritants; these criteria were used only in 46 patients (4%), primarily in the first years of the study period (due to lack of readily accessible equipment for pulmonary function tests); (2) reversibility in forced expiratory volume in 1 s (FEV_1), defined as ([FEV_1 after-FEV_1 before]/FEV_1 before) >15% (and an absolute increase of at least 150 mL) after a standard dose of inhaled Beta$_2$-agonist oral corticosteroid, or both (30 mg/d) for 14 days;[13,14] and/or (3) diurnal variability in peak expiratory flow (PEF) rate, defined as ([highest-lowest measurement during the observation period]/mean of measurements) >20% (and an absolute variation of at least 100 L/min).[15,16]

On referral to the clinic, the patients were tested for IgE-mediated allergy, and they were defined as having intrinsic asthma if they had normal concentrations of serum IgE[17] and no evidence of extrinsic asthma from history, skinprick tests, and—when the results of these were doubtful—radioallergosorbent tests (RAST) and specific bronchial provocation tests.[17-20] Patients with demonstrable IgE-mediated allergy were defined as having extrinsic asthma.

Nonasthmatic Patients (Controls)

Also studied were a group of controls matched for age (within 1 year), sex, and year of referral who had not attended the Allergy and Chest Clinic for asthma during the course of the study. Controls were randomly selected from all subjects who attended the clinic for suspected or known allergic diseases other than asthma (including allergic and nonallergic rhinitis, atopic dermatitis, and urticaria) after excluding those who were diagnosed as having asthma on referral to the clinic.

History

At the time of enrollment, i.e., the time of referral to the clinic, detailed history was obtained concerning known allergy, disposition to allergic diseases, allergic symptoms, e.g., rhinitis, eczema/atopic dermatitis, and urticaria, duration and frequency of respiratory symptoms (see below), triggering factors, use of antiasthma medication (drug and daily dose), and number of earlier emergency department visits and hospital admissions caused by asthma. At the first visit to the clinic, the patients' conditions were graded according to the frequency of symptoms within the preceding 8 months as follows: (1) grade 1: symptoms, on average, once a week; (2) grade 2: symptoms more than once a week but not daily; (3) grade 3: daily symptoms; and (4) grade 4: symptoms daily and at night. Furthermore, according to smoking habits, the patients were classified as current smokers, ex-smokers, and lifelong nonsmokers; for the first two categories, an estimate of their lifetime tobacco exposure was calculated as pack-years: (current tobacco consumption [g/dy]/20 x duration of smoking [years]).

Tests for IgE-Mediated Allergy, Etc.

Total IgE in serum was determined by PRIST (Pharmacia).[17] The standard skinprick test included the following allergens: birch, grass, mugwort, horse, dog, cat, house dust mite, (Dermatophagoides pteronyssinus and D farinae) and molds (Alternaria iridis and Cladosporium herbarum); further allergens were included if allergy was suspected from the history. The area of the weal produced by each antigen was compared with the area of the histamine weal, and the test was regarded as positive if at least one of the reactions was at least the same size as the histamine weal.[17] Tests for allergen-specific IgE (Al-RAST) were performed with the aluminum radioallergosorbent test kit according to the method of Weeke,[21] and evaluated according to Dirksen.[17] Specific bronchial provocations were carried out using the method described by Dirksen;[17] a positive reaction was defined as a fall in FEV_1 of 20% or more.[17] The blood eosinophilic count was routinely determined three times for each patient, and the most abnormal result was recorded.[17]

Spirometric Tests

Forced expiratory volume in one second, PEF, and forced vital capacity (FVC) were measured using a dry-wedge bellows spirometer (Vitalograph), and the best of three technically acceptable readings was recorded. The tests were repeated 15 to 20 min. after inhalation of a standard dose of bronchodilator; reversibility of FEV_1 was calculated as (FEV_1 after-FEV_1 before/FEV_1 before).[13] Predicted values for FEV_1, PEF, and FVC were calculated by using the regression of Quanjer.[22]

Mortality

The patients and the controls were enrolled in the study at the first visit at the Allergy Clinic (during the years 1974 to 1990) and followed up until the end of 1993. Notification of deaths was obtained from the Danish Death Register and death certificates from the Danish National Board of Health; in Denmark, causes of death were classified according to the eighth revision of the *International Classification of Diseases (ICD-8)* throughout 1974 to 1998. For the purpose of the present study, cause of death was classified according to *ICD-8* into five categories: (1) status asthmaticus; (2) chronic obstructive airways disease not classified as status asthmaticus; (3) cardiovascular diseases; (4) malignant neoplasms; and (5) other causes. To assess the accuracy of the cause of death, all death certificates in which the words "asthma" or "status asthmaticus" appeared in part 1 were further reviewed. Available data relating to the patients' visits at the Allergy Clinic and the terminal illnesses (medical records from our hospitals, other hospitals, or both) were evaluated by each of us. A decision was made by us as to whether asthma was appropriately listed as the cause of death, according to the definition given by the World Health Organization.[23]

Statistical Methods

Person years at risk were calculated for each individual from the date of entry into the study until the end of follow-up.[24] The end of follow-up was either (1) December 31, 1998, for subjects registered by the Danish Personal Identity Register as being alive, or (2) the date of death for subjects identified by the Danish Death Register as dead. The data were analyzed according to the methods described by Armitage and Berry.[24,25] The person years at risk provided the denominator of death rates in both asthmatics and controls, from which relative risks (RRs) of death were calculated. Deaths among the asthmatics were expressed as a proportion of all observed deaths and 95% confidence intervals (CIs) for this proportion were calculated.

The regression model of Cox[26] was used to identify variables related to the risk of death from asthma in patients with extrinsic and intrinsic asthma. If t is time, $x = x_1, x_2 \ldots x_r$ is a set of explanatory variables, and $a_1, a_2 \ldots a_r$, are regression coefficients, this model assumes that the intensity of death from asthma has a simple form: $(t,x) = (t) * \exp(a_1 x_1 + a_2 + \ldots a_1 x_r)$. Time was reckoned from enrollment until death from asthma (event), death from other causes (censoring), or until the end of the observation period. As suggested by Cox, the regression coefficients were estimated using the maximum likelihood method and the hypothesis of a significant effect of a variable on was evaluated by means of the likelihood ratio test. The results are given in terms of RR and 95% CI. For binary variables, RR is the risk among patients with a certain characteristic compared with the risk among patients without that characteristic. Variables with more than two levels were included using binary variables for the various levels. As the regression coefficients for men and women were very similar, only the model including both sexes is shown.

Results

Information concerning current status (dead or alive) at the end of follow-up (1993) was obtained for all the asthmatics (cases, n = 1,075) and the controls (n = 1,075). Each of the two groups of subjects studied (cases and controls) comprised 425 men and 650 women. The mean follow-up period was 8.6 years (SD 4.2 years) in cases and controls. The age distribution by sex of the asthmatics is given in Table 17.1.

Table 17.1. Age and Sex Distribution of Asthmatics (Case Population, n = 1,075)

Age, yr	Men, no. (%) (n = 425)	Women, no. (%) (n = 650)
<20	29 (7)	84 (5)
20-29	109 (26)	170 (26)
30-39	113 (27)	153 (24)
40-49	73 (17)	100 (15)
50-59	42 (10)	89 (14)
60-69	41 (10)	69 (11)
>70	18 (4)	35 (5)

Mortality from all causes was significantly increased among the asthmatic subjects compared with the control group, in that 93 (43 men) cases and 41 (15 men) controls died during the follow-up period (RR, 2.4; CI, 1.6 to 3.4). Mortality among the controls did not differ from the expected mortality in a sex- and age-matched sample of the Danish population, according to statistics published by the Danish National Board of Health. The increase in all-cause mortality occurred in both men and women, the RR in asthmatics compared with controls being 2.9 (CI, 1.6 to 5.3) and 2.0 (CI, 1.2 to 3.3), respectively. The predominant cause of excess mortality was obstructive pulmonary disease, that is, status asthmaticus (14 [7 men] vs. 0 deaths; RR, 8.2; CI, 1.9 to 70) and COPD not classified as status asthmaticus (19 [7 men] vs. 0 deaths; RR, 8.(3; CI, 1.2 to 55) (Table 17.2.). The subjects with asthma also showed a small nonsignificant increase in mortality from both circulatory diseases and malignant neoplasms.

Table 17.2. Cause of Death in Asthmatics (n = 1,075) and Controls (n = 1, 075)

Cause of Death (*ICD* Code)	Asthmatics	Controls	RR (95% CI)
All causes (000-999)	93	41	2.4 (1.6-3.4)
Status asthmaticus (493)	14	0	8.2 (1.9-70)
COPD not classified as status asthmaticus (490-496)	19	0	8.3 (1.2-55)
Circulatory diseases (390-459)	23	15	1.3 (0.9-1.8)
—Acute myocardial infarction (410)	12	4	
Malignant neoplasms (140-208)	17	14	1.1 (0.8-1.6)
—Malignant disease of trachea, bronchus, and lung (160-165)	4	5	
Other causes	20	12	

The comparison of the initial characteristics between the 33 patients who died from asthma during follow-up and the remaining patients are presented in Table 17.3. The mean follow-up time (years from inclusion to death) did not differ between the patients who died of acute (5.5 years [3.7]) and chronic (7.1 years [3.6]) asthma (p>0.5).

Table 17.3. Comparison between the Subjects Who Later Died from Asthma and Those Who Did Not*

	Died from Asthma			
	Acute (n = 14)		Chronic (n = 19)	
Age, yr	49.1	(13.0)	65.6	(8.6)
Smoking, pack-yr	6.9	(9.1)	13.3	(19.4)
Duration of asthma, yr	16.9	(17.9)	22.6	(18.2)
FEV_1, %pred	64.7	(15.7)	49.3	(9.4)
FEV_1/FVC	62.1	(13.1)	50.7	(9.5)
B-eosinophils, 10^9/L	0.61	(0.16)	0.61	(0.35)
Reversibility, [†] %	43.9	(15.3)	45.3	(22.9)

	Remaining Patients (n = 1, 042)	
Age, yr	37.6	(15.3)
Smoking, pack-yr	3.7	(7.3)
Duration of asthma, yr	9.0	(10.6)
FEV_1, %pred	87.7	(19.4)
FEV_1/FVC	75.5	(11.7)
B-eosinophils, 10^9/L	0.44	(0.36)
Reversibility, [†] %	28.0	(17.7)

Values are mean with SD in parentheses.
[†]*Defined as (FEV_1 after–FEV_1 before) * 100/FEV_1 before.*

The results of the regression analysis are shown in Table 17.4. The risk of subsequent death from asthma increased with presence of eosinophilia, reduction in FEV_1, advanced age, high degree of reversibility, and lifetime tobacco consumption. Eosinophilia and an increase in FEV_1 of more than 50% following administration of bronchodilator were highly significantly related to death from asthma.

No significant association could be demonstrated between previous hospital admissions for asthma, duration of asthma, self-reported frequency of symptoms, and reported triggering factors, e.g., dust, animals, and respiratory infections, and increased risk of subsequent death from asthma.

Introducing type of asthma (intrinsic asthma vs. extrinsic asthma) into the regression model showed that intrinsic asthma was highly significantly associated with death from asthma. Including interaction terms between type of asthma and age and FEV_1 percent predicted revealed, however, that this association was primarily due to the fact that the patients with intrinsic asthma were both older (mean age, 45 and 33 years, respectively) and had lower level of ventilatory function (mean FEV_1 percent predicted, 82 and 91, respectively) than the patients with extrinsic asthma. However, after allowing for differences in age and FEV_1 percent predicted, the risk of death from asthma was still higher (RR, 1.2), although statistically insignificant, in those with intrinsic asthma compared with those with extrinsic asthma.

A similar regression model in which FEV_1 percent predicted was substituted with the ratio between FEV_1 and FVC as the index of ventilatory function showed that patients with $FEV_1/FVC < 0.5$ had a

Table 17.4. Relative Risk of Death from Asthma According to Age, Smoking Habits, FEV_1 in Percent of Predicted (% pred), b-Eosinophils, and Degree of Reversibility (%) in FEV_1 Following Bronchodilator

Variable	RR	95% CI	Significance, p Value
Age, yr			<0.01
<39	1.0		
40-69	2.5	0.8-8.1	
>70	8.5	2.2-83.7	
Smoking habits			<0. 001
Never smokers	1.0		
<20 pack-yr	2.6	1.0-6.8	
>20 pack-yr	5.9	2.3-15.0	
B-eosinophils			<0. 001
<0.45 10^9/L	1.0		
>0.45 10^9/L	7.4	2.8-19.7	
FEV_1, % pred			<0.002
>70	1.0		
40-69	4.9	2.0-11.8	
<40	3.3	0.8-14.5	
Reversibility,* %			<0.002
15-24	1.0		
25-49	2.7	0.9-7.9	
>50	7.0	2.4-21.0	

*Defined as (FEV_1 after-FEV_1 before) * $100/FEV_1$ before.*

9.3 (CI, 2.9 to 29.8) higher risk of asthma death compared with patients with $FEV_1/FVC > 0.7$. However, this did not change the number or significance of the other evaluated potential predictors of increased risk of subsequent death from asthma.

Discussion

The present study revealed an excess mortality in asthmatics compared with matched controls primarily caused by death from acute and chronic asthma; and, furthermore, eosinophilia and high degree of reversibility following bronchodilator, together with age, level of pulmonary function, and smoking habits are predictors for an increased risk of death from asthma. These findings are of relevance both to epidemiologists who wish to investigate asthma mortality and to clinicians who wish to identify patients who are at increased risk of death from asthma. There are, however, a few precautions to take into account in the interpretation of the findings.

First, the group of patients studied were all referred from their general practitioner to the outpatient clinic for the purpose of diagnosis, institution of relevant therapy, or both. So, although the range of disease severity should be wide, the group of patients studied might not include those with the mildest cases. However, as soon as the disease had been turned into a stable phase by treatment and patient education, the patients were further attended by their general practitioner; most of the patients were seen only at the clinic over a period of a few months following their initial referral. We therefore assume that the asthmatics in the present study in several aspects are representative of the asthmatic population in general.

Second, the total number of deaths is relatively small and the RR estimates for especially other causes than asthma should therefore be interpreted with a little caution. However, the number of deaths from circulatory diseases, especially acute myocardial infarction, among the asthmatics compared with the controls merits a comment. It is well known that circulatory diseases, not the least ischemic heart disease, are related to tobacco smoking. In the present study, 9% of the asthmatics were ex-smokers and 27% were current smokers compared with 10% and 89%, respectively, among the controls (data not shown). Therefore, in contrast to what might have been expected, this finding may appear to confirm the previously reported excess risk of death from ischemic heart disease in male asthmatics.[27]

The excess mortality came mainly from acute and chronic asthma, and, compared with previous studies,[8] the large RR of death from asthma is not surprising. It should be emphasized that as much as 3% of the asthmatic cohort died from asthma over the 9-year follow-up period. Juel and Pedersen[28] have previously shown an increasing mortality from asthma in Denmark in the mid-1970s to 1988, which could not be explained by changes in coding practice as the eighth revision of the International Classification of Diseases was used in Denmark over the entire period. However, the data presented do not allow us to draw conclusions concerning changes in mortality rates from asthma.

The increased mortality from asthma in recent decades has caused great concern,[2] not the least because it comes at a time when mortality from most other causes is on the decline. However, there has been considerable controversy regarding the appropriate methods for investigating the causes of asthma mortality.[12] Case-control methods have been undertaken especially to investigate the possible role of prescribed drug treatment in asthma mortality,[29] but unlike the method used in the present study, most of these studies have been confined to patients with a recent hospital admission for asthma. The present study design, therefore, offered an opportunity to examine the association between several markers of asthma severity and risk of death from asthma.

Bronchial asthma is characterized by an inflammatory reaction in the airways presumably leading to nonspecific bronchial hyperresponsiveness and reversible airways obstruction. The degree of bronchial responsiveness is related to the clinical severity of asthma,[30] and previous studies have shown that bronchial responsiveness is inversely related to the number of eosinophils in bronchoalveolar lavage fluid.[31] The demonstrated relationship between eosinophilia and risk of death from asthma, therefore, indicates that eosinophil count should be taken into account in the management of asthma as an important marker for the degree of inflammatory reaction in the airways and, by that, the severity of asthma.

High degree of reversibility in pulmonary function following administration of bronchodilator, i.e., reduced baseline pulmonary function, is a known marker of poorly controlled asthma.[32] Furthermore, previous studies have shown that the response to an inhaled bronchodilator is correlated with the rate of decline of FEV_1 over the following years.[20,33] The observation that high degree of reversibility is a strong predictor for risk of subsequent death from asthma is therefore not surprising, although to our knowledge, this association has not been confirmed previously. From the combination of these findings, it might be reasonable to recommend that patients with asthma should be treated so that the baseline pulmonary function is also kept as near normal as possible.

References

1. Sly RM. Increases in deaths from asthma. *Ann Allergy* 1984; 53:20-5

2. Buist AS. Is asthma mortality increasing [editorial]? *Chest* 1988; 93 :449-50

3. Benatar SR. Fatal asthma. *N Engl J Med* 1986; 314:423-29

4. Gross M. What is this thing called love?—or, defining asthma [editorial]. *Am Rev Respir* Dis 1980; 121:203-04

5. British Thoracic Association Research Committee. Accuracy of death certificates in bronchial asthma. *Thorax* 1984; 39:505-09

6. Royal College of Physicians and Royal College of Pathologists. Medical aspects of death certification. *J R Coll Physicians Lond* 1982; 16:206-18

7. Sheffer AL, Buist AS, eds. Proceedings of the Asthma Mortality.: Task Force. *J Allergy Clin Immunol* 1987; 80:361-514

8. Markowe HLJ, Bulpitt CJ, Shipley MJ, et al. Prognosis in adult asthma: a national study. *BMJ* 1987; 295:949-52

9. Alderson M, Loy RM. Mortality from respiratory diseases and follow-up of patients with asthma. *Br J Dis Chest* 1977; 71:198-202

10. Almind M, Viskum K, Evald T, et al. A 7-year follow-up study of 343 adults with bronchial asthma. *Dan Med Bull* 1992; 39:561-65

11. Ulrik CS, Backer V, Dirksen A. Mortality and decline in lung function in 218 adults with bronchial asthma: a 10-year follow-up. *J Asthma* 1992; 29:29-38

12. Beasley R, Pearce N, Crane J. Use of near fatal asthma for investigating asthma deaths [editorial]. *Thorax* 1993; 48:1093-94

13. Ries AK. Response to bronchodilators. In: Clausen IL, ed. *Pulmonary function testing: guidelines and controversies*. New York: Academic Press, 1982; 215-21

14. Viljanen A. Reference values for spirometric, pulmonary diffusing capacity and body plethysmographic studies. *Scand J Clin Invest* 1982; 42(suppl 159):1-50

15. Clark TJH, Hetzel MR. Diurnal variation of asthma. *Br J Dis Chest* 1977; 71:87-92

16. Hetzel MR, Clark TJH. Comparison of normal and asthmatic circadian rhythms in peak expiratory flow rate. *Thorax* 1980; 35:732-38

17. Dirksen A. Clinical vs paraclinical data in allergy. *Dan Med Bull* 1982; 29(suppl 5):5-72

18. Koch C, Andersen P, Hertz JB, et al. Studies on hypersensitivity to bacterial antigens in intrinsic asthma. *Allergy* 1982; 37:191-201

19. Irani FA, Jones NL, Gent M, et al. Evaluation of disodium cromoglycate in intrinsic and extrinsic asthma. *Am Rev Respir Dis* 1972; 106:179-85

20. Ulrik CS, Backer V, Dirksen A. A 10-year follow up of 180 adults with bronchial asthma: factors important for the decline in lung function. *Thorax* 1992; 47:14-8

21. Weeke B. Aluminium hydroxide absorbed allergens used in a modified RAST (Al-RAST) [abstract]. *Allergol Immunopathol* 1977; 4:333

22. Quanjer Ph, ed. Standardized lung function testing. *Bull Eur Physiopathol Respir* 1985; 19(suppl 5):7-10

23. World Health Organization. *WHO international classification of diseases, 1965*. 8th ed rev. Geneva: World Health Organization, 1967; 3-231

24. Armitage P, Berry G. Survival analysis. In: Armitage P, Berry G, eds. *Statistical methods in medical research*. Oxford: Blackwell Scientific Publications, 1987; 421-39

25. Berry G. The analysis of mortality by the subject-years method. *Biometrics* 1983; 39:173-84

26. Cox DR. Regression models and life-tables. *J R Stat Soc* 1972; 34:187-220

27. Robinette CD, Fraumeni JF. Asthma and subsequent mortality in World War II veterans. *J Chronic Dis* 1978; 31:619-24

28. Juel K, Pedersen PA. Increasing asthma mortality in Denmark 1969-88 not a result of a changed coding practice. *Ann Allergy* 1992; 68:180-82

29. Pearce NE, Crane J, Burgess C, et al. Beta agonists and asthma mortality: deja vu. *Clin Exp Allergy* 1991; 21:401-10

30. Yan K, Salome CM, Woolcock AJ. Rapid method for measurement of bronchial hyperresponsiveness. *Thorax* 1983; 38:760-65

31. Gleich GJ. The eosinophil and bronchial asthma: current understanding. *J Allergy Clin Immunol* 1990; 85:422-36

32. Woolcock AJ. Inhaled drugs in the prevention of asthma. *Am Rev Respir Dis* 1977; 115:191-94

33. Vollmer WM, Johnson LR, Buist AS. Relationship of response to a bronchodilator and decline in forced expiratory volume in 1 second in population studies. *Am Rev Respir Dis* 1985; 132:1186-93

Chapter 18

Asthma Symptom Differences by Age and Sex

Introduction

Current data suggest there are age and gender differences in asthma. These differences have been demonstrated specifically for hospital admissions, quality of life, and use of metered dose inhalers (MDIs). Skobeloff and coworkers have demonstrated that hospital admission rates are higher for pre-pubertal boys than girls, yet higher in adult females than males[1]. Using the SF-36 questionnaire, Bousquet and colleagues have observed that males report significantly higher (better) QOL [(quality of life)] scores than females[2]. A recent study addressing use of MDIs concluded that females of all ages are more likely to have improper MDI technique than males. Such gender differences may reflect differences in biology, physiology, or exposures, or alternatively reflect behavioral differences or differences in asthma management[3]. Still missing, therefore, are adequate data about the natural history of asthma and other important characteristics of asthmatic patients, such as patterns of medication use, health care utilization, quality of life, symptom profiles, and how these characteristics

From "Characteristics of Patients with Asthma within a Large HMO: A Comparison by Age and Gender, " by Molly L. Osborne, William M. Vollmer, Kathryn P. Linton, and A. Sonia Buist, in *American Journal of Respiratory Critical Care Medicine Online,* Vol. 157, No. 1, January 1998, pp. 123-8. [Online] 1998. Available: http://www.ajrccm.org. © 1998 by the American Lung Association, 1740 Broadway, New York, NY 10019. Reprinted with permission. For complete contact information, please refer to Chapter 68, "Resources."

vary by age and gender. Such information will expand our understanding of this common and costly disease and provide information that is especially useful to those responsible for planning health care delivery within the managed care setting.

We report on data from 914 patients with asthma within a large health maintenance organization (HMO), Kaiser Permanente, NW Region [(KP)] who are participating in a longitudinal study of the risk factors for hospitalization. This paper presents descriptive data on characteristics of this population, including characteristics of asthma such as self-reported patterns of medication use, symptoms, exposure to aeroallergens, health care utilization, severity, and quality of life; as well as objective measures of lung function, skin test responsiveness, and observed use of MDIs. We also contrast the distribution of these characteristics by age and sex.

Methods

Sample and Research Setting

Participants were members of a large health maintenance organization (HMO), Kaiser Permanente, Northwest Region (KP), who were either hospitalized for asthma during the two years prior to recruitment or had at least two dispensings of anti-asthma medications in the year prior to recruitment. At the time of recruitment, all participants reported having physician-diagnosed asthma and indicated that they experienced ongoing symptoms consistent with asthma. By design, participants ranged from 3-55 yr of age. Our goal was to recruit approximately equal numbers of males and females in each of three age groups, approximately 266 in each age group. A total of 914 participants enrolled in the study.

Design

We report on baseline, cross-sectional data collected as part of a cohort study to characterize risk factors for episodes of hospital-based asthma care within an HMO. The baseline assessment included questionnaires to obtain information about characteristics of the participants and their asthma, skin prick testing to inhalant allergens, spirometry before and five minutes after administration of two puffs of isoproterenol, and observation of MDI use. Not everyone completed all aspects of the protocol. For example, we did not conduct spirometry on children under the age of six, or skin prick tests on children whose parents declined the skin prick tests for them.

Questionnaires

We developed two questionnaires: one for the 3-14 age group (completed by parents) and one for those aged 15-55 yr. The questionnaires included data on: respiratory symptoms, characteristics of asthma, demographic factors, tobacco use, allergen exposures, and medication use. Much of this information was obtained by incorporating relevant sections of the ATS-DLD 1978 respiratory symptom questionnaire[4] and the IUATLD bronchial symptoms questionnaire[5]. Questions about symptoms were adapted from the National Asthma Education Program (NAEP) Expert Panel Guidelines[6].

Each questionnaire included both a generic and a disease-specific measure of health status. For children, the pediatric questionnaire included the Rand Child Health Status scale[7] and Stein's Functional Status II-R scale[8]. The Rand scale is a seven-item scale that measures general well-being; the Stein scale asks about functional status in a general sense, but relates limitations to specific diseases. For those aged 15-55 yr, we used the SF-36 health status questionnaire[9] and the asthma quality of life questionnaire developed by Marks and coworkers[10]. Scores from the SF-36 questionnaire, a well-validated instrument for general health measures, have been shown to significantly correlate with severity of asthma, to have a high internal reliability (alpha = 0.91), and can be used to examine quality of life in asthma[2].

Spirometry and Use of MDI

Spirometry was performed using standardized methods with equipment that met or exceeded American Thoracic Society (ATS) requirements[11,12]. The best one-second forced expiratory volume (FEV_1) was chosen for analysis and expressed as percent predicted FEV_1 ($FEV_1\%$) using the prediction equations of Knudson and coworkers[13]. MDI use was observed and technique was evaluated according to a ten point scale developed by Manzella and colleagues[14]. If a participant did not use an MDI the observation was not done.

Skin Testing

We conducted skin prick testing using 13 inhalant allergens appropriate for the Pacific Northwest: alder; birch; juniper; grass; western weed; cat; dog; mite (*Dermatophagoides pteronyssinus* and *Dermatophagoides farinae*); alternaria; cladosporium; aspergillus; and penicillium (Hollister-Stier). We also included a positive control (histamine) and two negative controls (saline and a "dry" prick control). The allergens

171

were applied using standard prick test techniques[15]. Twenty minutes after the last prick, the technician carefully circled each wheal with an ink pen, placed cellotape over the mark, removed the tape, and placed it onto the data entry form. Two diameters were measured from the tape record: the widest diameter and the diameter at a right angle to the widest diameter.

Of those for whom skin prick test data are available, 99.5% had positive reactions (at least one diameter > 3 mm) to the histamine control. Only one percent of subjects responded to the dry prick control, which was applied following the final allergen (western weed mix). Responses to the saline control varied. Initially this was applied immediately following the dust mite (*D. pteronyssinus*) allergen. Following unusually high response rates, a second saline was added following the western weed mix. Response rates to these two saline controls were 27% and 8%, respectively. An analysis based on the difference of wheal-saline wheal gave the same results. Using a method patterned after that of Barbee and colleagues[16], we computed a continuous skin test score.

Statistical Methods

All analyses were performed using the Statistical Analysis System (SAS) statistical software package. We used standard methods for analyzing contingency tables. p values are based on the Pearson chi-square statistic and, for tests of trend, on the Mantel-Haenszel chi-square statistic[17]. Maximum likelihood methods for log-linear and logistic models were used to evaluate associations while controlling for other factors. We used analysis of covariance to examine the joint effects of multiple variables on the MDI use and quality-of-life scores. Unless otherwise stated, all p values are two-sided and the term "significant" indicates a p value < 0.05.

Results

Characteristics of the Sample

Table 18.1. demonstrates the demographics of the sample. There were approximately 60% males in the youngest age group (3-14 yr) and 60% females in the other two age groups. In all age groups, the percentage of nonwhites was small (6-13%), reflecting the low prevalence of minorities in the community. Compared to the population from which we attempted to recruit, study participants were older (28.7 versus 25.8 mean age p < 0.0001), but were similar in terms of gender or self-reported airflow obstruction (chronic bronchitis, emphysema, or chronic obstructive pulmonary disease). Response rates were 31% in the 3-14 age group, 30% in the 15-34 age group, and 43% in the 35-55 age group.

Table 18.1. Demographics of Sample

Age group (yrs)	3-14 (n = 271) (%)	15-34 (n = 226) (%)	35-55 (n = 417) (%)
Gender			
Male	58	39	41
Female	42	61	59
Household income			
<$30,000	23	20	21
$30-39,999	26	28	19
$40-49,999	17	21	18
$50-59,999	19	20	21
$60,000+	14	12	21
Race			
White	87	92	94
Other	13	8	6

Table 18.2. presents the distribution of smoking status for subjects aged 15-55 yr. As expected, the prevalence of ever having smoked increases with age, although the overall prevalence of current smoking (11%) was similar for subjects aged 15-34 yr and those aged 35-55 yr. After adjusting for age, reported smoking patterns differed significantly for males and females with current smoking twice as frequent in females as in males.

Characteristics of Asthma

Table 18.3. shows characteristics of asthma including prevalence of symptoms, pulmonary function, and skin test responsiveness. All

Table 18.2. Smoking Status by Age and Gender

| | Age Group (years) | | | | p Value for Sex Effect* | p Value for Age Effect* |
| | 15-34 | | 35-55 | | | |
	Males (n=89)	Females (n=137)	Males (n=171)	Females (n=243)		
Never smoked (%)	82	69	54	56	0.009	<0.001
Ex-smoker (%)	12	15	39	31		
Current smoker (%)	6	16	7	13		

*Two-sided p values simultaneously adjusting for age (as a continuous factor) and sex via maximum likelihood estimation of the log-linear model with smoking status as the response.

differed significantly by age and sex. For self-reported prevalences of daytime and/or nocturnal symptoms, younger participants reported fewer symptom days than older participants and males reported fewer symptom days than females. About half of the younger participants (3-14 yr) reported 0-1 symptom d/wk, whereas at least two-thirds of women aged 15-55 and men aged 35-55 reported 2 or more days with symptoms per week. One third of the men aged 35-55 reported daily symptoms whereas almost half the women did. Specifically, men 15-34 yr reported fewer symptoms than women ($p < 0.001$) and, a similar trend was seen in the 35-55 yr old group, but did not reach significance ($p = 0.083$).

For pulmonary function, expressed as prebronchodilator FEV_1, % predicted, and bronchodilator response, both the percent of participants with an $FEV_1 < 80\%$ predicted and the bronchodilator response increased with age. Less than 15% of participants under 35 yr had an $FEV_1 < 80\%$. There were differences between men and women in $FEV_1\%$ predicted, with men having a lower $FEV_1\%$ predicted than women. After bronchodilator, however, there were no differences between the two.

Finally, approximately 80% of the subjects had at least one positive skin test (> 3 mm). The skin test score, a measure of the size of the reaction, increased with age in both males and females ($p < 0.01$).

Table 18.3. Characteristics of Asthma

	3-14 M	3-14 F	15-34 M	15-34 F	35-55 M	35-55 F	p Value* for Sex Effect
Prevalence of symptoms (day and/or night) in last month	(n = 156)	(n = 115)	(n = 89)	(n = 137)	(n = 171)	(n = 246)	
< 1/wk, %	56	48	48	27	32	27	0.002
2-6/wk, %	31	37	36	42	32	28	
Daily, %	13	16	16	31	36	45	
Pulmonary function	(n = 120)	(n = 85)	(n = 88)	(n = 137)	(n = 161)	(n = 240)	
Pre-bronchodilator							
FEV_1, % ≥80%	80	89	85	81	51	63	0.034
FEV_1, % 60-80%	16	11	11	15	25	18	
FEV_1, %<60%	4	0	3	4	24	19	
Post-bronchodilator	(n = 126)	(n = 82)	(n = 86)	(n = 133)	(n = 157)	(n = 237)	
% change in FEV_1, mean ± SD	7.5 ± 10.6	6.9 ± 7.1	6.7 ± 7.0	8.2 ± 9.1	11.4 ± 14.0	13.7 ± 19.9	0.306
Skin prick test responsiveness	(n = 131)	(n = 94)	(n = 88)	(n = 136)	(n = 165)	(n = 237)	
Skin test score							
0-2, %	21	34	14	20	19	32	0.011
3-10, %	37	30	27	21	19	22	
11-22, %	26	21	31	26	25	22	
23+, %	16	15	28	32	36	25	
% positive skin test	86	76	88	85	90	79	0.002

*Two-sided p values, simultaneously adjusting for age (as a continuous factor) and sex, via maximum likelihood estimation of the log-linear model for prevalence of symptoms, pre-bronchodilator response skin score; via analysis of variance for post-bronchodilator response; and via logistic regression per positive skin test.

175

However, the increase in males was significantly greater (p < 0.011) than that in females such that in the 35-55 yr range, more than one third of males comprised the upper quartile (wheal size) as compared to one fourth of females.

Medication Use and Health Care Utilization for Asthma

Table 18.4. presents data on medications used for asthma within the last 12 mo and self-reported health care utilization (HCU). Virtually all individuals reported using beta agonist medications. Significantly more older participants (about 10%) reported using > 8 puffs

Table 18.4. Patterns of Medication Use and Health Care Utilization

| | Age Group (years) | | | | | | p Value for Sex Effect* | p Value for Age Effect* |
| | 3-14 | | 15-34 | | 35-55 | | | |
	M	F	M	F	M	F		
Medication in last 12 mo	(n = 156)	(n = 115)	(n = 89)	(n = 137)	(n = 171)	(n = 246)		
β-agonist %	97	97	97	97	87	95	0.025	<0.001
>8 puffs/d of MDI β-agonist %	4	2	2	6	8	13	0.123	<0.001
Cromolyn %	19	15	17	14	9	8	0.365	<0.001
Inhaled corticosteroids %	20	19	24	36	50	67	0.002	<0.001
Oral steroids %	30	27	20	25	15	30	0.020	0.194
Anticholinergic %	0	1	0	1	4	7	0.088	<0.001
Theophylline %	6	4	24	18	21	30	0.330	<0.001
Health care utilization	(n = 156)	(n = 115)	(n = 89)	(n = 137)	(n = 171)	(n = 246)		
Treated in ER %	54	50	56	56	47	61	0.112	0.944
Hospitalized for asthma %	26	19	31	24	19	34	0.336	0.136
Hospitalized in last year %	5	3	2	3	1	2	0.695	0.163

*Two-sided p values, simultaneously adjusting for age (as a continuous factor) and sex, via logistic regression.

daily. Of interest, there were wide variations in the use of non-beta agonist medication. About two thirds of participants were using anti-inflammatory agents, although the type of anti-inflammatory agent varied with age. Younger participants were significantly more likely to use cromolyn ($p < 0.001$), whereas older participants were more likely to use inhaled corticosteroids, ($p < 0.001$) particularly older females. These differences persisted even after adjusting for smoking status (never versus current/ex) ($p < 0.05$). "Oral steroids" refers primarily to the use of corticosteroids for exacerbations of asthma. Only 11 participants reported taking daily oral steroids. Very few individuals reported taking anticholinergic medication for asthma.

Over 50% of participants reported ever having had emergency room treatment for asthma, and up to one-third reported a previous asthma-related hospitalization, although less than 5% reported being hospitalized within the last year. In general, these patterns did not differ based on age or gender. In the 35-55 yr old age group, however, significantly more females than males reported emergency room visits ($p < 0.007$).

Quality of Life

Table 18.5. demonstrates quality of life reported by adult participants in the study according to both the Asthma Quality of Life score (AQLS) and the SF-36 score. The AQLS ranges from 1-10, with 1 being the best quality of life score, whereas the SF-36 score ranges from 0-100 with 100 being the best quality of life score. On both scales, younger individuals (15-34 yr) reported a better quality of life than those who were older (35-55 yr), and a better quality of life was reported by males than females for both age ranges. The gender differences were seen in all four subscales of the AQLS (p values ranging from < 0.001 to 0.006). The SF-36 score showed similar results. Men report significantly better quality of life than women on all but the "role emotional," "mental health," and "change in health" scales. For the latter two scales the trend was in the same direction. In children (3-14 yr), in contrast, two quality of life assessment instruments did not reveal significant gender differences (data not shown).

Ability to Use Metered Dose Inhaler

MDI use scores were compared according to age and sex. The potential range of scores is 0-10. The overall score for use of the MDI suggests that about 71% of the activities required for successful use were done properly. There was no difference in use across the three age ranges 3-14, 15-34, and 35-55 (data not shown). The gender differences were very small, with lower scores among males ($p < 0.005$).

Table 18.5. Asthma Quality of Life Scores

	Age Group (years)				p Value for Sex Effect*	p Value for Age Effect*
	Males		Females			
	15-34 (n=80)	35-55 (n=171)	15-34 (n=129)	35-55 (n=246)		
Asthma specific QOL scores: (lower value indicates quality of life)						
Breathlessness	1.8±1.6	2.0±1.6	2.6±1.8	3.0±2.0	<0.001	0.011
Mood	1.9±1.4	1.9±1.8	2.2±1.9	2.4±2.0	0.005	0.258
Social	1.1±1.4	1.2±1.6	1.5±1.8	1.6±1.9	0.003	0.140
Concerns	1.2±1.2	1.5±1.5	1.6±1.6	1.9±1.9	0.006	0.015
Total	1.5±1.2	1.7±1.4	2.1±1.5	2.3±1.7	<0.001	0.026
SF-36 scores: (higher value indicates better quality of life)						
Physical functioning	90±12	85±18	77±16	71±23	<0.001	<0.001
Social functioning	78±15	77±20	75±18	73±21	0.016	0.562
Role physical	78±32	69±39	70±38	61±41	0.015	0.008
Role emotional	79±34	75±38	74±37	75±37	0.483	0.523
Mental health	75±15	76±18	71±18	74±18	0.083	0.288
Vitality	61±16	58±22	53±21	51±22	<0.001	0.020
Bodily pain	76±18	72±24	68±23	63±27	<0.001	0.007
General health	70±15	66±22	59±22	60±22	<0.001	0.631
Change in health	62±23	55±19	63±24	58±23	0.148	0.001

*Two-sided p values, simultaneously adjusting for age (as a continuous factor) and sex, via analysis of covariance.

Discussion

We have described 914 patients with asthma within a large HMO, a predominantly Caucasian middle class population recruited through a pharmacy database. The most important findings are that women with asthma report more symptoms and poorer quality of life than do men, although measures of airflow obstruction are comparable. It is important to point out that these findings are generalizable specifically to patients with asthma who require anti-asthma medications. It is very likely that the patients in our study have more severe asthma than patients who do not require asthma medications. We chose this group deliberately, recognizing that very little information is available on characteristics of such patients, yet they require significant health care resources[18].

Since interpretation of these findings could be limited by generalizability of the data, we specifically have addressed several potential limitations. First, we compared the study participants to all potential participants on anti-asthma medications with doctor-diagnosed asthma who refused to participate in the study. Compared with all potential participants, study participants were older, but were similar in terms of gender or self-reported airflow obstruction. Second, although we deliberately tried to recruit equal numbers of participants in each age-sex subgroup, differential response rates resulted in substantially more participants in the 35-55 yr old group and an unequal gender distribution across the three age groups with more males in the 3-14 age range, and more females in the 15-55 age range. This gender distribution, however, is consistent with the distribution of asthma prevalence in the U.S.: in children, asthma is more prevalent in boys than in girls with the gender ratio changing in the adult years. Since several hundred participants were recruited in each age category, we remain confident that the data are generalizable.

We acknowledge that our findings in the older group may be limited by the overlap between asthma and chronic obstructive pulmonary disease (COPD). Asthma in older adults is a poorly understood condition that seems, in many, to combine the classic features of asthma (reversible airflow obstruction) with features more common to chronic obstructive pulmonary disease (irreversible airflow obstruction)[19]. Consequently, following asthma is difficult in the elderly because of the misclassification of smoking-related COPD. In a previous study, we performed a chart review of asthma contacts within this HMO and found that COPD/asthma accounted for about 12% of all charts listing asthma as a diagnosis[20]. To minimize overlap in the current study, we required all participants to have physician-diagnosed asthma[21]. We felt this definition of asthma was well-accepted and appropriate for a cross-sectional analysis of patients with asthma within this HMO.

Our results indicate that women report more symptoms, and experience poorer quality-of-life than do men. One possible interpretation for these results is that women have more severe disease than males. However, several pieces of evidence suggest this is not the case. First, males had a lower prebronchodilator $FEV_1\%$ predicted than females; there was no difference between men and women in postbronchodilator FEV_1. Although the FEV_1 is a single snapshot in time, we would have expected to see a lower baseline $FEV_1\%$ predicted in females than males if women had more severe disease than males. Second, self-reported symptoms did not correlate with either $FEV_1\%$ predicted or use of "burst" oral steroids, both accepted measures of asthma severity.

Another interpretation is that the gender difference is due to a questionnaire bias. Since there is no gold standard for symptom scores or quality of life in asthma, we have only indirect ways to address this. First the symptom questionnaires are standard and identical for men and women. Also, there is internal consistency in the quality of life data in that the SF-36 showed a pattern of impaired health between males and females similar to the disease-specific instrument.

Yet another interpretation of these results is that for the same level of airflow obstruction, women seek medical attention more frequently than do men. Consistent with this hypothesis, women tend to make more office visits, receive greater numbers of medical tests, and are prescribed more medications than are men across all diseases[24]. Also, adult women tend to be more frequently hospitalized than men across all diseases[25], and for asthma[1,3]. If women seek more medical attention than men for the same level of air flow obstruction, one explanation is that women actually experience greater discomfort and as a consequence report more symptoms, take more anti-asthma medication, and seek more health care than men. The fact that women report poorer quality of life than men across several dimensions of the RAND SF-36 suggests that women perceive the same level of airflow obstruction differently than men, and that this impacts their daily living. Although less likely, it is possible that men perceive their asthma similarly to women, yet do not seek medical attention for it with the frequency that women do, nor report worse quality of life.

Our data demonstrated that older asthmatics, particularly females, reported using inhaled corticosteroids and beta agonists more than younger asthmatics. The fact that 9% of all participants aged 3-55 reported using more than 8 puffs/day of MDI beta agonists raises concern about possible patient misuse of medications and/or over-prescription.

It is possible that the increased medication use by females reflects the inability to correctly use an MDI as compared to males. However, females were observed to use MDIs at least marginally better than males according to a 10-point observational scale developed by Manzella and colleagues[14]. Although, Goodman and coworkers have demonstrated poorer MDI technique by females than males[26], their study population which included patients with COPD was different from ours, and their methodology was different, perhaps more accurate. Goodman and associates used a miniature sensing system to define an acceptable maneuver by four components: (1) inspiratory flow at actuation, (2) actuation during early inspiration, (3) adequate breath holding time, and (4) a deep inhalation. We simply do not have enough information to distinguish between these possibilities.

Our data demonstrated that skin test responsiveness increased with age. These data are consistent with the concept that asthma is more severe and is correlated with greater allergic responsiveness in older patients compared to younger patients. It is not clear why skin prick test responsiveness should increase with age, although it may simply reflect increasing lifetime exposure to environmental antigens. It is well established that skin test responsiveness wanes later in life (> 55 yr) as has been corroborated by large epidemiological studies in this country and abroad[27,28].

Although our data do not address the best ways to minimize symptoms and improve quality of life, they do suggest several important implications for practice guidelines. The lack of agreement between symptoms and objective measures of severity, particularly in females, underscores the importance of clearly documenting both symptoms and the extent of airflow obstruction in asthma. The use of a peak flow meter or an asthma diary might be particularly helpful in women who report frequent symptoms as a way of allowing them to monitor their asthma and adjust their medication, thereby allowing them to feel more in control. Second, the overuse of beta-agonists could be used to identify a subgroup of patients in which asthma is under-treated with anti-inflammatory agents. Third, it is essential to insure that all patients use MDIs correctly, since this might also decrease medication usage. Fourth, allergen avoidance should be routinely discussed with patients and their specific allergen sensitivities should be targeted. Fifth, specific action plans to manage changes in asthma symptoms and signs should be introduced to decrease unscheduled health care utilization.

Although there are no data confirming that focusing asthma education on women decreases health care utilization, it seems a reasonable first step. Also, it may be appropriate to consider use of peak flow meters in patients whose symptoms do not seem to correlate with the degree of airflow obstruction. Finally, asthma education programs might be particularly helpful in women. Guidelines are being developed for such programs[6,29]. A recent study of patients with moderate to severe asthma demonstrated that self-management education programs were associated with significant improvements in control of asthma symptoms, MDI technique, and environmental control practices[30]. In summary, we have demonstrated important differences in the characteristics of asthma among men and women of a large health maintenance organization. These differences may have implications for asthma management in a managed care setting.

References

1. Skobeloff, E. M., W. H. Spivey, S. S. St. Clair, and J. M. Schoffstall. 1992. The influence of age and sex on asthma admissions. *J.A.M.A.* 268: 3437-3440.

2. Bousquet, J., J. Knani, H. Dhivert, A. Richard, A. Chicoye, J. E. Ware Jr., and F.-B. Michel. 1994. Quality of life asthma: I. Internal consistency and validity of the SF-36 questionnaire. *Am. J. Respir. Crit. Care Med* 149: 371-375.

3. Redline, S., and D. Gold. 1994. Challenges in interpreting gender differences in asthma. *Am. J. Respir. Crit. Care Med* 150: 1219-1221.

4. Burney, P. G. J., S. Chinn, J. R. Britton, A. E. Tattersfield, and A. O. Papacosta. 1989. What symptoms predict the bronchial response to histamine? Evaluation in a community survey of the bronchial symptoms questionnaire (1984) of the international union against tuberculosis and lung disease (IUATLD). *Int. J. Epidemiol. 1989a* 18: 165-173.

5. Burney, P. G. J., L. A. Laitinen, S. Perdrizet, H. Huckauf, A. E. Tattersfield, S. Chinn, N. Poisson, A. Heeren, J. R. Britton, and J. Jones. 1989. Validity and repeatability of the IUATLD (1984) bronchial symptoms questionnaire: an international comparison. *Eur. Respir. J. 1989b* 2: 940-945.

6. National Asthma Education Program (NAEP). 1991. Guidelines for the diagnosis and management of asthma. National Institutes of Health (NIH), Bethesda, MD. Publication No. 91-3042.

7. Eisen, M., J. E. Ware, C. A. Donald, *et al.* 1979. *Measuring components of children's health status*. RAND Corporation, Santa Monica, CA.

8. Stein, R. E. K., and D. J. Jessop. 1990. Functional status II(R): a measure of child health status. *Med. Care* 28: 1041-1055.

9. Ware, J. E., C. A. Sherbourne, and A. R. Davies. 1988. A short-form general health survey. Corporation Publication Number P-7444, Santa Monica, CA.

10. Marks, G. B., S. M. Dunn, and A. J. Woolcock. 1992. A scale for the measurement of quality of life in adults with asthma. *J. Clin. Epidemiol* 45: 461-472.

11. Becklake, M., and R. O. Crapo. 1991. Lung function testing. Selection of reference values and interpretive strategies. *Am. Rev. Respir. Dis* 144: 1202-1218.

12. Enright, P. L., L. F. Johnson, J. E. Connett, *et al.* 1991. Spirometry in the Lung Health Study: I. Methods and quality control. *Am. Rev. Respir. Dis* 143: 1215-1223.

13. Knudson, R. J., M. D. Lebowitz, C. J. Holberg, and B. Burrows. 1983. Changes in the normal maximal expiratory flow-volume curve with growth and aging. *Am. Rev. Respir. Dis* 127: 725-734.

14. Manzella, A. B., C. M. Brooks, J. M. Richards Jr., R. A. Windsor, S. Soong, and W. C. Bailey. 1989. Assessing the use of metered dose inhalers by adults with asthma. *J. Asthma* 26: 223-230.

15. Ten, R. M., J. S. Klein, and E. Frigas. 1995. Allergy skin testing. *Mayo Clin. Proc.* 70: 783-784.

16. Barbee, R. A., M. D. Leibowitz, H. C. Thompson, and B. Burrows. 1976. Immediate skin-test reactivity in a general population sample. *Ann. Int. Med* 84: 129-133.

17. Mantel, N., and W. Haenszel. 1959. Statistical aspects of the analysis of data from retrospective studies of disease. *J. Natl. Cancer Inst* 22: 719-748.

18. Weiss, K. B., P. J. Gergen, and T. A. Hodgson. 1992. An economic evaluation of asthma in the United States. *N. Engl. J. Med* 326: 862-866.

19. Braman, S. S., J. T. Kaemmerlen, and S. M. Davis. 1991. Asthma in the elderly: a comparison between patients with recently acquired and long-standing disease. *Am. Rev. Respir. Dis* 143: 336-340.

20. Osborne, M. L., W. M. Vollmer, and A. S. Buist. 1992. Diagnostic accuracy of asthma within a health maintenance organization. *J. Clin. Epidemiol* 45: 403-411.

21. Evans, R. III, D. I. Mullally, R. W. Wilson, P. F. Gergen, H. M. Rosenberg, J. S. Grauman, F. M. Chevarley, and M. Feinleib. 1987. National trends in the morbidity and mortality of asthma in the U.S.: prevalence, hospitalization and death from asthma over two decades, 1976-1984. *Chest* 91: 65S-74S.

22. U.S. Public Health Service. 1965. Health Interview Responses Compared with Medical Records. U.S. Government Printing Office, Washington, DC. DHEW Series 2, No. 7.

23. U.S. Public Health Service. 1967. Interview Data on Chronic Conditions Compared with Information Derived from Medical Records. U.S. Government Printing Office, Washington, DC. DHEW Series 2, No. 23.

24. Council on Ethical and Judicial Affairs, American Medical Association. 1991. Gender disparities in clinical decision making. *J.A.M.A* 266: 559-562.

25. 1988 Summary: National Hospital Discharge Survey. 1990. Washington, DC, U.S. Department of Health and Human Services. 185:1-12.

26. Goodman, D. E., E. Israel, M. Rosenberg, R. Johnston, S. T. Weiss, and J. Drazen. 1994. The influence of age, diagnosis, and gender on proper use of metered-dose inhalers. *Am. J. Respir. Crit. Care Med* 150: 1256-1261.

27. Dodge, R., M. G. Cline, M. D. Lebowitz, and B. Burrows. 1994. Findings before the diagnosis of asthma in young adults. *J. Allergy Clin. Immun* 94: 831-835.

28. Sears, M. R., B. Burrows, E. M. Flannery, G. P. Herbison, C. J. Hewitt, and M. D. Holdaway. 1991. Relation between airway responsiveness and serum IgE in children with asthma and in apparently normal children. *N. Engl. J. Med* 325: 1067-1071.

29. Kohler, C. L., S. L. Davies, and W. C. Bailey. 1995. How to implement an asthma education program. *Clin. Chest Med* 16: 557-565.

30. Li, D., D. German, S. Lulla, R. G. Thomas, and S. R. Wilson. 1995. Prospective study of hospitalization for asthma: a preliminary risk factor model. *Am. J. Respir. Crit. Care Med* 151: 647-655.

Chapter 19

Asthma in the Workplace

While some traditional dust-related diseases may be waning, concerns are rising about more subtle but expensive respiratory illnesses hitting the workplace.

Silicosis, asbestosis, coal workers' pneumoconiosis, byssinosis. A decade ago, those were the occupational respiratory diseases of chief concern to health officials such as Dr. Gregory Wagner, director of the Division of Respiratory Disease Studies at the National Institute for Occupational Safety and Health (NIOSH). But with progress in combating illness among workers in the "dusty trades" has come an increasing awareness of other, more subtle, respiratory conditions due in whole or part to exposures in the workplace.

"When you look at what is causing people to be sick as well as dying, you see the emergence of nondust diseases for lungs taking increasing prominence in the statistics," says Wagner. For example, data from the Bureau of Labor Statistics (BLS) show that occupational respiratory conditions due to toxic agents increased from 11,500 cases in 1973 to 18,300 in 1991. Over the same period, dust-related diseases increased from 1,500 to 2,500 cases. While this new wave of occupational diseases—asthma, bronchitis, chronic obstructive pulmonary disease, emphysema, respiratory irritation—in many cases is not as deadly, it does have a substantial impact on workers' health and

From "The Changing Face of Respiratory Illness," by Stephen G. Minter, in *Occupational Hazards,* Vol. 57, No. 2, February 1995, pp. 43-4. © 1995 by Penton Publishing Inc., 1100 Superior Ave., Cleveland, OH 44114. Reprinted with permission.

health care costs. "The obstructive lung diseases may shorten the life some, but the more important issue is the 20-30 years prior to death that an individual will have increased health care needs, diminished productivity at work, increased absenteeism, and generally poorer quality of life inside and outside of work," said Wagner. "The same is true with asthma and the infectious diseases."

Asthma

Heading the list of occupational respiratory illnesses receiving increased scrutiny is asthma. Some 10 to 20 million Americans suffer from asthma, with estimates of occupational asthma accounting for anywhere from 2 to 15 percent of the total. In fact, the increasing prevalence of asthma is a worldwide phenomenon, and workplace and environmental conditions are being explored more intensively as part of the effort to find the cause, notes Wagner.

Occupational asthma, as defined by the American Lung Association (ALA), is a lung disease in which the airways overreact to dusts, vapors, gases, or fumes. When these irritants are inhaled, the airway muscles tighten, the tissues swell, and excess mucous is produced, all of which make breathing difficult.

Asthma can be divided into allergic and nonallergenic categories. For allergic asthma, sensitization usually occurs gradually. In the early stages of the disease, says ALA, symptoms such as coughing, wheezing, or tightness in the chest occur during the workweek, and decrease or even disappear during weekends or vacations. Later, symptoms may persist and show up when workers are exposed to common lung irritants such as cigarette smoke or house dust. For nonallergenic asthma, generally caused by a high-level exposure to irritants, permanent airway reactivity occurs in most cases and reaction time can be immediate.

Well over 300 sensitizing agents or jobs have been associated with the development of occupational asthma, Wagner noted. Moreover, health researchers have recognized that a specific sensitizer may not be needed to cause asthma. Instead, overexposure to irritants in the workplace can create asthma in an individual who previously did not have the disease.

Wagner said that specific sensitizers are just like other toxic chemicals in that dose-response relationships exist. "The higher the exposure, the more people will become sensitized," he explained, adding that there will be variations among individuals as to how resistant or sensitive they are to the effects of a particular toxin. But Wagner noted that once sensitized, an employee undergoes a permanent change and may become extraordinarily sensitive to a particular agent.

Employers thus need two strategies: prevent workers who are not sensitized from becoming sensitized, and reduce or eliminate exposure among sensitized individuals. "The scientific evidence is good that the more you let somebody who is sensitized continue to be exposed to something, the more likely he or she is to suffer permanent impairment," said Wagner.

Similarly, he said, eight-hour time-weighted average exposure limits may not be appropriate for controlling asthma resulting from irritant exposures because the asthma may be induced by transient peak exposures rather than sustained exposure levels. "The complexity of the relationship among workplace exposures, home exposures, general environmental exposures, and personal health habits is clearly difficult to unravel," said Wagner. "That complexity has tended to obscure relationships between workplace exposures and the development of these conditions in the past."

Table 19.1. Occupational Respiratory Conditions Due to Toxic Agents: The 10 Industries with the Highest Incidence Rates (1991)

Industry	Rate
Miscellaneous petroleum and coal products	46.8
Secondary nonferrous metals	31.9
Ship and boat building and repair	24.8
Ophthalmic goods	21.9
Primary nonferrous metals	17.3
Motor vehicle and equipment	13.4
Paperboard mills	13.4
Pulp mills	13.0
Miscellaneous manufacturing	12.4
Flat glass manufacturing	10.9
Overall	2.4

Source: "Work-Related Lung Disease Surveillance Report 1994," National Institute for Occupational Safety and Health (NIOSH).

Table 19.2. Occupational Dust Diseases of the Lungs: The 10 Industries with the Highest Incidence Rates (1991)

Industry	Rate
Coal mining	36.8
Plastics materials and synthetics	3.5
Ship and boat building and repair	3.3
Pottery and related products	2.3
Nonmetallic mineral mining, except fuels	1.8
Petroleum refining	1.8
Grain mill products	1.7
Metal mining	1.6
Nonferrous rolling and drawing	1.3
Household furniture	1.3
Overall	0.3

Source: "Work-Related Lung Disease Surveillance Report 1994," National Institute for Occupational Safety and Health (NIOSH).

More than a Nuisance

A number of studies conducted to assess the health effects of air pollution on various cities or communities around the world have turned up an unexpected finding—an increase in the risk of airway disease among residents exposed to dust or fumes at work.

Dr. Margaret Becklake, a professor in the departments of medicine and epidemiology and biostatistics at McGill University, Montreal, said air pollution studies in the U.S., Poland, Norway, and Italy provide important evidence of the role that all dusts, not just specific dusts such as silica, play in the causation of occupational disease.

"The old concept was that there were nuisance dusts that didn't matter too much. We regarded them as harmless because they didn't have specific effects like silica or asbestos," said Becklake. "We should get rid of that concept. Global exposure, the importance of everything you breathe in, not just individual agents, is an important concept to recognize."

One reason the community-based studies are so valuable, asserts Becklake, is that there is self-selection in the workplace. She said studies indicate that smokers tend to have both bigger lungs and lungs that are less reactive to tobacco smoke irritation. "If you do cross-sectional studies of young smokers from 18 to their early 20s, you find often that lung function is better in smokers than nonsmokers," said Becklake. "It was the fact of their better lung status that allowed them to take up smoking."

Similarly, she believes, workers who are very reactive to airway irritants tend to drop out of industries quickly, leaving only the well (and not coincidentally a high percentage of smokers) employed and thus masking the effect of occupation in workplace studies. She also said that workers who are more sensitive to airway irritation probably tend to find ways within their jobs to minimize their exposure. "It is internal avoidance within the job," she said.

Old and New

While NIOSH is looking beyond the traditional dust diseases, Wagner said lung diseases in miners and in workers exposed to crystalline silica require a "sustained public health preventive focus to continue our progress."

"We have a concerted silicosis control and elimination activity that has been going on for a number of years now. That is focused on a single hazardous exposure where there are a diversity of controls that are available," he said. "We can sub-segment the workforce and say, for example, 'Abrasive blasting with crystalline silica is still an extreme hazard that needs to be controlled.' Many industries have proven their ability to control this, so it is a matter of applying what is known in situations where there may not be that same level of awareness or commitment to prevention."

Respiratory problems such as asthma present a whole different set of problems. "On their face, these conditions are indistinguishable to a primary care physician from diseases of everyday life," said Wagner. They also arise from a tremendous variety of agents, occupations, and industries. "We're at a much earlier stage of understanding how to have a comprehensive preventive effort there," Wagner admits.

Still, surveillance efforts underway through state health departments and the Association of Occupational and Environmental Clinics are starting to unravel the asthma puzzle. For example, isocyanates account for a quarter of the occupational asthma exposures reported in Michigan and 10 percent of those in New Jersey.

Other leading causes of asthma on the job include machining coolants/ oil mists, aldehydes, epoxy resins, tungsten carbide/cobalt, acrylates, chlorine, acids, and diesel exhaust.

NIOSH is wrapping up field work on a major asthma study of workers at a USDA insect rearing facility. Analysis of the data, said Wagner, will help the agency understand how to promote asthma prevention in the workplace.

Part Three

Theories about the Causes of Asthma

Chapter 20

Genetics of Asthma

Approximately 5,000 people, many of them children, will die of asthma this year. Scientists have long known that allergic reactions to environmental irritants such as dust, pollen, and other allergens, air pollution, and cigarette smoke trigger asthma attacks. They have now identified a gene that may contribute to susceptibility to asthma attacks by telling the body to overproduce a receptor for immunoglobulin E (IgE), an antibody involved in allergies.

Asthma Facts

- Asthma affects as many as 15 million persons in the United States.

- After hay fever, asthma is the most frequent chronic condition in persons under age 18. Nearly 5.1 million Americans under age 18 have asthma.

- Asthma was the underlying cause of 5,106 deaths in the United States in 1991 and the number is growing.

From "Asthma Gene Is Nothing to Sneeze At," in *Environmental Health Perspectives,* Vol. 102, No. 12, [Online] December 1994; "Allergy Receptor Pictured," in *Environmental Health Perspectives,* Vol. 107, No. 6, [Online] June 1999; and "Genes and Ozone," in *Environmental Health Perspectives,* Vol. 106, No. 3, [Online] March 1998. Available: http://ehpnet1.niehs.nih.gov/. Produced by the National Institute of Environmental Health Sciences (NIEHS), P.O. Box 12233, Research Triangle Park, NC 27709. For complete contact information, please refer to Chapter 68, "Resources."

- Blacks with asthma are about three times as likely to die of asthma as are whites. Inner city black children are more likely to develop asthma than white children in suburban areas, and are less likely to receive treatment.

- The 1991 National Center for Health Statistics National Hospital Discharge Survey indicates that asthma was the first-listed diagnosis in 490,000 hospital admissions.

- In 1990, the cost for treatment of asthma was estimated at $6.2 billion. Forty-three percent of asthma's economic impact was associated with emergency room use, hospitalization, and death.

Source: National Institute of Allergy and Infectious Diseases

Researchers led by William Cookson of John Radcliffe Hospital and Julian Hopkin of Churchill Hospital, both in Oxford, England, presented the new research in the June [1991] issue of *Nature Genetics.* When IgE binds to a protein receptor in cells lining the airways of the nose and chest, it sets off a series of events leading to an allergy attack. The gene found in the study contains the information for making part of the IgE receptor. The researchers found that people with a particular variant of the gene were likely to have high levels of IgE in their blood, an indicator of a tendency to allergy attacks. The researchers studied 60 families in which 10 had at least one person who had inherited both the variant and the allergic reaction. Of the 12 children who had the variant, all had allergic reactions, compared to only 2 of the children who did not inherit the variant.

The researchers stressed that the association was found only in a minority of the families, and that other genes may be implicated in asthma as well. Still, in an article by the Associated Press, Marshall Plaut, chief of the asthma and allergy branch of the National Institute of Allergy and Infectious Diseases, said, "I think they might have at least a partial answer, and it could be very important."

Any answers as to how and why people develop asthma would be good news to the 15 million Americans who suffer from it. But answers to these questions alone will not stop the increasing rates of asthma, which has become a major environmental health threat, particulary among inner-city children who are more often exposed to allergens and air pollution and may be especially sensitive to them. Misdiagnosis, mismedication or lack of treatment, and lack of the means to remove environmental contributors to asthma are common in inner cities. Answers to these problems are also needed to prevent the increasing numbers of childhood deaths from asthma.

Recent studies sponsored by NIH and the National Center for Health Statistics (NCHS) show that African-American children who live in urban areas are more likely to develop asthma than white children who live in the suburbs and more likely to die from it due to a lack of diagnosis or treatment. In an article in the *Washington Post,* epidemiologist Diane Wagener of the NCHS said, "Deaths due to asthma among children should not happen, because it's a preventable situation." Public health officials say that although genetic research may help to identify individuals who may be susceptible to developing asthma, without adequate prevention and treatment measures the information has little worth.

Allergy Receptor Pictured

For many people, the rites of spring have historically involved stocking up on plenty of antihistamines and tissue, but that may not be the case in the future. Researchers at Northwestern University in Chicago and Harvard Medical School in Boston have determined the precise shape of the receptor protein for immunoglobin E (IgE), the antibody that is responsible for the springtime sniffles and other allergic symptoms that afflict some 20% of the U.S. population. This may be the first step toward developing an allergy medication that stops the allergic response before it happens, rather than merely treating the symptoms.

The study was reported in the 23 December 1998 issue of *Cell.* Theodore S. Jardetzky, an assistant professor in the Department of Biochemistry, Molecular Biology, and Cell Biology at Northwestern, was the principal investigator for the team. His collaborators were Jean-Pierre Kinet, a professor of pathology at Harvard Medical School who first cloned the gene for the IgE receptor in 1986, and Scott Garman, a postdoctoral fellow in the Northwestern Department of Biochemistry, Molecular Biology, and Cell Biology.

About 50 million people in the United States have some form of allergy. Many allergies, such as hay fever and eczema, are more inconvenient than life-threatening, but some allergic responses, such as anaphylaxis, can result in death. Allergies are also strongly suspected of playing a role in asthma. According to the National Institute of Allergy and Infectious Diseases, 90% of asthmatic children and 50% of asthmatic adults also have allergies. According to the Centers for Disease Control and Prevention, asthma accounts for almost

500,000 hospitalizations each year and is the foremost reason that children miss school. And the problem is growing—asthma prevalence in the United States is expected to rise by 5% each year.

Allergic responses are mediated by IgE, which is one of five classes of antibodies. As IgE circulates through the blood and the lymph, it binds to receptors found on the surface of mast cells (a type of white blood cell). There, IgE acts as an antenna, patrolling its airspace for allergens. When an antibody picks up the signal of a nearby allergen, the mast cell responds by releasing histamine and other powerful chemicals that cause an inflammatory response in surrounding tissues.

Mast cells are found throughout the body but are most highly concentrated in tissues that are exposed to the outside world, such as the skin and nasal and lung linings. So when an allergic response occurs, those tissues are most likely to be affected, resulting in the rashes, welts, runny noses, and watery eyes traditionally associated with allergies.

The IgE receptor had previously defied imaging because it has a heterogenous sugar coating that solubilizes the receptor and prevents it from crystallizing into a structure that can be examined through X-ray diffraction. To counteract this problem, the scientists expressed the human IgE receptor gene in cultured insect cells from the cabbage looper and the fall armyworm, which attach fewer sugars to the molecule. Next, they applied a technique called multiple isomorphous replacement, in which IgE receptor crystals were soaked in one of two solutions containing either gold or platinum. The large, heavy atoms of the metals were absorbed into the crystals, adding mass in the form of electrons to the receptor at key points and making it possible to calculate its image. According to Jardetzky, by comparing data that correspond to the receptor by itself to another set of data that reflects the changes effected by the binding of one of these heavy metals to the receptor, the researchers can calculate the structure of the receptor.

The researchers then used the very high intensity X rays of the Advanced Photon Source at Argonne National Laboratory in Illinois to scrutinize the IgE crystals. The Advanced Photon Source is a synchrotron, which uses magnetic fields to maintain charged particles in an orbit. The orbiting particles give off energy in the form of X rays. Special detectors measure the X rays as they bounce off the crystal being analyzed, and computers convert the data into an image of the crystal.

The researchers found that the receptor has an inverted "V" shape. At one end of the V is a spike that attaches the receptor to the cell membrane. The IgE antibody binds at the upward-pointing elbow of the V shape. Jardetzky and colleagues are currently investigating several potential inhibitors and are working on capturing an image of IgE bound to its receptor. "It may be more fruitful for drug development if we can get a picture of this 'lock and key' mechanism," says Jardetzky. "From that, it may emerge that it is better to design an inhibitor for the antibody than for the receptor."

Because allergic responses result only from IgE binding to the IgE receptor, therapeutic strategies aimed at inhibiting IgE-receptor interactions could provide a single treatment to fight multiple conditions such as asthma and sinusitis. The researchers believe that blocking the IgE receptor from binding the IgE antibody will short-circuit the allergy cycle.

Because the IgE-receptor interaction controls only the allergy branch of the body's immune response, it could be inhibited without compromising the entire immune response, says Kinet. The IgE receptor is thought to play some as-yet undefined role in immunity to parasitic infections. Jardetzky allows that inhibition of the IgE-receptor interaction may result in susceptibility to parasitic infections, particularly in developing nations, where such diseases are endemic. However, notes Kinet, IgE is not the only natural defense the body has against parasites. The advantages offered by such an inhibitor, he says, would far outweigh the disadvantages.

Genes and Ozone

New research suggests that whether or not a person reacts to toxic levels of ozone in the air depends upon their genes. If the animal studies that support this association are confirmed in humans, this newest example of the interaction between genes and the environment could have untold implications for industry, insurance, and health.

Researchers believe that knowing they are susceptible could help people protect themselves on bad ozone days, and they hope that clinical genetic therapies might also eventually be developed. Others say information on susceptibility could lead to stricter government regulation of air quality to reduce nitrogen oxides from car exhausts, which combine with oxygen and sunlight to form ozone.

Yet another view is that such information could create a subpopulation of people at risk for discrimination on the basis of their genetic makeup. "It could be a sticky issue if the gene ran in certain ethnic or racial groups, or if disclosure of the gene could risk insurance coverage," says pulmonologist Jeffrey Drazen of the Harvard Medical School in Cambridge, Massachusetts.

"This could become quite a societal issue," acknowledges Steven Kleeberger, one of the scientists who reported the link in the December 1997 issue of *Nature Genetics*. Kleeberger, a researcher at the Johns Hopkins University department of environmental health sciences, predicts that, given genetic susceptibility, the health effects of ozone will become even more of a regulatory and political issue in the future. The findings of Kleeberger's research, along with those of a second study by George Leikauf and colleagues from the University of Cincinnati that were published in the same issue, move the field of air pollution genetics solidly forward. Now, scientists don't talk about if such susceptibility genes are identified in humans, but when.

Both studies used strains of inbred mice with differing responses to ozone. Kleeberger's team selected one strain of mice that was resistant to ozone and one strain that was very responsive. They crossbred the groups, then bred the groups' offspring to select for expression of genes on chromosome 11 and chromosome 17 that control responsivity to ozone. The Cincinnati researchers also found a locus on chromosome 11 that broadly overlapped with Kleeberger's area, indicating the two teams may be honing in on the same gene.

There was significant activity in the segment on chromosome 17, and in searching the mouse genome database for this chromosome, Kleeberger and his team identified several candidate genes that may be causing the activity. One, the tumor necrosis factor alpha (*TNF-α*) gene, seems a highly logical candidate, Kleeberger says. TNF is a pro-inflammatory cytokine that influences genes in the immune response cascade. To test their hypothesis, Kleeberger's team treated the susceptible strain of mice with antibodies that neutralized the *TNF-α* protein. The reaction of these mice to ozone was similar to that of the resistant mice. Although Kleeberger calls this evidence "intriguing," it is not proof that *TNF-α* is the controlling gene in ozone susceptibility, he says. More linkage and physical map studies are needed to identify what he suspects may be a bevy of major and contributing genes associated with differing susceptibilities to ozone.

Indeed, Aravinda Chakravarti, a professor of genetics and medicine at Case Western Reserve University in Cleveland, Ohio, questions the use of mice as surrogates for how ozone affects human biology. The inbred mice used in the studies surely have less genetic variation in their reaction to ozone than that found in humans, he says, and moreover, humans metabolize oxygen differently.

But Kleeberger points out that the "mouse represents a unique model to study genes in their most simple representation." Michael Blaese, chief of the clinical gene therapy branch at the National Human

Genome Research Institute in Bethesda, Maryland, says it makes sense that *TNF*-α may be in some way linked to ozone susceptibility because it is involved in so many important biological activities.

Even so, Blaese believes that any effort to clinically correct or repair susceptibility genes will be a long time in coming because of the inherent difficulties of gene therapy. More likely, he says, researchers will search for clinical ways to interfere with the protein encoded by the gene.

This work offers hope to millions of asthmatics, says Sharon Hipkins, director of programs and policy at the Asthma and Allergy Foundation of America in Washington, DC. It highlights "clinical recognition that there probably is a familial trait that mediates reaction to high ozone levels and that, likely, many asthmatics are affected," she says. But Kleeberger says that asthma is a very complex disorder with a number of different phenotypes and that the association between ozone and asthma susceptibility is not completely understood.

"What is most interesting about these studies is that we have always viewed air pollution as having adverse effects on society as a whole," says Drazen. "Like reactions to medications, we are learning we might be able to identify selected individuals who are affected."

Chapter 21

Environmental Genome Project

Human health is determined by the complex interplay between genetic susceptibility and environmental exposures.

Rapid advances in molecular genetic technologies are providing new opportunities to understand the genetic basis for individual differences in susceptibility to environmental exposures.

NIEHS is expanding its research program on genetic susceptibility to environmentally-associated diseases such as asthma through the new Environmental Genome Project initiative.

This project, which will make use of technology developed by the NIH Human Genome Project, is aimed at:

- the identification of allelic variants (polymorphisms) of environmental disease susceptibility genes in the U.S. population,

- developing a central database of polymorphisms for these genes,

- fostering population-based studies of gene-environment interaction in disease etiology.

By identifying those genes and functional allelic variants that affect individual response to environmental agents, scientists can better

Excerpted from "Asthma Genetics: The Human Genome Project," [Online] February 12, 1999; and from "Environmental Genome Project Overview," [Online] March 15, 2000. Available: http://www.niehs.nih.gov/. Produced by the National Institute of Environmental Health Sciences (NIEHS), P.O. Box 12233, Research Triangle Park, NC 27709. For complete contact information, please refer to Chapter 68, "Resources."

predict health risks and assist regulatory agencies in the development of environmental protection policies.

Environmental Genome Project Overview

The human health/disease condition is determined by the complex interplay between genetic susceptibility, environmental exposures, and aging. The rapid advances in molecular genetic technologies is providing us with new opportunities to understand the genetic basis for individual differences in susceptibility to environmental exposure. The NIEHS is expanding its research program on genetic suscepti- bility to environmentally-associated diseases through a new Environ- mental Genome Project. This project, which will make use of technology developed by the Human Genome Project, is aimed at the identification of allelic variants (polymorphisms) of environmental disease susceptibility genes in the U.S. population, developing a cen- tral database of polymorphisms for these genes, and fostering popu- lation-based studies of gene-environment interaction in disease etiology. By identifying those genes and allelic variants that affect individual response to environmental agents, scientists can better predict health risks and assist regulatory agencies in the development of environmental protection policies.

While a host of genes that play a role in susceptibility to environ- mental exposure have been identified, the polymorphisms of these genes have not been systematically sought, identified, or reported. The identification of polymorphisms that confer altered sensitivity or re- sistance to specific exposures will be the foundation of the Environ- mental Genome Project. The Environmental Genome Project was granted Concept Clearance by the National Advisory Environmental Health Sciences Council on February 4, 1998.

The NIEHS Environmental Genome Project will be a multi- disciplinary, collaborative effort, involving several other NIH insti- tutes as well as the Department of Energy (DOE) and other federal agencies. Examples of categories of genes that include environmen- tal response genes are: xenobiotic metabolism and detoxification genes; hormone metabolic genes; receptor genes; DNA repair genes; cell cycle genes; cell death control genes; genes mediating immune and inflammatory responses; genes mediating nutritional factors; genes involved in oxidative processes and, genes for signal transduction sys- tems. A central database of the polymorphisms will be made available. This database will in turn support both functional studies of alleles and population-based studies of disease risk. Such population-based epidemiological studies are central to the identification of both the alleles and the environmental exposure that cause disease, and represent an integral component of the Environmental Genome Project. The Project will include additional susceptibility genes as they are discovered.

Working with genetically susceptible (sub)populations will allow the more precise identification of environmental agents that cause disease and the true risks of exposure. However, it is of paramount importance to emphasize that identification of polymorphism(s) in an individual does not predict that individual's risk to exposure because of complex, multiple interactions. An individual's complete exposure risk can only be determined by consideration of additional exposure history, nutritional status, age and developmental changes, gender, and other factors. It is our intention that the Environmental Genome Project will generate data that will be utilized in epidemiological studies to enhance our understanding of environmental association with disease. As susceptible (sub)populations are identified, they must be distinguished from susceptible individuals within that population. Some individuals within the susceptible population will be at increased risk for specific exposures while some individuals in that population will have no increase in exposure risk.

The Environmental Genome Project will provide information for future research on molecular mechanisms of susceptibility gene products and of genetic responses to environmental exposure. The Project will foster development of new high-throughput technology for a broader application of molecular genetics in epidemiology as a function of environmental exposure.

Why an Environmental Genome Project

Understanding genetic susceptibility to environmental agents will allow more precise identification of the environmental agents that cause disease and the true risks of exposures. This can lead to more aggressive disease prevention and the improvement of public health by allowing individuals to make better informed decisions regarding environmental exposures they allow/tolerate.

The mission of NIEHS is to understand the impact of environmental exposures on human health and disease. In keeping with our stated mission, the ultimate aim of the EGP is to understand the impact and interaction of environmental exposures on human disease. Human disease states are ultimately the result of interactions between intrinsic genetic susceptibility, age of the affected individual(s), and environmental exposures. The determining factors in a long and healthy life are directly related to environmental exposures with respect given to the cumulative dose of the exposure. Sensitivity to exposures is also a component of the complex interaction of factors that contribute to the health and disease status of an individual. Another equally important component to the disease status of an individual is aging. The longer one lives, the greater the possibility of succumbing to disease. By bettering the understanding of environmental exposures' impacts on human health and disease, work can be done to improve public health by implementing preventative measures.

Goals

The two major goals of the Environmental Genome Project are:

- To facilitate identification of functionally important polymorphisms in environmental response genes that may determine differences in disease risks to environmental exposures.
- To facilitate epidemiological studies of gene-environment interactions in disease etiology through:
  1. Improving technologies for genetic analysis
  2. Optimizing study designs
  3. Developing sample repositories
  4. Addressing social, legal, and ethical implications of common polymorphisms

The specific goals requisite to accomplishing the two major goals are:

To establish a catalog of polymorphisms in environmental response genes based upon resequencing of selected genes in this project.

The first phase of the EGP will select target genes for resequencing; utilize the high throughput technologies developed by the Human Genome Project for rapid sequence analysis; utilize a national repository for analyzing sequence variation in the U.S. population; and make this data available to the scientific community via a centralized database.

To establish paradigms for elucidating functionally important polymorphisms in environmental response genes.

The next phase in the Environmental Genome Project will be to define functionally important polymorphisms. There is a multiplicity of approaches possible for the elucidation of functionally important polymorphisms. The NIEHS Environmental Genome Project will encourage and support research that will define models of functionally important polymorphisms.

Functional analysis in model organisms becomes a priority once sequence variations have been identified. Inquiries about how sequence variations impact on protein-protein and protein-chemical interactions are important to explore. The EGP will encourage and support combinatorial approaches in the determination of functionally important polymorphisms. After sequence variations have been confirmed and functionally important polymorphisms defined, the role of the epidemiologists in executing population-based studies becomes crucial.

To facilitate epidemiological studies of gene-environment interactions in disease etiology.

An ultimate goal of the Environmental Genome Project will be to facilitate epidemiological studies of gene-environment interactions in disease etiology. To this end it is imperative that the EGP associated efforts improve technologies for genetic analyses in population-based studies; optimize study designs; develop population-based resources; and address the ethical, legal, and social implications associated with common polymorphisms and genetic susceptibility to environmental exposures. It is of paramount importance to emphasize that identification of polymorphism(s) in an individual does not predict that individual's risk to exposure because of complex multiple interactions. An individual's risk to an environmental agent is influenced not only by genetic determinants but also by co-exposures, diet, age-related changes, gender, and other factors. It is intended that the data gathered from the Environmental Genome Project will be used in epidemiological studies to improve the understanding of environmental factors in disease. As susceptible subgroups are identified they must be distinguished from susceptible individuals within that population. Some individuals in the susceptible population will be at an increased risk from specific exposures while some individuals will have no increase in exposure risk. At the opposite end of the spectrum will be those individuals in the susceptible population with a reduced exposure risk. This outlines the characteristics of genetic sensitivity which is markedly different than the situation that exists with predisposing genes.

Chapter 22

Asthma Clinical Genetics Network

Glaxo Wellcome launched today a unique initiative that promises real hope of unravelling the genetic basis of asthma and discovering better treatments for the 100 million sufferers of the disease around the world. The Asthma Clinical Genetics Network brings together academic physicians, expert in the diagnosis of asthma and care of patients, with a centre skilled at marrying genetic and clinical data. This international network will conduct a study into the genetic basis of asthma that is unprecedented in scale and design.

Asthma tends to run in families and thus has a significant genetic component. The six European clinical sites and one U.S. clinical site in the Network will enroll 100 families that have at least one asthma sufferer plus affected or unaffected siblings and natural parents. Participants will be recruited either from patients at the Network clinics or through GP referrals.

The Network centres will conduct standard clinical tests for asthma with all the family, including skin prick allergy tests and airway responsiveness tests, and also collect blood samples for DNA analysis from each patient and his or her family members. The genetic and clinical information will be collated in a database in the U.S.

From "Long-Term Hope for Asthma Sufferers Lies in Their Genes: Glaxo Wellcome Establishes Asthma Clinical Genetics Network," [Online] September 28, 1998. Available: http://www.aanma.org/pr092898.html. Produced by Allergy and Asthma Network—Mothers of Asthmatics, Inc. (AANMA), 2751 Prosperity Ave., Ste. 150, Fairfax, VA 22031. Reprinted with permission. For complete contact information, please refer to Chapter 68, "Resources."

and the results analysed to find regions of the genome that are altered in asthma sufferers.

"With 700 families involved, this will be by far the biggest coordinated sample collection and gene screening effort ever in asthma," said Glaxo Wellcome's Worldwide Director of Genetics, Dr. Allen Roses. "This scale and the comparative data we will be getting from family members who are unaffected by asthma are vital if we are to uncover the genetic clues that matter most in asthma. We hope that within four years the Network will have identified regions of the genome that will eventually tell us more about what causes asthma, about inherited predispositions to developing asthma, and how we at Glaxo Wellcome can find new therapies to treat asthma."

"This research should provide answers to some of the questions clinicians have about asthma," said Professor Peter Helms, at the Department of Child Health at Aberdeen University. "It is clear that the genetics of asthma are complicated. We still don't know why asthma is associated with allergy or hay fever in some patients and not in others, or why some asthma sufferers appear to inherit asthma from their parents yet others with no family history develop it."

The seven clinical centres taking part in the Asthma Network are:

- Medical School, University of Aberdeen, UK

- Department of Child Health, University of Leicester, UK

- Medical School, University of Sheffield, UK

- Beatrix Children's Hospital, Groningen University Hospital, the Netherlands

- Paediatric Respiratory Unit, Hippokration General Hospital, Greece

- Vokestoppen Children's Asthma and Allergy Centre, Oslo, Norway

- Duke University Medical Center, Durham, North Carolina, United States.

The Center for Human Genetics at Duke University Medical Center will serve as the screening and epidemiology centre for the Network. "The establishment of the Asthma Network has demonstrated a real spirit of collaboration between the sponsor, Glaxo Wellcome, and all the centres", said Dr. Margaret Pericak-Vance, Head of the Center for Human Genetics at Duke University Medical Center. We are really pleased to be able to use our genome screening, genetic epidemiology, and informatics expertise for such a worthwhile cause."

Glaxo Wellcome has plans to establish further clinical genetics networks for other diseases which will be announced at a later date.

Glaxo Wellcome is a research-based pharmaceutical company whose people are committed to fighting disease by bringing innovative medicines and services to patients throughout the world, and to the healthcare providers who serve them.

For further information, please contact:

Allergy and Asthma Network—Mothers of Asthmatics, Inc.
2751 Prosperity Avenue, Suite 150
Fairfax, VA 22031
Phone: (800)878-4403 or (703)641-9595
Fax: (703)573-7794

Chapter 23

Asthma and Race

In the early 1980s, studies were published showing a relationship between race and environmental risk, raising concerns that minority populations were being unfairly affected by pollution. Around this time, researchers also began to notice that asthma prevalence was significantly higher in minority communities. In one 1990 study published in the *American Review of Respiratory Disease,* asthma prevalence in black children was found to be 7.2%, as compared with 3.0% among white children. A 1994 study published in *Pediatrics* found extraordinarily high rates of asthma in New York City's minority Bronx neighborhoods—as high as 12.8%.

For many, the relationship between race and asthma seemed to be clear evidence that the health of minorities was being compromised by inequitable environmental practices. A study published in the 23 October 1996 issue of the *American Journal of Public Health* suggests, however, that differences in asthma prevalence may be due as much to differences in diagnosis as to differences in environment.

Excerpted from "The Question of Asthma and Race," in *Environmental Health Perspectives,* Vol. 105, No. 4, [Online] April 1997. Available: http://ehpnet1.niehs.nih.gov/docs/1997/105-4/NIEHSnews.html. Produced by the National Institute of Environmental Health Sciences (NIEHS), P.O. Box 12233, Research Triangle Park, NC 27709; and from "Asthma: A Concern for Minority Populations," [Online] August 1996. Available: http://www.niaid.nih.gov/factsheets/minorasthma.htm. Produced by the Office of Communications and Public Liaison, National Institute of Allergy and Infectious Diseases (NIAID). For complete contact information, please refer to Chapter 68, "Resources."

This study by Joan Cunningham, Douglas W. Dockery, and Frank E. Speizer of the Harvard School of Public Health focused on the prevalence of asthma and persistent wheeze among 1,416 black and white Philadelphia school children age 9-11. Wheezing is one of the primary symptoms of asthma. The study found, as most previous studies had, that black race was a significant predictor of diagnosed asthma; 9.4% of black children were reported to be asthmatic, while only 5.2% of white children were reported to be diagnosed with the disease. However, when the prevalence of persistent wheeze in the two groups was analyzed, no statistically significant difference was found (9.1% prevalence for black children versus 6.8% for white children). These results led the researchers to conclude that part of the discrepancy in asthma prevalence between races could be explained by differences in diagnosis. "The issue that we're raising is that blacks tend to get the diagnosis of asthma more than whites," Dockery said.

Why symptomatic blacks are diagnosed with asthma more often than symptomatic whites is puzzling, Dockery said, but he offers one scenario that may explain the difference: "It may be that low-income minorities are less likely to have a general practitioner that they visit regularly. Instead, they are more likely to seek emergency room care. If these children come into the hospital on an emergency basis with a breathing problem, . . . and if they respond to a bronchiodilator, they are very likely to be labeled as asthmatic." On the other hand, Dockery said, more affluent children may be treated for breathing problems, including persistent wheeze, by a family doctor, but because this type of care is less episodic, doctors don't feel pressured to make an immediate asthma diagnosis. An editorial by Peter Gergen, a health scientist administrator at the Agency for Health Care Policy Research, that also appears in the 23 October 1996 *American Journal of Public Health* supports this explanation, pointing out that studies have shown that poor children are more likely to use emergency rooms as their principal source of health care. "We are faced with the paradox that inadequate care can contribute to increased diagnostic labeling of wheezing episodes among poor children," Gergen writes.

The Harvard group is not the first to propose that differences in asthma prevalence across races is due in part to differences in diagnosis; a similar conclusion was proposed in the 1994 article in the journal *Pediatrics*. However, the authors of the Harvard study point out that these results do not imply that there are no other factors influencing the higher rates of asthma seen in minorities. For example, low socioeconomic status may increase the prevalence of asthma diagnosis among minority children in two ways—first, by exposing them to harmful agents that actually cause the condition and, second, by forcing them into the type of sporadic health care that results in a quick diagnosis.

"Part of this seems to be difference in diagnosis, but we still think there is . . . some environmental factor that these studies have not brought out that is contributing [to asthma]," Dockery said. Research is now uncovering how exposure to dust mites, cockroaches, pets, mold spores, and endotoxins might contribute to the disease, he said. Several intervention trials are now taking place to see if healthy environments can reduce a person's chances of developing asthma symptoms.

Studies on the Genetic Basis of Asthma

In collaboration with the National Heart, Lung, and Blood Institute (NHLBI), NIAID is funding a cooperative study at four centers (Johns Hopkins University, Baltimore, MD; University of Chicago, Chicago, IL; University of Maryland, Baltimore, MD; and University of Minnesota, Minneapolis, MN) to explore the genetic basis of asthma. This study is enrolling asthmatic patients and their families (many of whom are from ethnic minorities) in order to identify genes for asthma and for responsiveness to allergens. This study has identified several candidate genes for asthma, some of which may be more common in African-American populations. In other studies, investigators supported by NIAID have identified a genetic change in interleukin-4 (IL-4), an immune-signaling molecule involved in asthma and allergic responses, that correlates with asthma severity. This change appears to be several-fold more common among African Americans than among whites. Studies of such genes should facilitate development of new and more potent and selective therapies, and may help to identify patient populations who might respond best to a particular drug.

Chapter 24

Interleukin-11 and Asthma

Respiratory syncytial virus (RSV), rhinovirus, and parainfluenza virus type 3 often are associated with exacerbations of asthma and airways hyperreactivity.[1,2] Their effects are thought to be mediated by direct airway injury and in part by the local inflammatory response.[3] However, the cellular events that mediate these processes are understood poorly. Interleukin-11 (IL-11) is a newly appreciated pleiotropic cytokine [regulates immune responses] of the IL-6 family.[4] Early studies focused on its roles in hematopoiesis [process of formation and development of various types of blood cells], ability to stimulate the acute phase response, and inhibit adipocyte [fat cell] differentiation. There are, however, a number of features that make it particularly relevant to asthma. First IL-11 is known to be a T-cell-dependent stimulator of B-cell immunoglobulin production[5] and activated T cells are believed to play an important role in the pathogenesis of asthma.[6,7] Secondly, IL-11 is a member of the IL-6-type cytokine family and members of this family, in particular leukemia inhibitory factor, have the ability to induce cholinergic [relating to nerve cells that employ

From "Asthma-Associated Viruses Specifically Induce Lung Stromal Cells to Produce Interleukin-11, A Mediator of Airways Hyperreactivity," (The Thomas L. Petty 37th Aspen Lung Conference: Asthma—Structure and Function) by Oskar Einarsson, Gregory P. Geba, James R. Panuska, Zhou Zhu, Mary Landry, and Jack A. Elias, in *Chest*, Vol. 107, No. 3, March 1995, pp. 132S-133S. © 1995 by American College of Chest Physicians, 3300 Dundee Rd., Northbrook, IL 60062. Reprinted with permission. For complete contact information, please refer to Chapter 68, "Resources."

acetylcholine as their neurotransmitter] neuronal differentiation and neuronal tachykinin [any of a group of polypeptides that have in common 4 or 5 amino acids] production.[6,7] Cholinergic hyperactivity and increased tachykinin production could contribute to the airways hyperresponsiveness and bronchospasm characteristic of the asthmatic diathesis [inborn state].[9,10] The third feature is its highly cationic nature [referring to positively charged ions and their properties] (pI>-11), which is unusual among cytokines. Cationic molecules such as eosinophil major basic protein (pI=10.9) are believed to play a potential role in asthma since they induce bronchospasm and hyperresponsiveness in vivo.[11] Lastly, work from our laboratories has demonstrated IL-11 production by lung fibroblasts and epithelial cells in response to IL-1, transforming growth factor beta (TGF-[beta]), histamine, and major basic protein. We, therefore, hypothesized that respiratory viruses could also induce IL-11 production and that IL-11 might play an important role in viral-induced airways hyperresponsiveness.

To test this hypothesis, we determined whether viruses that are associated with asthmatic exacerbations induce stromal cell IL-11 production, investigated the specificity of this response, and characterized the effects of IL-11 on the physiology of the mouse airway. Uninfected human lung fibroblasts [cells present in connective tissue, capable of forming collagen fibers] (CCL-202, MRC-5), type 2 alveolar epithelial-like cells (A549), and transformed human tracheal epithelial cells (9HTE) produced quantities of IL-11 that were barely detectable by enzyme-linked immunosorbent assay. Respiratory syncytial virus was a potent stimulator of lung fibroblast IL-11 production, causing a 50- to 100-fold increase within 48 h after infection. This was associated with proportionate changes in IL-11 messenger RNA as assessed by Northern blot analysis. Similar results of less magnitude were obtained using the epithelial cell lines. Parainfluenza virus type 3 and rhinovirus were found to induce IL-11 production in an identical fashion. The ability to induce IL-11 production was, at least partially, specific for these viruses since influenza virus A, adenovirus, and cytomegalovirus were only marginal stimulators, and herpes simplex type 2 virus, Streptococcus pneumoniac, Staphylococcus aureus, and Mycobacterium aviumintracellulare did not induce IL-11 production despite visible cytopathic effects in similar culture systems.

To determine if the ability of viruses to stimulate IL-11 production in vitro was relevant to the in vivo state, studies were undertaken to determine if IL-11 could be detected in the airway secretions from patients with upper respiratory tract infections. To accomplish this, we measured the IL-11 levels in nasal samples sent for RSV isolation and/or antigen detection during the 1993 to 1994 RSV season. The IL-11 levels in secretions from children with upper respiratory tract symptoms were compared with those from children whose nasal aspirates were done for surveillance purposes. IL-11 levels in nasal aspirates from children lacking upper respiratory tract symptoms were below the level of detectability of our assay. In contrast, most children with upper respiratory tract symptoms had levels of IL-11 that were elevated. Interestingly, a similar pattern could be seen when the children were grouped according to the presence of bronchospasm.

To understand its potential in vivo effects, we administered rhIL-11 (10,[mu]g) to BALB/C mice by nasal inhalation. The animals subsequently were anesthetized with pentobarbital, tracheostomized [making a permanent opening into the trachea through the neck], and respiratory system resistance was determined via body plethysmography [measuring and recording changes in volume of organ by a plethysmograph]. Airway responsiveness was assessed by determining the concentration of nebulized methacholine [parasympathomimetic agent used as a vasodilator] that produced a 100% increase in respiratory system resistance (PC 100). No difference was noticed in baseline resistance between test or control animals. However, animals receiving rhIL-11 demonstrated a significant lower log PC 100, thus more reactivity to methacholine, at 24 h (0.51 [+ or -] 0.15 vs 2.45 0.32 mg/mL, p<0.005) and 48 h (0.49 [+ or -] 0.20 vs 3.0 [+ or -] 0.1 mg/mL, p<0.005) after administration.

These studies demonstrate that RSV, parainfluenza virus type 3, and rhinovirus are not only potent but are also, in part, specific inducers of IL-11 production in lung stromal cells [framework usually of connective tissue of an organ, gland, or other structure]. Furthermore, IL-11 can be detected in nasal secretions of children presenting with viral-like upper respiratory tract symptoms, Finally IL-11 can induce airway hyperresponsiveness when administered locally to the airways of BALB/C mice. We therefore conclude that IL-11 may be an important mediator of airway hyperresponsiveness associated with viral infections of the respiratory tract.

References

1. Pattemore PK, Johnston SL, Bardin PG. Viruses as precipitants of asthma symptoms: I. Epidemiology. *Clin Exp Allergy* 1992; 22:325-36

2. Cypcar D, Stark J, Lemanske RF. The impact of respiratory infections on asthma. *Pediatr Clin North Am* 1992; 39:1259-76

3. Bardin PG, Johnston SL, Pattemore PK. Viruses as precipitants of asthma symptoms, II. Physiology and mechanisms. *Clin Exp Allergy* 1992; 22:809-22

4. Du XX, Williams DA. Interleukin-11: a multifunctional growth factor derived from the hematopoietic microenvironment. *Blood* 1994; 83:1023-30

5. Yin T, Schendel P, Yang YC. Enhancement of in vitro and in vivo antigen-specific antibody responses by interleukin-11. *J Exp Med* 1992; 175:211-16

6. Corrigan CJ, Kay AB. T cells and eosinophils in the pathogenesis of asthma. *Immunol Today* 1992; 13:501-07

7. Robinson DS, Hamid Q, Ying S, et al. Predominant T_2-like bronchoalveolar T-lymphocyte population in atopic asthma. *N Engl J Med* 1992; 326:298-304

8. Patterson P, Nawa H. Neuronal differentiation factors/ cytokines and synaptic plasticity. *Cell* 1993; 72 (suppl):123-37

9. Nadel JA. Regulation of neurogenic inflammation by neutral endopeptidase. *Am Rev Respir Dis* 1992; 145:S48-S52

10. Ihre E, Larsson K. Airways responses to ipratropium bromide do not vary with time in asthmatic subjects: studies of inter-individual and intraindividual variation of bronchodilatation and protection against histamine-induced bronchoconstriction. *Chest* 1990; 97:46-51

11. Gundel RH, Letts LG, Gleicb GJ. Human eosinophil major basic protein induces airway constriction and airway hyperresponsiveness in primates. *J Clin Invest* 1991; 87:1470-73

—by Oskar Einarsson, Gregory P. Geba,
James R. Panuska, Zhou Zhu,
Mary Landry, and Jack A. Elias

Chapter 25

Infectious Asthma

Asthma, an important cause of respiratory morbidity and mortality, is an inflammatory condition of the airways whose underlying etiology is not completely understood. Recognition of the significance of inflammation in asthma has led to recommendations for more widespread use of anti-inflammatory therapy.[1] It is important to acknowledge, however, that current asthma therapies are palliative, not curative. Research into new possible underlying causes for asthma are therefore warranted.

Earlier in this century, many clinicians believed that respiratory infection played a significant role in asthma etiology.[2-5] Recent clinical studies have also suggested that bronchitis and pneumonia are associated with subsequent asthma.[6-8] Results of cross-sectional[9-12] and prospective[13,14] epidemiologic studies have found that preceding respiratory illnesses, including bronchitis, chronic bronchitis, and pneumonia, are associated with subsequent asthma in both children[9,12-14] and adults.[9,10] Smith[15] has recently proposed a viral hypothesis for the onset of allergic diseases and asthma. Busse,[16-18] Bardin, et al,[19] and Sheth and Busse[20] have reviewed potential mechanisms whereby infection may exacerbate and possibly even initiate asthma. It has further been suggested that the adult acute asthmatic bronchitis syndrome may be a risk factor for the subsequent development of asthma.[21]

From "Infectious Asthma: A Reemerging Clinical Entity?" by David L. Hahn, M.D., in *The Journal of Family Practice*, Vol. 41, No. 2, August 1995, pp. 153-7. © 1995 by Dowden Publishing Co., Inc., 110 Summit Ave., Montvale, NJ 07645. Reprinted with permission.

Discovery of bacterial etiologies for some diseases of previously unknown origin (for example, *Helicobacter pylori* in peptic ulcer disease) have led to greater acceptance of the concept that infection might be involved in the etiology of other chronic inflammatory conditions of unknown cause.[22] Acute respiratory infection is acknowledged as a common cause for asthma exacerbations, but there is less evidence that infection is the *initiating* event for asthma. Since the etiology for asthma remains unknown, it is reasonable to ask whether further clinical definition of infectious asthma (reflecting infection associated with the *initiation* of asthma rather than solely with later exacerbations) will advance our understanding of the underlying cause and optimal management of this disease. This report describes clinical and spirometric findings in a consecutive series of 92 primary care outpatients with a diagnosis of chronic asthma who had pulmonary function tests recorded, and compares the clinical and spirometric findings in patients with chronic asthma classified as infectious and noninfectious.

Methods

Study Setting and Patients

The study site was a community-based primary care (family practice) office affiliated with a multisite, multispecialty group practice located in and around a mid-sized midwestern city, the population of which is predominantly white and middle class. Between 1988 and 1993, inclusive, the author recorded encounters with 97 patients who had a clinical diagnosis of symptomatic chronic asthma. Following each encounter, clinical data from the medical record and results of pulmonary function, if available, were entered into a database for later analysis. The goal was to record data for all encountered patients who reported symptomatic asthma. Whether any such patients were missed is unknown.

This case series includes 92 (95%) patients for whom baseline pulmonary function testing was also recorded. For this group, previous medical records were available for 89 (97%) group practice patients. Three (3%) patients were referred from outside the group practice, and they provided copies of medical records for review.

Pulmonary Function Measurements

Spirometric testing was performed according to American Thoracic Society guidelines,[23] using a Gould spirometer (System 21, Gould

Medical Products, Inc., Dayton, Ohio). Baseline testing was performed for all 92 study group patients and in 84 (91%) patients after treatment with inhaled albuterol or a course of oral steroids. In most cases, the author performed spirometric testing. Sometimes pulmonary function was performed elsewhere in the medical center using a comparable apparatus and technique.

Classification of Asthma Syndromes

Patients with intermittent or persistent wheeze, cough, and dyspnea triggered by a variety of stimuli, who responded to inhaled beta-adrenergics and/or oral or parenteral steroids, received a diagnosis of chronic asthma based on clinical criteria of the American Thoracic Society.[24] Patients reporting that initial asthma symptoms were associated with an acute respiratory illness (usually bronchitis, pneumonia, or an influenza-like illness) were classified as infectious. Patients with atopic, occupational, and exercise-induced asthma, who did not report associations with respiratory infection when symptoms were first noticed, were classified as noninfectious. This classification refers only to associations with respiratory infection at the time asthma symptoms first began and does not refer to later exacerbations of asthma symptoms caused by respiratory infections. Some patients could not be classified because of lack of recall, unavailability of relevant medical records, or both.

Classification as infectious or noninfectious asthma was based on medical record evidence and patient recall of respiratory illness at the time asthma symptoms (usually wheeze and dyspnea) first occurred, regardless of whether a diagnosis of asthma was made at that time or later. As part of the typical patient workup, the author asked questions regarding possible infectious initiation of asthma. First, an open-ended question ("Tell me about the *very first time* you ever noticed any of your symptoms of asthma") was asked. Second, a more specific confirmatory probe ("So when you noticed your very first symptoms, they happened/did not happen after respiratory illness?") was used. Medical record data pertaining to initial recorded symptoms were often shared with the patient during this interview process.

Statistical Methods

Fisher's exact test was used to analyze 2 x 2 tables. Analysis of variance (ANOVA) was used to test for subgroup differences in means of continuous variables. A multivariate regression model was used to test for subgroup differences in pulmonary function values, while simultaneously controlling for the effects of current smoking and the reported duration of asthma symptoms. Two-sided P values of $<.05$ were reported as significant.

Results

Table 25.1. summarizes the clinical findings for the 92 study-group patients with chronic asthma encountered during the 6-year study period. Seventy-eight (85%) patients were over 20 years of age, 46% were male, and 25% were current smokers; data concerning previous smoking were not recorded. Age-of-onset data were available for 89 (97%) patients: 27 (30%) reported onset before age 20, 40 (45%) between ages 20 and 40, and 22 (25%) after age 40. Calculated asthma duration (current age minus age at onset) varied as follows: 5 years or less (45%), 5 to 15 years (30%), and more than 15 years (25%). Current age, age at onset, and asthma duration were significantly intercorrelated as follows: R (age vs age at onset)=.81 ($P<.001$), R (age vs duration) =.22 ($P=.036$), and R (age at onset vs duration)=-.40 ($P<.001$).

Based on available information, 77 (84%) patients could be classified as either infectious or noninfectious (Table 25.1.). Patients with infectious asthma tended to be older than those with noninfectious asthma (41.7 vs 35.9 years of age, P=NS), were older when asthma began (36.1 vs 22.3 years of age, $P<.001$), and had a much shorter duration of symptoms (5.6 vs 13.3 years, $P=.001$). Patients with infectious asthma were also more likely to be current smokers (40% vs 15%, $P=.03$), but the sex distributions were approximately equal (44% male). Of the 41 subjects with infectious asthma, 14 (34%) reported some clinical history of allergy not associated with asthma initiation (mostly allergic rhinitis or allergic triggers for subsequent asthma episodes).

There were no significant differences for any of the variables reported in Table 25.1. between the 92 patients in the study group and the 5 patients who were excluded because they had not had pulmonary function tests.

Pulmonary Function Test Results

Table 25.2. presents pre- and post-bronchodilator pulmonary function results (as percentage of predicted FEV_1 and $FEF_{25\%-75\%}$) for the entire study group and for the subgroups of patients with and without infectious asthma. Twenty-eight (30.4%) patients had moderately severe baseline pulmonary function as indicated by a pre-bronchodilator

Table 25.1. Clinical Characteristics of Patients Classified as Infectious and Noninfectious Asthmatics

	Total group (N=92)	Infectious* (n=41)	Noninfectious† (n=36)	P value‡
Age, y [mean (SD)]	37.7 (15.4)	41.7 (14.1)	35.9 (17.1)	NS
Male, %	46	44	44	NS
Current smoker, %‡	25	40	15	.03
Age when asthma symptoms first reported, y [mean (SD)]	28.9 (16.4)	36.1 (15.8)	22.3 (14.5)	<.001
Duration of asthma symptoms, y [mean (SD)]	8.9 (9.9)	5.6 (6.6)	13.3 (12.5)	.001

*Infectious asthma: first symptoms of asthma reported following a respiratory illness (usually bronchitis, pneumonia, or an influenza-like illness).

†Noninfectious asthma: atopic, occupational, or exercise-induced asthma without an infectious presentation. Classification was not possible for 15 (16.3%) patients for whom sufficient clinical history was unavailable.

‡Data on current smoking status were available for 81 (88%) patients, including 35 infectious and 33 noninfectious asthmatics.

SD denotes standard deviation; NS, not significant.

FEV_1 of less than 65% of the predicted value. Pre-bronchodilator FEV_1 of less than 65% predicted was present in 42% of infectious asthmatics and in 22% of noninfectious asthmatics (P=NS). When analyzed as continuous variables, pre- and post-bronchodilator FEV_1 and $FEF_{25\%-75\%}$ were all significantly worse for patients with infectious asthma as compared with those with noninfectious asthma. These differences remained significant after simultaneous adjustment for current smoking and asthma duration (Table 25.2.).

For the total study group, post-bronchodilator FEV_1 increased 21.8%. There were no significant differences in bronchodilator response for patients with infectious and noninfectious asthma or for the degree of fixed obstruction, as measured by the ratio of FEV_1, to FVC (forced vital capacity) (Table 25.2.).

Discussion

Acute respiratory infections preceding asthma have been frequently documented, but pathogenetic mechanisms remain speculative.[13] Possible initiation of asthma by a variety of agents including respiratory syncytial virus,[20] adenovirus,[25] *Mycoplasma pneumoniae*,[26] and *Chlamydia pneumoniae*[27] has been discussed. Chronic infection as a cause for persistent asthma symptoms has also been suggested for adenovirus[25] and chlamydia species.[27,28]

This study reported primarily on adult patients with chronic asthma drawn from a primary care population. The age distribution of asthma patients was a function of the practice, which contained fewer childhood asthmatics than one would expect from sampling the general population. Therefore, study results may not apply to childhood-onset asthma. Compared with patients having noninfectious asthma, infectious asthmatics developed symptoms at a later age and had worse baseline and post-bronchodilator pulmonary function, despite a much shorter duration of symptomatic disease. This pattern resembles previous descriptions of adult-onset asthma, which is associated with worse symptoms and a poorer prognosis when compared with asthma in younger patients.[5,29]

Several limitations of this study require comment. This was a clinical descriptive study in a single primary care practice, and as such, is subject to selection bias. Classification bias cannot be ruled out. Classification as infectious or noninfectious was made independently of knowledge of pulmonary function test results, and no a priori hypothesis was made regarding the significant association between infectious asthma and worse pulmonary function. Recall bias is a serious

Table 25.2. Pulmonary Function Test Results for Patients Classified as Infectious and Noninfectious Asthmatics

	Total group (N=92)		Infectious* (n=41)		Noninfectious† (n=36)		P value‡
FEV$_1$, % predicted (SD)							
Pre-bronchodilator	74.4	(20.2)	67.7	(15.4)	77.9	(21.8)	.016
Post-bronchodilator§	90.6	(14.4)	86.5	(10.4)	94.9	(15.1)	.047
FEF$_{25-75\%}$, % predicted (SD)							
Pre-bronchodilator	50.2	(27.6)	41.8	(19.7)	52.4	(28.1)	.044
Post-bronchodilator§	64.7	(25.4)	61.4	(19.1)	72.8	(27.6)	.040
FEV$_1$/FVC, % (SD)	77.9	(8.6)	77.1	(7.7)	78.4	(9.1)	NS

*Infectious asthma: first symptoms of asthma reported following a respiratory illness (usually bronchitis, pneumonia, or an influenza-like illness).

†Noninfectious asthma: atopic, occupational, or exercise-induced asthma without an infectious presentation. Classification was not possible for 15 (16.3%) patients for whom sufficient clinical history was unavailable.

‡Adjusted for asthma duration and current smoking.

§Post-bronchodilator results were available for 84 (91.3%) patients with chronic asthma, 40 (97.6%) patients with infectious asthma, and 32 (88.9%) patients with noninfectious asthma.

FEV$_1$ denotes forced expiratory volume in 1 second; FEF, forced expiratory flow; FVC, forced vital capacity; SD, standard deviation; NS, not significant.

consideration, with patients ill for a shorter period possibly having a better recollection of the antecedent event. This limitation was overcome partially by the availability of previous medical records for some patients, and addressed by adjusting for asthma duration. Patient recall was supported by medical records, which often spanned decades, or occasionally a lifetime, representing one of the advantages of performing retrospective clinical research in a family practice setting. Results remained significant after controlling for duration of disease in a multivariate model. It is possible that smoking was related to worse pulmonary function in infectious asthmatics. Since smoking is known to be associated with chronic obstructive pulmonary disease (COPD), it is possible that smoking contributed to lower FEV_1 in infectious asthmatics, who had a higher prevalence of current smoking. There was no difference, however, between patients in the infectious and noninfectious groups in the ratio of FEV_1 to FVC (a measure of fixed obstruction in COPD). Furthermore, patients with a clinical diagnosis of COPD who also had asthma were excluded from this report. Finally, results remained significant after controlling for smoking in the multivariate model. Pulmonary function test results (as percentages of predicted values) are already normalized by age, sex, race, and body mass index. Therefore, in the author's opinion, further controlling for these variables in the multivariate model used in this analysis was not indicated.

This study found that infectious asthma had worse baseline pulmonary function compared with other forms of asthma, despite a significantly shorter duration of symptoms for infectious asthma (5.6 v 13.3 years). This pattern of findings could be explained by worse pulmonary function at the time infectious asthma became symptomatic, by a greater rate of loss of function after symptoms began, or by a combination of these mechanisms. Regarding a possible accelerated loss of function, infectious asthma could be associated with a severe acute insult, which is stable and unchanged over time, or with a continuing, progressive loss of function. Concern has been raised recently over the long-term use of inhaled steroids for asthma whose cause might involve chronic persistent infection.[28] These issues can be resolved only by means of prospective longitudinal studies.

This cross-sectional clinical study can offer only hypotheses for future research, not conclusive proof. The classification of infectious asthma, as employed here, is novel and its association with worse pulmonary function requires confirmation. Since causative factors of asthma are unknown, and inhaled corticosteroid therapy is now being advocated[1] despite the therapy's unknown effects on ultimate pulmonary function,[30] it is worthwhile to perform further studies on the reemerging clinical entity of infectious asthma. If this avenue of research proves fruitful and treatable infectious causes of asthma are identified, the possibility of "cure" may exist for some asthma patients for whom only palliative therapies are currently available.

References

1. National Asthma Education Program. Guidelines for the diagnosis and management of asthma. *J Allergy Clin Immunol* 1991; 88 (suppl):425-534.

2. Bivings L. Asthmatic bronchitis following chronic upper respiratory infection. *JAMA* 1940; 115:1434-6.

3. Chobot R, Uvitsky IH, Dundy H. The relationship of the etiologic factors in asthma in infants and children. *J Allergy* 1951; 22:106-10.

4. Fox JL. Infectious asthma treated with triacetyloleandomycin. *Penn Med J* 1961; 64:634-5.

5. Ogilvie AG. Asthma: a study in prognosis of 1,000 patients. *Thorax* 1962; 17:183-9.

6. Hallett JS, Jacobs RL. Recurrent acute bronchitis: the association with undiagnosed bronchial asthma. *Ann Allergy* 1985; 55:568-70.

7. Williamson HA, Schultz P. An association between acute bronchitis and asthma. *J Fam Pract* 1987; 24:35-8.

8. Kolnaar BGM, van den Bosch WJHM, van den Hoogen HJM, van Weel C. The clustering of respiratory diseases in early childhood. *Fam Med* 1994; 26:106-10.

9. Burrows B, Lebowitz M. Characteristics of chronic bronchitis in a warm, dry region. *Am Rev Respir Dis* 1975; 112:365-70.

10. Burrows B, Knudson RJ, Leibowitz M. The relationship of childhood respiratory illness to adult obstructive airway disease. *Am Rev Respir Dis* 1977; 115:751-60.

11. Dodge RR, Burrows B. The prevalence and incidence of asthma and asthma-like symptoms in a general population sample. *Am J Resp Dis* 1980; 122:567-75.

12. Infante-Rivard C. Childhood asthma and indoor environmental factors. *Am J Epidemiol* 1993; 137:834-44.

13. Sherman GB, Tosteson TD, Tager IB, Speizer FE, Weiss ST. Early childhood predictors of asthma. *Am J Epidemiol* 1990; 132:83-95.

14. Dodge RR, Burrows B, Lebowitz MD, Cline MG. Antecedent features of children in whom asthma develops during the second decade of life. *J Allergy Clin Immunol* 1993; 92:744-9.

15. Smith JM. Asthma and atopy as diseases of unknown cause. A viral hypothesis possibly explaining the epidemiologic association of the atopic diseases and various forms of asthma. *Ann Allergy* 1994; 72:156-62.

16. Busse WW. Respiratory infections and bronchial hyperreactivity. *J Allergy Clin Immunol* 1988; 81:770-5.

17. Busse WW. The relationship between viral infections and onset of allergic diseases and asthma. *Clin Exp Allergy* 1989; 19:1-9.

18. Busse WW. Role and contribution of viral respiratory infections to asthma. *Allergy* 1993; 48:57-64.

19. Bardin PG. Johnston SL, Pattemore PK. Viruses as precipitants of asthma symptoms II. Physiology and mechanisms. *Clin Exp Allergy* 1992; 22:809-22.

20. Sheth KK, Busse WW. Respiratory tract infections and asthma. In: Gershwin ME, Halpern GM, eds. *Bronchial asthma. Principles of diagnosis and treatment.* Totowa, New Jersey: Humana Press, 1994:481-512.

21. Hahn DL. Acute asthmatic bronchitis: a new twist to an old problem. *J Fam Pract* 1994; 39:431-5.

22. Blaser MJ. Bacteria and diseases of unknown cause. *Ann Intern Med* 1994; 121:144-5.

23. American Thoracic Society. Recommended standardized procedures for pulmonary function testing. *Am J Resp Dis* 1978; 118:55-77.

24. American Thoracic Society. Standards for the diagnosis and care of patients with chronic obstructive pulmonary disease (COPD) and asthma. *Am J Resp Dis* 1987; 136:225-44.

25. Macek V, Sorli J, Kopriva S, Marin J. Persistent adenoviral infection and chronic airway obstruction in children. *Am J Respir Crit Care Med* 1994; 150:7-10.

26. Yano T, Ichikawa Y, Komatu S, Arai S, Oizumi K. Association of *Mycoplasma pneumoniae* antigen with initial onset of bronchial asthma. *Am J Respir Crit Care Med* 1994; 149:1348-53.

27. Hahn DL, Dodge R, Golubjatnikov R. Association of *Chlamydia pneumoniae* (strain TWAR) infection with wheezing, asthmatic bronchitis and adult-onset asthma. *JAMA* 1991; 266:225-30.

28. Hahn DL. Clinical experience with anti-chlamydial therapy for adult-onset asthma. *Am Rev Respir Dis* 1993; 147:A297.

29. Burrows B. The natural history of asthma. *J Allergy Clin Immunol* 1987; 80:375S-7S.

30. Hahn DL, van Schayck CP, Dompeling E, Folgering H. Effect of inhaled steroids on the course of asthma. *Ann Intern Med* 1993; 119:1051-2.

Part Four

Triggers and Risk Factors Associated with Asthma

Chapter 26

Targeting Asthma Triggers

Asthma Alert

Asthma is one of our nation's most common chronic health conditions and is on the rise. It can start in childhood, resolve, recur, or develop in adulthood. Many people have both asthma and allergies. Unlike an allergy, asthma is an inflammatory disease of the lung. Since your nose connects to your lung, the inflammatory process can occur along the entire airway. Once the airway begins to swell, breathing becomes difficult. Asthmatics are often short of breath and have a feeling of tightness in the chest. All asthmatics should be under a doctor's care to manage their disease, to keep it under control and to keep them healthy.

Common Triggers

- Cigarette smoke
- Cockroaches
- Dust mites
- Mold
- Pets and animals
- Pollen
- Cold air
- Exercise
- Stress
- Respiratory infections

From "Asthma and Allergy Prevention," [Online] February 12, 1999. Available: http://www.niehs.nih.gov/airborne/prevent/alert/html. Produced by the National Institute of Environmental Health Sciences (NIEHS), P.O. Box 12233, Research Triangle Park, NC 27709. For complete contact information, please refer to Chapter 68, "Resources."

If your asthma attacks:

- Don't panic
- Breathe deep, slow, and easy
- Rest
- Take your prescribed asthma medication
- Call for help
- Get to a doctor

Allergy Prevention

The best way to prevent an allergy is to recognize that you have one (see "Signs of an Allergy" below). Often people confuse an allergy with a cold or flu. Remember colds are short-lived and passed from person to person, whereas allergies are immune system reactions to normally harmless substances. Allergies are best prevented by avoiding exposure to allergens in the first place. A good first step to avoiding allergens is to follow the various PREVENTIVE STRATEGIES outlined for each allergen or irritant.

Signs of an Allergy

- Sneezing, watery eyes, or cold symptoms that last more than 10 days without a fever.
- Repeated ear and sinus infections.
- Loss of smell or taste.
- Frequent throat clearing, hoarseness, coughing, or wheezing.
- Dark circles under the eyes caused by increased blood flow near the sinuses (allergic shiners).
- A crease just above the tip of the nose from constant upward nose wiping (allergic salute).

Cigarette Smoke

Cigarette smoke contains a number of toxic chemicals and irritants. People with allergies may be more sensitive to cigarette smoke than others and research studies indicate that smoking may aggravate allergies.

Smoking does not just harm smokers but also those around them. Research has shown that children and spouses of smokers tend to have more respiratory infections and asthma than those of non-smokers.

In addition, exposure to secondhand smoke can increase the risk of allergic complications such as sinusitis and bronchitis.

Common symptoms of smoke irritation are burning or watery eyes, nasal congestion, coughing, hoarseness, and shortness of breath presenting as a wheeze.

Preventive Strategies

- Don't smoke and if you do, seek support to quit smoking. Contact Puff-Free Partners, such as:

  1. Nicotine Anonymous, Ph: (415)750-0328, http://www.nicotine-anonymous.org

  2. American Lung Association, Ph: (800)LUNG-USA, http://www.lungusa.org/tobacco

  3. American Cancer Society, Ph: (800)ACS-2345, http:/www.cancer.org/tobacco

- Seek smoke-free environments in restaurants, theaters, and hotel rooms.

- Avoid smoking in closed areas like homes or cars where others may be exposed to secondhand smoke.

Cockroaches

Cockroaches are one of the most common and allergenic of indoor pests.

Recent studies have found a strong association between the presence of cockroaches and increases in the severity of asthma symptoms in individuals who are sensitive to cockroach allergens.

These pests are common even in the cleanest of crowded urban areas and older dwellings. They are found in all types of neighborhoods.

The proteins found in cockroach saliva are particularly allergenic but the body and droppings of cockroaches also contain allergenic proteins.

Preventive Strategies

- Limit the spread of food around the house and especially keep food out of bedrooms.

- Keep food and garbage in closed containers. Never leave food out in the kitchen.

- Mop the kitchen floor and wash countertops at least once a week.

- Eliminate water sources that attract these pests, such as leaky faucets and drain pipes.
- Plug up crevices around the house through which cockroaches can enter.
- Use bait stations and other environmentally safe pesticides to reduce cockroach infestation.

Dust Mites

Dust mites are tiny microscopic relatives of the spider and live on mattresses, bedding, upholstered furniture, carpets, and curtains.

These tiny creatures feed on the flakes of skin that people and pets shed daily and they thrive in warm and humid environments.

No matter how clean a home is, dust mites cannot be totally eliminated. However, the number of mites can be reduced by following the suggestions below.

Preventive Strategies

- Encase your mattress and pillows in dust-proof or allergen impermeable covers (available from specialty supply mail order companies, bedding, and some department stores).
- Wash all bedding and blankets once a week in hot water (at least 130-140° F) to kill dust mites.
- Replace wool or feathered bedding with synthetic materials and traditional stuffed animals with washable ones.
- If possible, replace wall-to-wall carpets in bedrooms with bare floors (linoleum, tile, or wood).
- Use a damp mop or rag to remove dust. Never use a dry cloth since this just stirs up mite allergens.
- Use a dehumidifier or air conditioner to maintain relative humidity at about 50% or below.
- Use a vacuum cleaner with either a double-layered microfilter bag or a HEPA filter to trap allergens that pass through a vacuum's exhaust.

Food Allergies

Our consumption of food nearly triples during the holiday season. With the scrumptious variety of foods available during the holidays, a food allergy can easily present itself.

Symptoms of a food allergy can be as simple as skin problems (itchiness, rashes, or hives) or intestinal troubles (abdominal pain, diarrhea, or vomiting), or as dangerous as swelling of the respiratory passages, shortness of breath, fainting, or anaphylactic shock.

The more common food allergens are egg, milk, shellfish, peanuts, soy, and wheat. These foods are often hidden as ingredients in casseroles or desserts. You should be aware of what you are eating, but don't limit your diet to only a few foods since a well balanced diet is best.

Preventive Strategies

If you have a food allergy:

- Beware of foods that cause you symptoms.
- If you have had severe reactions to a food, talk to your doctor about carrying an epinephrine injector.
- Learn to read food labels carefully.
- When dining out, ask about the ingredients used in preparing the dish before tasting the food.
- If you experience symptoms, avoid any further contact with that food item, rinse your mouth, and see a doctor.

Grass Pollen

As with tree pollen, grass pollen is regional as well as seasonal. In addition, grass pollen levels can be affected by temperature, time of day, and rain.

Of the 1,200 species of grass that grow in North America, only a small percentage of these cause allergies. The most common grasses that can cause allergies are Bermuda grass, Johnson grass, Kentucky bluegrass, Orchard grass, Sweet vernal grass, and Timothy grass.

Preventive Strategies

Specifically:

- If you have a grass lawn, have someone else do the mowing. If you must mow the lawn yourself, wear a mask.
- Keep grass cut short.
- Choose ground covers that don't produce much pollen, such as Irish moss, bunch, and dichondra.

In general:

- Avoid the outdoors between 5-10 AM. Save outside activities for late afternoon or after a heavy rain, when pollen levels are lower.

- Keep windows in your home and car closed to lower exposure to pollen. To keep cool, use air conditioners and avoid using window and attic fans.

- Be aware that pollen can also be transported indoors on people and pets.

- Dry your clothes in an automatic dryer rather than hanging them outside. Otherwise pollen can collect on clothing and be carried indoors.

House Dust

House dust is a component of who you are. House dust is not just dirt but a mixture of potentially allergenic materials, such as fibers, food particles, mold spores, pollens, dust mites, plant and insect parts, hair, animal fur and feathers, dried saliva and urine from pets, and flakes of human and animal skin.

The more time you spend indoors, particularly in the fall and winter, the greater your exposure to house dust allergens.

Preventive Strategies

- Dust rooms thoroughly with a damp cloth at least once a week.

- Wear protective gloves and a dust mask while cleaning to reduce exposure to dust and cleaning irritants.

- Use electric and hot water radiant heaters to provide a cleaner source of heat than "blown air" systems.

- Reduce the number of stuffed animals, wicker baskets, dried flowers, and other dust collectors around the house.

- Replace heavy drapes and blinds with washable curtains or shades.

- Replace carpets with washable scatter rugs or bare floors (wood, tile, or linoleum).

Mold Spores

Mold spores are allergens that can be found both indoors and outdoors. There is no definite seasonal pattern to molds that grow indoors.

However outdoor molds are seasonal, first appearing in early spring and thriving until the first frost.

Indoor molds are found in dark, warm, humid, and musty environments such as damp basements, cellars, attics, bathrooms, and laundry rooms. They are also found where fresh food is stored, in refrigerator drip trays, garbage pails, air conditioners, and humidifiers.

Outdoor molds grow in moist shady areas. They are common in soil, decaying vegetation, compost piles, rotting wood, and fallen leaves.

Preventive Strategies

- Use a dehumidifier or air conditioner to maintain relative humidity below 50% and keep temperatures cool.
- Air out closed spaces such as closets and bathrooms.
- Vent bathrooms and clothes dryers to the outside.
- Check faucets, pipes, and ductwork for leaks.
- When first turning on home or car air conditioners, leave the room or drive with the windows open for several minutes to allow mold spores to disperse.
- Remove decaying debris from the yard, roof, and gutters.
- Avoid raking leaves, mowing lawns, or working with peat, mulch, hay, or dead wood. If you must do yard work, wear a mask and avoid working on hot, humid days.

Pets and Animals

Many people think animal allergies are caused by the fur or feathers of their pet. In fact, allergies are actually aggravated by:

- proteins secreted by oil glands and shed as dander
- proteins in saliva (which stick to fur when animals lick themselves)
- aerosolized urine from rodents and guinea pigs

Keep in mind that you can sneeze with and without your pet being present. Although an animal may be out of sight, their allergens are not. This is because pet allergens are carried on very small particles. As a result pet allergens can remain circulating in the air and remain on carpets and furniture for weeks and months after a pet is gone.

Preventive Strategies

- Remove pets from your home if possible.
- If pet removal is not possible, keep them out of bedrooms and confined to areas without carpets or upholstered furniture.
- Wear a dust mask and gloves when near rodents.
- After playing with your pet, wash your hands and clean your clothes to remove pet allergens.
- Avoid contact with soiled litter cages.
- Dust often with a damp cloth.

Ragweed Pollen

Ragweed and other weeds such as curly dock, lambs quarters, pigweed, plantain, sheep sorrel, and sagebrush are some of the most prolific producers of pollen allergens.

Although the ragweed pollen season runs from August to November, ragweed pollen levels usually peak in mid-September in many areas in the country.

In addition, pollen counts are highest between 5-10 AM and on dry, hot, and windy days.

Preventive Strategies

- Avoid the outdoors between 5-10 AM. Save outside activities for late afternoon or after a heavy rain, when pollen levels are lower.
- Keep windows in your home and car closed to lower exposure to pollen. To keep cool, use air conditioners and avoid using window and attic fans.
- Be aware that pollen can also be transported indoors on people and pets.
- Dry your clothes in an automatic dryer rather than hanging them outside. Otherwise pollen can collect on clothing and be carried indoors.

Tree Pollen

Trees are the earliest pollen producers, releasing their pollen as early as January in the Southern states and as late as May or June in the Northern states.

Trees can aggravate your allergy whether or not they are on your property, since trees release large amounts of pollen that can be distributed miles away from the original source.

Of the 50,000 different kinds of trees, less than 100 have been shown to cause allergies. Most allergies are specific to one type of tree such as ash, box elder, cottonwood, elm, hickory, maple, olive, pecan, poplar, sycamore, walnut, and willow.

However, people do show cross-reactivity among trees in the alder, beech, birch, and oak family, and the juniper and cedar family.

Preventive Strategies

- If you buy trees for your yard, look for species that do not aggravate allergies such as catalpa, crape myrtle, dogwood, fig, fir, palm, pear, plum, redbud, and redwood trees.

- Avoid the outdoors between 5-10 AM. Save outside activities for late afternoon or after a heavy rain, when pollen levels are lower.

- Keep windows in your home and car closed to lower exposure to pollen. To keep cool, use air conditioners and avoid using window and attic fans.

- Be aware that pollen can also be transported indoors on people and pets.

- Dry your clothes in an automatic dryer rather than hanging them outside. Otherwise pollen can collect on clothing and be carried indoors.

Chapter 27

Nitrogen Dioxide and Allergic Asthma

Over the past few decades many countries have experienced an increase in both morbidity and mortality from asthma. Air pollution is a possible culprit, and researchers have paid special attention to NO_2 [nitrogen dioxide] concentrations, which have risen steadily as the result of burning of fossil fuels, mainly from motor vehicle engines. Epidemiological and clinical studies have addressed the effects of exposure to low concentrations of NO_2 on respiratory health indoors and outdoors. Most of the studies assessing the relation between indoor NO_2 and respiratory health have been conducted in children and the results are inconsistent.[1] In adults, many experimental studies have been conducted, showing on average a small increase in airways reactivity to NO_2 by comparison with clean air.[2] However, the approach of exposing subjects to individual pollutants bears little resemblance to the complexities of atmospheric pollution. Molfino, et al.,[3] used a different approach—low concentrations of ozone—to test and corroborate the hypothesis that air pollution enhances airways responsiveness to ragweed and grass allergens. Two recent reports in *The Lancet* show that NO_2 alone[4] and in combination with SO_2 [sulphur dioxide],[5] at concentrations that may be encountered in daily life, enhance the bronchoconstrictive response to inhaled house dust mites in patients with mild asthma. Neither of these latest experimental studies allows estimation of the clinical magnitude of the reported functional change, although Tunnicliffe, et al.,[4] suggest that these effects are likely to be small.

Increased airways reactivity is not the only effect induced by low levels of NO_2. Devalia, et al.,[6] in an in-vitro study, found that exposure to 400-800 ppb [parts per billion] of NO_2 caused bronchial epithelial cell dysfunction. Whether the enhanced airway reactivity to inhaled allergens is the consequence of cellular damage remains unclear. Aris, et al.,[7] showed that exposure of healthy subjects to 200 ppb of ozone was followed by an influx of inflammatory cells into the airway, although there was no correlation with spirometric changes. Concurrent exposure to different air pollutants could induce significant inflammation and enhance the reactivity of asthmatics to a wide range of asthma triggers. Devalia, et al.,[5] showed that joint exposure to NO_2 and SO_2 led to increased bronchial reactivity to allergens whereas NO_2 alone did not. The more complex mixtures of pollutants likely to be present in urban air could induce even larger inflammatory and functional changes than the ones reported so far. Thus, the effect of air pollution on allergic asthma could be larger than that seen in the experimental studies.

From a public health perspective, we need to know the size of the population at risk; and to determine that we need to integrate the individual opportunities for exposure at specific time-space ordinates. Here both indoor and outdoor sources of NO_2 are relevant. In a U.S. study, cooking with a gas stove generated concentrations of 200 to 400 ppb of NO_2, with transient peaks as high as 1000 ppb.[8] In a study of children in New Mexico, Samet, et al.,[1] found that, in 30% of their bimonthly calls, children reported having been in the kitchen while meals were being cooked during the previous 24 hours, for an average of 20 minutes. However, frequency and characteristics of these indoor exposures to NO_2 probably differ from one country to another. Outdoor levels of NO_2 around 400 ppb are reached only during the severe air pollution episodes that occur sporadically. Peak hourly levels of 382-423 ppb were recorded during a pollution episode in London in December, 1991.[9] Thus, while it is clear that allergic asthmatics can experience cellular and functional damage if exposed to levels of NO_2 of 400 ppb or higher, we do not know either the magnitude of the subsequent clinical effects or the prevalence of exposure of asthmatics to such levels of pollution. This lack of knowledge hinders a more precise evaluation of the problem from a public health perspective.

Increasing levels of NO, over recent decades could have influenced asthma in two ways: (a) by decreasing the threshold of allergen exposure needed to develop sensitisation and allergic asthma; and (b) by increasing morbidity of existing asthma. There is growing evidence for the latter possibility.[4,5] By contrast, evidence for an increased incidence of asthma due to air pollution has not yet been provided. However, if NO_2 and other air pollutants increase the permeability of bronchial mucosa to allergens,[5] the threshold for allergen exposure to produce sensitisation may decrease and the incidence of allergic asthma may increase.

Until lately the association between NO_2 and asthma was inconsistent. The studies reported by Tunnicliffe, et al.,[4] and by Devalia, et al.,[5] confirm the findings reported by Molfino, et al.,[3] for ozone and should stimulate further research to characterise the synergism between NO_2 and aeroallergens as causal or contributory factors in asthma.

References

1. Samet JM, Lambert WE, Skipper BJ, et al. Nitrogen dioxide and respiratory illnesses in infants. *Ant Rev Respir Dis* 1993;148:1258-65.

2. Folinsbee LJ. Does nitrogen dioxide exposure increase airways responsiveness? *Toxicol Indust Health* 1992;8:273-83.

3. Molfino NA, Wright SC, Katz I, et al. Effect of low concentrations of ozone on inhaled allergen responses in asthmatics subjects. *Lancet* 1991;338:199-203.

4. Tunnicliffe WS, Burge PS, Ayres JG. Effect of domestic concentrations of nitrogen dioxide on airway responses to inhaled allergen in asthmatic patients. *Lancet* 1994;344:1733-36.

5. Devalia JL, Rusznack C, Herdman MJ, Trigg CJ, Tarraf H, Davies RJ. Effect of nitrogen dioxide and sulphur dioxide on airway response of mild asthmatic patients to allergen inhalation. *Lancet* 1994;344:1668-71.

6. Devalia JL, Sapsford RJ, Cundell DR, Rusznak C, Campbell AM, Davies RJ. Human bronchial epithelial cell dysfunction following in vitro exposure to nitrogen dioxide. *Eur Respir J* 1993;6:1308-16.

7. Aris PM, Christian D, Hearne PQ, Finkbeiner WE, Balmes JR. Ozone-induced airway inflammation in human subjects as determined by airway lavage and biopsy. *Am Rev Respir Dis* 1993;148:1363-72.

8. Harlos DP. Acute exposure to nitrogen dioxide during cooking or commuting. Dissertation. Boston, MA: Harvard School of Public Health, 1988.

9. Brought GFJ. Air quality in the UK: a summary of results from instrumented air monitoring networks in 1991-92. Warren Spring Laboratory, report LR 941. Stevenage: WSL, 1993.

—by Josep M Anto and Jordi Sunyer,
Institut Municipal d'Investigacio Medica, (IMAS),
Universitat Autonoma de Barcelona, Barcelona, Spain

Chapter 28

Ozone and Your Health

On a hot, smoggy summer day, have you ever wondered: Is the air safe to breathe? Should I be concerned about going outside?

In fact, breathing smoggy air can be hazardous because smog contains ozone, a pollutant that can harm our health when there are elevated levels in the air we breathe. This [chapter] will tell you what kinds of health effects ozone can cause, when you should be concerned, and what you can do to avoid dangerous exposures.

What Is Ozone?

Ozone is an odorless, colorless gas composed of three atoms of oxygen. Ozone occurs both in the Earth's upper atmosphere and at ground level. Ozone can be good or bad, depending on where it is found:

- *Good Ozone.* Ozone occurs naturally in the Earth's upper atmosphere—10 to 30 miles above the Earth's surface—here it forms a protective layer that shields us from the sun's harmful ultraviolet rays. This "good" ozone is gradually being destroyed by manmade chemicals. An area where ozone has been most significantly

Excerpted from "Smog—Who Does It Hurt?" [Online] July 27, 1999. Available: http://www.epa.gov/airnow/health/smog1.html; and from "Fact Sheet: Health and Environmental Effects of Ground-Level Ozone," [Online] July 17, 1997. Available: http://www.epa.gov/ttn/oarpg/naaqsfin/o3health.html. Produced by the Office of Air Quality Planning and Standards (OAQPS), U.S. Environmental Protection Agency (EPA). For complete contact information, please refer to Chapter 68, "Resources."

depleted—for example, over the North or South pole—is sometimes called a "hole in the ozone."

- *Bad Ozone.* In the Earth's lower atmosphere, near ground level, ozone is formed when pollutants emitted by cars, power plants, industrial boilers, refineries, chemical plants, and other sources react chemically in the presence of sunlight.

The booklet *Ozone: Good Up High, Bad Nearby,* which can be found on the web at http://www.epa.gov/oar/oaqps/gooduphigh, contains additional information about both good and bad ozone.

This [chapter] focuses on bad ozone—that is, ozone that occurs at ground level and can affect the health of people who breathe it.

Should I Be Concerned about Exposure to Ground-Level Ozone?

That depends on who you are and how much ozone is in the air. Most people only have to worry about ozone exposure when ground-level concentrations reach high levels. In many U.S. communities, this can happen frequently during the summer months. In general, as ground-level ozone concentrations increase, more and more people experience health effects, the effects become more serious, and more people are admitted to the hospital for respiratory problems. When ozone levels are very high, *everyone* should be concerned about ozone exposure.

Scientists have found that about one out of every three people in the United States is at a higher risk of experiencing ozone-related health effects (see [below] "Who Is Most at Risk from Ozone?"). If you are a member of a "sensitive group," you should pay special attention to ozone levels in your area. This [chapter] describes several tools that the U.S. Environmental Protection Agency (EPA), in partnership with state and local agencies, has developed to inform the public about local ozone levels. These tools provide the information you need to decide whether ozone levels on any particular day may be harmful to you. When ozone concentrations reach unhealthy levels, you can take simple precautions (described [below] in "What Can I Do to Avoid Unhealthy Exposure to Ozone?") to protect your health.

How Might Ozone Affect My Health?

Scientists have been studying the effects of ozone on human health for many years. So far, they have found that ozone can cause several types of short-term health effects in the lungs:

- *Ozone can irritate the respiratory system.* When this happens, you might start coughing, feel an irritation in your throat, and/ or experience an uncomfortable sensation in your chest. These symptoms can last for a few hours after ozone exposure and may even become painful.

- *Ozone can reduce lung function.* When scientists refer to "lung function," they mean the volume of air that you draw in when you take a full breath and the speed at which you are able to blow it out. Ozone can make it more difficult for you to breathe as deeply and vigorously as you normally would. When this happens, you may notice that breathing starts to feel uncomfortable. If you are exercising or working outdoors, you may notice that you are taking more rapid and shallow breaths than normal. Reduced lung function can be a particular problem for outdoor workers, competitive athletes, and other people who exercise outdoors.

- *Ozone can aggravate asthma.* When ozone levels are high, more asthmatics have asthma attacks that require a doctor's attention or the use of additional medication. One reason this happens is that ozone makes people more sensitive to allergens, which are the most common triggers for asthma attacks. (Allergens come from dust mites, cockroaches, pets, fungus, and pollen.) Also, asthmatics are more severely affected by the reduced lung function and irritation that ozone causes in the respiratory system.

- *Ozone can inflame and damage the lining of the lung.* Some scientists have compared ozone's effect on the lining of the lung to the effect of sunburn on the skin. Ozone damages the cells that line the air spaces in the lung. Within a few days, the damaged cells are replaced and the old cells are shed—much in the way that skin peels after a sunburn. If this kind of damage occurs repeatedly, the lung may change permanently in a way that could cause long-term health effects and a lower quality of life.

- *Scientists suspect that ozone may have other effects on people's health.* Ozone may aggravate chronic lung diseases, such as emphysema and bronchitis. Also, studies in animals suggest that ozone may reduce the immune system's ability to fight off bacterial infections in the respiratory system.

Most of these effects are considered to be short-term effects because they eventually cease once the individual is no longer exposed to elevated levels of ozone. However, scientists are concerned that repeated

251

short-term damage from ozone exposure may permanently injure the lung. For example, repeated ozone impacts on the developing lungs of children may lead to reduced lung function as adults. Also, ozone exposure may speed up the decline in lung function that occurs as a natural result of the aging process. Research is underway to help us better understand the possible long-term effects of ozone exposure.

Who Is Most at Risk from Ozone?

Four groups of people, described below, are particularly sensitive to ozone. These groups become sensitive to ozone when they are active outdoors, because physical activity (such as jogging or outdoor work) causes people to breathe faster and more deeply. During activity, ozone penetrates deeper into the parts of the lungs that are more vulnerable to injury. Sensitive groups include:

- *Children.* Active children are the group at highest risk from ozone exposure. Such children often spend a large part of their summer vacation outdoors, engaged in vigorous activities either in their neighborhood or at summer camp. Children are also more likely to have asthma or other respiratory illnesses. Asthma is the most common chronic disease for children and may be aggravated by ozone exposure.

- *Adults who are active outdoors.* Healthy adults of all ages who exercise or work vigorously outdoors are considered a "sensitive group" because they have a higher level of exposure to ozone than people who are less active outdoors.

- *People with respiratory diseases, such as asthma.* There is no evidence that ozone causes asthma or other chronic respiratory disease, but these diseases do make the lungs more vulnerable to the effects of ozone. Thus, individuals with these conditions will generally experience the effects of ozone earlier and at lower levels than less sensitive individuals.

- *People with unusual susceptibility to ozone.* Scientists don't yet know why, but some healthy people are simply more sensitive to ozone than others. These individuals may experience more health effects from ozone exposure than the average person.

Scientists have studied other groups to find out whether they are at increased risk from ozone. So far there is little evidence to suggest that either the elderly or people with heart disease have heightened sensitivity to ozone. However, like other adults, elderly people will be at higher risk from ozone exposure if they suffer from respiratory disease, are active outdoors, or are unusually susceptible to ozone as described above.

How Can I Tell If I Am Being Affected by Ozone?

Often, people exposed to ozone experience recognizable symptoms, including coughing, irritation in the airways, rapid or shallow breathing, and discomfort when breathing or general discomfort in the chest. People with asthma may experience asthma attacks. When ozone levels are higher than normal, any of these symptoms may indicate that you should minimize the time spent outdoors, or at least reduce your activity level, to protect your health until ozone levels decline.

Ozone damage also can occur without any noticeable signs. Sometimes there are no symptoms, or sometimes they are too subtle to notice. People who live in areas where ozone levels are frequently high may find that their initial symptoms of ozone exposure go away over time—particularly when exposure to high ozone levels continues for several days. This does not mean that they have developed resistance to ozone. In fact, scientists have found that ozone continues to cause lung damage even when the symptoms have disappeared. The best way to protect your health is to find out when ozone levels are elevated in your area and take simple precautions to minimize exposure even when you don't feel obvious symptoms.

How Do Scientists Know about the Health Effects of Ozone?

EPA has gathered a great deal of information about the health effects of ozone. This information comes from a number of sources, including animal research, studies that compare health statistics and ozone levels within communities, and controlled testing of human volunteers to determine how ozone affects lung function. In these studies, volunteers are exposed to ozone in specially designed chambers where their responses can be carefully measured. Volunteers are prescreened in medical examinations to determine their health status, and they are never exposed to ozone levels that exceed those found in major cities on a very smoggy day.

Though our understanding of ozone's effects has increased substantially in recent years, many important questions still remain to be investigated. For example, does repeated short-term exposure to high

253

levels of ozone cause permanent lung damage? Does repeated exposure during childhood to high levels of ozone cause reduced lung function in adults? Scientists are continuing to study these and other questions to gain a better understanding of ozone's effects.

How Can I Find Out about Ozone Levels in My Area?

EPA and state and local air agencies have developed a number of tools to provide people with information on local ozone levels, their potential health effects, and suggested activities for reducing ozone exposure.

Air Quality Index. EPA has developed the Air Quality Index, or AQI, (formerly known as the Pollutant Standards Index) for reporting the levels of ozone and other common air pollutants. The index makes it easier for the public to understand the health significance of air pollution levels. Air quality is measured by a nationwide monitoring system that records concentrations of ozone and several other air pollutants at more than a thousand locations across the country. EPA "translates" the pollutant concentrations to the standard AQI index, which ranges from 0 to 500. The higher the AQI value for a pollutant, the greater the danger. An AQI value of 100 usually corresponds to the national ambient air quality standard (NAAQS) for the pollutant. These standards are established by EPA under the Clean Air Act to protect public health and the environment.

The AQI scale has been divided into distinct categories, each corresponding to a different level of health concern. In Table 28.1 the AQI ranges are shown in the middle column and the associated air quality descriptors are shown in the right column. The left column shows the ozone concentrations, measured in parts per million (ppm), that correspond to each category.

Though the AQI scale extends to 500, levels above 300 rarely occur in the United States. This publication and most other references to the AQI do not list health effects and cautionary statements for levels above 300. If ozone levels above 300 should ever occur, everyone should avoid physical exertion outdoors.

When pollutant levels are high, states are required to report the AQI in large metropolitan areas (populations over 350,000) of the United States. You may see the AQI for ozone reported in your newspaper, or your local television or radio weathercasters may use the AQI to provide information about ozone in your area. Here's the type of report you might hear: "The Air Quality Index today was 160. Air

Table 28.1. Air Quality Index (AQI) Categories

Ozone Concentration (ppm) (8-hour average, unless noted)	Air Quality Index Values	Air Quality Descriptor
0.0 to 0.064	0 to 50	Good
0.065 to 0.084	51 to 100	Moderate
0.085 to 0.104	101 to 150	Unhealthy for Sensitive Groups
0.105 to 0.124	151 to 200	Unhealthy
0.125 (8-hr.) to 0.404 (1-hr.)	201 to 300	Very Unhealthy

quality was unhealthy due to ozone. Hot, sunny weather and stagnant air caused ozone in Center City to rise to unhealthy levels."

AQI Colors. To make it easier for the public to quickly understand the air quality in their communities, EPA has assigned a specific color to each AQI category. You will see these colors when the AQI is reported in a color format—such as in a color-print newspaper, on television broadcasts, or on your state or local air pollution agency's web site. This color scheme can help you quickly determine whether air pollutants are reaching unhealthy levels in your area. For example, the color orange means that conditions are "unhealthy for sensitive groups," the color red means that conditions are "unhealthy" for everyone, and so on.

Ozone Maps. In many areas of the country, measurements of ozone concentrations are converted into color contours of the AQI categories and displayed on a map to show ozone levels in the local area. The map is updated throughout the day and shows how ozone builds during hot summer days. In some areas, ozone maps are used to show a forecast of ozone levels for the next day. Once you understand the color scheme, you can use the maps to quickly determine whether ozone concentrations are reaching unhealthy levels in your area. Ozone maps appear on some televised weather broadcasts and are also available from EPA's web site at http://www.epa.gov/airnow.

What Can I Do to Avoid Unhealthy Exposure to Ozone?

You can take a number of steps. Table 28.2, "Health Effects and Protective Actions for Specific Ozone Ranges," tells you what types of health effects may occur at specific ozone concentrations and what you can do to avoid them. If you are a parent, keep in mind that your children are likely to be at higher risk, particularly if they are active outdoors. You may therefore want to pay special attention to the guidance for sensitive groups.

In general, when ozone levels are elevated, your chances of being affected by ozone increase the longer you are active outdoors and the more strenuous the activity you engage in. Scientific studies show that:

- At ozone levels above 0.12 ppm, heavy outdoor exertion for short periods of time (1 to 3 hours) can increase your risk of experiencing respiratory symptoms and reduced lung function.

- At ozone levels between 0.08 and 0.12 ppm, even moderate outdoor exertion for longer periods of time (4 to 8 hours) can increase your risk of experiencing ozone-related effects.

EPA recommends limiting outdoor activities as ozone levels rise to unhealthy levels. You can limit the amount of time you are active outdoors or your activity level. For example, if you're involved in an activity that requires heavy exertion, such as running or heavy manual labor (see [below] "What Does Exertion Have to Do with Ozone-Related Health Effects?"), you can reduce the time you spend on this activity or substitute another activity that requires less exertion (e.g., go for a walk rather than a jog). In addition, you can plan outdoor activities when ozone levels are lower, usually in the early morning or evening.

What Does Exertion Have to Do with Ozone-Related Health Effects?

Exercise and outdoor activities can play an important role in maintaining good health. Physical exertion helps build up strength in the heart and lungs. But exerting yourself outdoors can actually increase your chances of experiencing health effects when ozone concentrations are at unhealthy levels. Why is this true? Think of it this way: Exertion generally causes you to breathe harder and faster. When this happens, more ozone is taken into your lungs, and ozone reaches tissues that are susceptible to injury. Research has shown that respiratory effects are observed at lower ozone concentrations if either the level or duration of exertion is increased. This is why EPA recommends decreasing the level or duration of exertion to avoid ozone health effects.

Examples of typical daily activities that involve **moderate exertion** include climbing stairs, light jogging, easy cycling, playing tennis or baseball, and stacking firewood. Outdoor occupational activities such as simple construction work, pushing a wheelbarrow with a load, using a sledgehammer, or digging in your garden, would also involve moderate exertion. Activities that involve **heavy exertion** include vigorous running or cycling, playing basketball or soccer, chopping wood, and heavy manual labor. Because fitness levels vary widely among individuals, what is moderate exertion for one person may be heavy exertion for another. No matter how fit you are, cutting back on the level or duration of exertion when ozone levels are high will help protect you from ozone's harmful effects.

What Can I Do to Reduce Ozone Levels?

Ground-level ozone is created when certain pollutants, known as "ozone precursors," react in heat and sunlight to form ozone. Cars and other vehicles are the largest source of ozone precursors. Other important sources include industrial facilities, power plants, gasoline-powered mowers, and evaporation of cleaners, paints, and other chemicals.

We can all help reduce ozone levels by taking the following steps:

- Drive less. For example, instead of using a car, you may want to walk, use mass transit, or ride a bike.

- Carpool.

- Make sure your car is well-tuned.

- Take care not to spill gasoline when you fill the tank of your car or lawn or recreation equipment.

- Make sure that you tightly seal the lids of chemical products— such as solvents, garden chemicals, or household cleaners—to keep evaporation to a minimum.

Summary

Why Are We Concerned about Ground-Level Ozone?

- Ozone is the prime ingredient of smog in our cities and other areas of the country. Though it occurs naturally in the stratosphere to provide a protective layer high above the earth, at ground-level it is the prime ingredient of smog.

Table 28.2. Health Effects and Protective Actions for Specific Ozone Ranges

Ozone Level	Health Effects and Protective Actions
Good	**What are the possible health effects?** — No health effects are expected.
Moderate	**What are the possible health effects?** — Unusually sensitive individuals may experience respiratory effects from prolonged exposure to ozone during outdoor exertion. **What can I do to protect my health?** — When ozone levels are in the "moderate" range, consider limiting prolonged outdoor exertion if you are unusually sensitive to ozone.
Unhealthy for Sensitive Groups	**What are the possible health effects?** — If you are a member of a sensitive group,[1] you may experience respiratory symptoms (such as coughing or pain when taking a deep breath) and reduced lung function, which can cause some breathing discomfort. **What can I do to protect my health?** — If you are a member of a sensitive group,[1] limit prolonged outdoor exertion. In general, you can protect your health by reducing how long or how strenuously you exert yourself outdoors and by planning outdoor activities when ozone levels are lower (usually in the early morning or evening). — You can check with your state air agency to find out about current or predicted ozone levels in your location. This information on ozone levels is available on the Internet at http://www.epa.gov/airnow.
Unhealthy	**What are the possible health effects?** — If you are a member of a sensitive group,[1] you have a higher chance of experiencing respiratory symptoms (such as aggravated cough or pain when taking a deep breath), and reduced lung function, which can cause some breathing difficulty. — At this level, anyone could experience respiratory effects. **What can I do to protect my health?** — If you are a member of a sensitive group,[1] avoid prolonged outdoor exertion. Everyone else—especially children—should limit prolonged outdoor exertion.

Table 28.2. (continued) Health Effects and Protective Actions for Specific Ozone Ranges

Ozone Level	Health Effects and Protective Actions
Unhealthy	**What can I do to protect my health? (continued)** — Plan outdoor activities when ozone levels are lower (usually in the early morning or evening). — You can check with your state air agency to find out about current or predicted ozone levels in your location. This information on ozone levels is available on the Internet at http://www.epa.gov/airnow.
Very Unhealthy	**What are the possible health effects?** — Members of sensitive groups[1] will likely experience increasingly severe respiratory symptoms and impaired breathing. — Many healthy people in the general population engaged in moderate exertion will experience some kind of effect. According to EPA estimates, approximately half will experience moderately reduced lung function; one-fifth will experience severely reduced lung function; 10 to 15 percent will experience moderate to severe respiratory symptoms (such as aggravated cough and pain when taking a deep breath). — People with asthma or other respiratory conditions will be more severely affected, leading some to increase medication usage and seek medical attention at an emergency room or clinic. **What can I do to protect my health?** — If you are a member of a sensitive group,[1] avoid outdoor activity altogether. Everyone else—especially children—should limit outdoor exertion and avoid heavy exertion altogether. — Check with your state air agency to find out about current or predicted ozone levels in your location. This information on ozone levels is available on the Internet at http://www.epa.gov/airnow.

[1]*Members of sensitive groups include children who are active outdoors; adults involved in moderate or strenuous outdoor activities; individuals with respiratory disease, such as asthma; and individuals with unusual susceptibility to ozone.*

- When inhaled, even at very low levels, ozone can:

  1. cause acute respiratory problems;

  2. aggravate asthma;

  3. cause significant temporary decreases in lung capacity of 15 to over 20 percent in some healthy adults;

  4. cause inflammation of lung tissue;

  5. lead to hospital admissions and emergency room visits [10 to 20 percent of all summertime respiratory-related hospital visits in the northeastern U.S. are associated with ozone pollution]; and

  6. impair the body's immune system defenses, making people more susceptible to respiratory illnesses, including bronchitis and pneumonia.

Who Is Most at Risk from Exposure to Ground-Level Ozone?

- Children are most at risk from exposure to ozone:

  1. The average adult breathes 13,000 liters of air per day. Children breathe even more air per pound of body weight than adults.

  2. Because children's respiratory systems are still developing, they are more susceptible than adults to environmental threats.

  3. Ground-level ozone is a summertime problem. Children are outside playing and exercising during the summer months at summer camps, playgrounds, neighborhood parks, and in backyards.

- Asthmatics and Asthmatic Children:

  1. Asthma is a growing threat to children and adults. Children make up 25 percent of the population and comprise 40 percent of the asthma cases.

  2. Fourteen Americans die every day from asthma, a rate three times greater than just 20 years ago. African-Americans die at a rate six times that of Caucasians.

  3. For asthmatics having an attack, the pathways of the lungs become so narrow that breathing becomes akin to sucking a thick milk shake through a straw.

4. Ozone can aggravate asthma, causing more asthma attacks, increased use of medication, more medical treatment and more visits to hospital emergency clinics.

- Healthy Adults:

  1. Even moderately exercising healthy adults can experience 15 to over 20 percent reductions in lung function from exposure to low levels of ozone over several hours.

  2. Damage to lung tissue may be caused by repeated exposures to ozone—something like repeated sunburns of the lungs—and this could result in a reduced quality of life as people age. Results of animal studies indicate that repeated exposure to high levels of ozone for several months or more can produce permanent structural damage in the lungs.

  3. Among those most at risk to ozone are people who are outdoors and moderately exercising during the summer months. This includes construction workers and other outdoor workers.

How Does Ground-Level Ozone Harm the Environment?

- Ground-level ozone interferes with the ability of plants to produce and store food, so that growth, reproduction, and overall plant health are compromised.

- By weakening sensitive vegetation, ozone makes plants more susceptible to disease, pests, and environmental stresses.

- Ground-level ozone has been shown to reduce agricultural yields for many economically important crops (e.g., soybeans, kidney beans, wheat, cotton).

- The effects of ground-level ozone on long-lived species such as trees are believed to add up over many years so that whole forests or ecosystems can be affected. For example, ozone can adversely impact ecological functions such as water movement, mineral nutrient cycling, and habitats for various animal and plant species.

- Ground-level ozone can kill or damage leaves so that they fall off the plants too soon or become spotted or brown. These effects can significantly decrease the natural beauty of an area, such as in national parks and recreation areas.

- One of the key components of ozone, nitrogen oxides, contributes to fish kills and algae blooms in sensitive waterways, such as the Chesapeake Bay.

What Improvement Would Result from EPA's New Standards?

EPA's new ozone standards will provide increased protection beyond that provided by the previous standard from the following effects:

- Reduced risk of significant decreases (15% to over 20%) in children's lung functions (such as difficulty in breathing or shortness of breath), approximately 1 million fewer incidences each year, which can limit a healthy child's activities or result in increased medication use, or medical treatment, for children with asthma

- Reduced risk of moderate to severe respiratory symptoms in children, hundreds of thousands of fewer incidences each year of symptoms such as aggravated coughing and difficult or painful breathing

- Reduced risk of hospital admissions and emergency room visits for respiratory causes, thousands fewer admissions and visits for individuals with asthma

- Reduced risks of more frequent childhood illnesses and more subtle effects such as repeated inflammation of the lung, impairment of the lung's natural defense mechanisms, increased susceptibility to respiratory infection, and irreversible changes in lung structure. Such risks can lead to chronic respiratory illnesses such as emphysema and chronic bronchitis later in life and/or premature aging of the lungs

- Reduce the yield loss of major agricultural crops, such as soybeans and wheat, and commercial forests by almost $500,000,000.

Background: What Is Ground-Level Ozone?

- Ozone is not emitted directly into the air, but is formed by gases called nitrogen oxides (NOx) and volatile organic compounds (VOCs) that in the presence of heat and sunlight react to form ozone. Ground-level ozone forms readily in the atmosphere, usually during hot weather.

- NOx is emitted from motor vehicles, power plants, and other sources of combustion. VOCs are emitted from a variety of sources, including motor vehicles, chemical plants, refineries, factories, consumer and commercial products, and other industrial sources.

- Changing weather patterns contribute to yearly differences in ozone concentrations from city to city. Also, ozone and the pollutants that cause ozone can be carried to an area from pollution sources located hundreds of miles upwind.

Chapter 29

How Energy Policies Affect Public Health

One of the largest and most cost-effective sets of investments aimed at improving public health through a prevention-based approach is being made by neither the Department of Health and Human Services nor the Environmental Protection Agency (EPA). The Department of Energy's (DOE) Office of Energy Efficiency and Renewable Energy each year invests more than half a billion dollars in the development and deployment of technologies to prevent pollution. Energy choices made in the United States over the last several decades in manufacturing, transportation, and construction are having a significant effect on today's air quality. Likewise, the energy choices and investments that we make today will have profound consequences for future environmental quality, which should be of great concern to public health professionals.

In the past few years, a number of major studies and survey reports have documented the growing body of evidence establishing the link between air pollution and public health. What is less well known is that the vast majority of the pollutants most clearly linked to increased morbidity and mortality are energy related. In 1994, energy-related emissions—such as those from power plants, vehicles, and industry—accounted for more than 90% of emissions of sulfur dioxide, carbon monoxide, nitrogen oxides and volatile organic compounds, and for most of the smallest particulates (under 2.5 microns in diameter).[1,2]

Excerpted from "How Energy Policies Affect Public Health," by Joseph J. Romm and Christine A. Ervin, in *Public Health Reports,* Vol. 111, No. 5, September-October 1996, pp. 390-9. © 1996 by U.S. Department of Health and Human Services. Reprinted with permission.

The production and use of energy does more environmental damage than any other economic activity. In a world of ever-increasing population seeking an ever-increasing standard of living, reconciling environmental, public health, and economic goals will require that we use our resources much more efficiently. Instead of controlling the effects of pollution after it is already generated, we must take a new approach to pollution, one that is familiar to the public health community but has not been the traditional approach in the environmental field: prevent it from occurring in the first place.

DOE has the single largest set of resource efficiency and pollution prevention investments in the world. These investments not only help the environment by preventing the emission of millions of tons of pollution, they lower the cost of using energy, thereby saving consumers and businesses billions of dollars a year. In other words, these technologies achieve net economic savings for society, and we get emission reductions and improved public health as a free benefit.

The first half of this article will examine the connections between air pollution and respiratory health problems, and the second half will discuss what DOE is doing to prevent air pollution now and for the future.

The Relationship between Air Pollution and Respiratory Health Problems

Lung disease, which affects more than 10% of the population, is the third leading cause of death in the United States and among the fastest growing.[3] Annual deaths from lung cancer increased nearly 20% from 1979 to 1992.[3] Studies have confirmed the link between air pollution, and increases in respiratory-related hospitalizations and visits to doctors.[4,5]

The direct health care costs of respiratory disease combined with the indirect costs (such as lost productivity) are staggering. The total annual cost for lung disease has been estimated to exceed $60 billion.[3] Urban areas are especially hard hit. In Los Angeles alone, the cost of air pollution is estimated at $9.8 billion per year in medical expenditure and lost time from work.[6] And the costs are rising. Total estimated costs of asthma-related illnesses have more than doubled since 1985, from $4.5 billion to $9.5 billion.[3,7]

The 1970 Clean Air Act and its amendments establish a set of health-related national ambient air quality standards for six air pollutants (sometimes called criteria pollutants) that are persistent and widespread: particulate matter, sulfur dioxide (SO_2), nitrogen dioxide and related compounds (NO_x), ozone, carbon monoxide, and lead. This article focuses on the first five.

Particulates. A number of recent epidemiological studies on the health effects of air pollution involve the effects of particulates, a broad term encompassing thousands of types of chemicals. The particulates most widely studied are those particles with an aerodynamic diameter of 10 microns or less (PM10) and those with a diameter of 2.5 microns or less (PM2.5). Also known as fine particles, PM2.5 includes sulfate and nitrate aerosols. Fine particles are capable of getting through the natural filtering system of the nose and throat and can penetrate deep into the human lung and do serious damage.[2] Although chemically heterogeneous, particulates as a group are generally acidic. Sulfate aerosols, which make up the largest percentage of fine particles in the eastern United States, come from sulfur dioxide produced by coal and oil combustion.[8] Nitrate aerosols which comprise about one-third of fine particulates in Los Angeles come from vehicle emissions.[9]

In 1993, Harvard researchers published results of a 16-year, six-city study that tracked the health of over 8,000 individuals for a period of 14 to 16 years. Researchers observed a nearly linear relationship between particle concentrations in the air and increased mortality rates, indicating that even relatively low levels of air pollution (fine particles) contributed to adverse health effects. The risk of early death in high-level areas was 26% higher than in areas with the lowest levels of pollution, even after controlling for other risk factors such as smoking and occupation The study found that the risk of cardiopulmonary disease in high level areas was 37% higher than in low level areas.[10]

In 1995, another study by the American Cancer Society and Harvard Medical School, involving over 550,000 people living in 151 cities tracked for more than seven years, found a 17% increase in mortality risks in areas with higher concentrations of fine particles relative to those in areas with lower concentrations. Researchers also found a 15% increase in mortality risks in areas with higher concentrations of sulfite aerosols. The risk of death from cardiopulmonary disease was 31% higher in the most polluted cities. For subjects who had never smoked, the increased risk of premature death from cardiopulmonary disease was 43%. For women who resided in the more polluted cities and had never smoked, the risk of cardiopulmonary disease increased 57%.[11]

A 1996 meta-analysis by the Natural Resources Defense Counsel (NRDC) extrapolated the results of the earlier epidemiological studies to estimate the extent of premature death due to particulate air pollution in 239 U.S. cities. The NRDC study estimated that 64,000 people may die prematurely from heart and lung disease attributable to particulate air pollution, with lives being shortened an average of one to two years in the most polluted cities.[11]

In their gaseous state, SO_2 and NO_x also have adverse health impacts.[9] Oxides of sulfur can cause injury to the respiratory system.[12] It is well documented that asthmatics are especially sensitive to even relatively low SO_2 exposure, as measured by increased airway resistance and reduced lung function.[9] Nitrogen dioxide can irritate the lungs and lower resistance to respiratory infections.[1,13] Children exposed to high levels of nitrogen dioxide may be more susceptible than other children to respiratory tract infections.[13,14] Nitrogen oxides are also an important precursor to both ozone and acid rain.[15]

Ozone. Ozone was first identified as a key component of urban air pollution (smog) in Southern California in the 1950s. Today, ozone (O_3) is one of our most prevalent air pollution problems. Ozone is an example of a class of pollutants called photochemical oxidants that result from chemical reactions driven by heat and sunlight. Ozone concentrations tend to peak daily in the afternoon, and seasonally during the late spring and summer. The primary precursor pollutants are NO_x and volatile organic hydrocarbons. Combined with summertime stagnation of air masses, the pollutants cook into a chemical atmospheric "soup" and form dangerous levels of ozone.

Ozone is capable of destroying organic matter, including lung and airway tissue. Ozone acts as a powerful respiratory irritant at the levels frequently found in most of the nation's urban areas during the summer months.[9] More than 50 million Americans live in 82 ozone nonattainment areas according to the latest EPA data.[1,16] Nonattainment areas are geographic areas that do not meet the health-related primary national ambient air quality standards set by the EPA under the Clean Air Act and its amendments. According to an American Lung Association committee,[8]

"During years with particularly hot summers (e.g., 1988), rates of ozone generation increase and violations of the ozone national ambient air quality standard occurred in counties with a population totaling 135 million."[14,17]

The adverse impact of ozone on health has been understood for more than a quarter of a century. In 1970, the Council on Environmental Quality reported that an increased frequency of asthma attacks occurs in some patients even on those days when hourly concentrations of ozone are well within air quality standards.[18] A growing number of studies have linked short-term ozone exposure to hospital admissions and doctor visits for asthma and other respiratory problems.[21] A June 1996 study by the Harvard School of Public Health for the American Lung Association found that exposure to ozone was linked to 10,000 to 15,000 hospital admissions and between 30,000 to 50,000 emergency room visits in 13 U.S. cities during 1993 and 1994.[4]

Other recent findings warn of increased health effects from ozone air pollution:

- Asthma attacks increase substantially with ozone levels.[19]
- Above average ozone levels increase death rates.[20]
- Ozone exacerbates allergies.[21]
- Long-term exposure to ozone may affect the severity of asthma.[22]

A 1993 study by the American Lung Association estimated children with asthma and more than eight million people with chronic obstructive pulmonary disease lived in areas that exceeded the federal health standard for ozone. As many as 27 million children under the age of 13 and nearly two million children with asthma are exposed to potentially unhealthful levels of ozone.[14]

While exposure to ozone air pollution causes adverse health effects in most people, children are especially susceptible to these effects. The rate of asthma in children under 18 jumped 79% between 1982 and 1993.[23] Inner-city children suffer from asthma at twice the national average, and minorities suffer a disproportionate amount as well (see "Groups at Special Risk" at end of article).[16]

The cost to the nation is great, in terms of lives as well as economic costs. Deaths from asthma have increased more than 90% since 1979. The annual direct health care cost of asthma is approximately $6.9 billion.[3] Indirect costs, such as lost productivity, have been quantified at about $2.6 billion, with asthma accounting for an estimated three million lost work days annually.[7]

Carbon monoxide. When carbon monoxide is inhaled, it is absorbed by the blood more readily than oxygen and causes body tissues to be deprived of oxygen. Carbon monoxide (CO) combines chemically with hemoglobin, the oxygen-transporting element of human blood, at a rate far greater than that of oxygen itself.[24,25] At high

269

levels, death is certain.[9] Studies show that exposure to 10 parts per million of CO for approximately eight hours may dull mental performance.[18] Such levels of CO are commonly found in cities throughout the world. In heavy traffic situations, levels of 70, 80, or 100 parts per million are not uncommon.

Nearly 20 million people are exposed to harmful, nonfatal levels of CO, causing a wide variety of ailments including headaches, nausea, fatigue, dizziness, and exacerbation of various heart conditions including the onset of heart attacks.[8] Moreover, it is believed to impose an extra burden on those already suffering from anemia and chronic lung disease.[8,9]

Multiple pollutants. While each of the above pollutants have been documented to cause adverse health impacts in isolation, most of the time people will be exposed to more than one of them at a time. Indeed, in urban settings in the summer, one might well be subjected to all of them simultaneously. One would expect that the negative health effects of multiple exposure would at the very least be additive, and it would certainly not be surprising if there were a more negative synergistic effect. Only a limited number of studies have been done in this area, but those results are ominous.[9] One clinical study exposed asthmatic young women to ozone, to sulfur dioxide, and to both sequentially. It was the third condition, in which ozone exposure was followed by sulfur dioxide exposure, that triggered bronchial reactions.[26]

The Energy Solution: Pollution Prevention

Our energy choices in a number of sectors of the economy have had a profound effect on air quality and public health. Consider transportation. An average car travels some 100,000 miles over its life, consuming over 3,000 gallons of gasoline and discharging tons of air pollutants. Vehicles are responsible for a large fraction of the air pollution in urban areas around the world. That will only worsen as the world's fleet of 500 million cars doubles to one billion cars by 2030.

At the turn of the century, steam, electric, and internal combustion engines were all competing for the emerging automobile market. If large quantities of oil had not been discovered at the same time, it is quite possible that alternative kinds of fuels and propulsion would have emerged. Vehicle exhaust controls helped curb emissions, as did federal fuel efficiency standards. But those gains have been outstripped by trends of more cars being owned per household and cars being driven longer. Clean fuels and technologies still struggle in a market dominated by cheap gasoline and a political environment that is ambivalent about the federal government's role in encouraging technology innovation.

In the early 1980s, the Reagan Administration cut funding for the renewable energy program by 90%, slowing down the development and introduction of nearly pollution-free power generation technologies immeasurably. Similarly, deep cuts in federal funding for energy-efficient transportation, industrial, and budding technologies delayed or killed the introduction of hundreds of clean technologies into the marketplace. Federal funding for pollution prevention did not begin to increase again until the early 1990s.

Many other national decisions have had adverse consequences for the environment. For example, regulatory choices in the 1970s slowed the expansion of natural gas as a fuel for electric power generation. This delayed the more widespread use of the cleanest fossil fuel.

Given our past energy choices, we are faced today with a tremendous burden of energy-related pollution. Fine particles, 2.5 microns or less in size, are chiefly produced by coalfired power plants and by combustion of fossil fuels in transportation and manufacturing. More than 90% of sulfur dioxide emissions are energy related, coming primarily from the burning of coal and oil in utility and industrial operations. Nearly 90% of carbon monoxide emissions are energy related, mostly from vehicular traffic. More than 95% of nitrogen dioxide emissions are derived from fossil fuel combustion arising principally from motor vehicles, power plants, and industrial sources. Ozone is not emitted directly but is a byproduct, principally of emissions of volatile organic compounds (more than 90% of which are energy related, mostly from vehicles and industrial processes) and of oxides of nitrogen.[1]

The conclusions are clear. Air pollution has numerous and severe adverse public health impacts. If we are to prevent those impacts, we must make our energy production and consumption more efficient and cleaner. Moreover, we must act soon. While energy use was flat in the 1980s, and some energy-related emissions (such as SO_2 emissions) have declined due to the Clean Air Act, U.S. energy consumption has risen 15% since 1990, fueled by population and economic growth, and some energy-related emissions (for example, NO_x) have begun to rise. The Energy Information Administration projects that U.S. energy consumption will rise by a third over the next two decades. Globally, population growth, urbanization, and industrialization, especially in the developing world, are combining to create an explosion in energy consumption and energy-related emissions. Worldwide energy use could double over the next three to four decades.

In the face of such growth in energy demand, we can no longer pursue only the traditional approach to the environment: cleaning up pollution after the fact or safely disposing of it in the land, water, or atmosphere. We need to dramatically reduce or prevent pollution from occurring in the first place, in the generation of electricity and in the use of energy in transportation, industry, and buildings. The DOE is responsible for 72% of the federal investment in the research, development, and demonstration of pollution prevention technologies.[27]

The largest set of these programs are in the Office of Energy Efficiency and Renewable Energy. Over the next decade and a half, these programs hold the prospect of preventing a significant amount of pollution while dramatically lowering the nation's energy bill (see Table 29.1.). The full spectrum of DOE programs aimed at reducing air pollution cover a broad range of supply and demand technologies.

Clean energy supply. Clearly fossil fuel use is going to increase globally for decades under even the most optimistic scenarios for the use of alternative energy sources. Therefore we need to develop and deploy technologies for burning fossil fuels more cleanly and expand the use of the cleanest burning fossil fuel, natural gas. Natural gas is the premier hydrocarbon in our country's fossil-based energy portfolio, in part because of the efficiency and economic and environmental benefits of natural gas, but also as part of our effort to reduce our rising national dependence on imported oil. For these reasons, the

Table 29.1. Estimated Pollution Prevented with Technologies Sponsored by the Office of Energy Efficiency and Renewable Energy, Department of Energy

Pollutant	Annual Reductions (U.S. tons) 2000	Annual Reductions (U.S. tons) 2010	Cumulative Reductions (U.S. tons) 1997-2010
SO_2	70,000	370,000	2.1 million
NO_x	270,000	1,290,000	7.4 million
CO	1,100,000	5,400,000	31 million

Source: Office of Energy Efficiency and Renewable Energy, U.S. Department of Energy

Department has been a leader in supporting increased natural gas use in electric generation, in industrial cogeneration and process systems, in residential and commercial heating and cooling technologies, and in transportation. Particularly promising are fuel cells, which are compact modular devices that generate electricity and heat with high efficiency and virtually no pollution. Fuel cells run on hydrogen converted primarily from natural gas. Together with small gas-fired turbines, they will help lead the expanded use of natural gas and are essential for the growth of a more distributed and cleaner global electricity system.

At the same time, the prospects for renewable energy resources—such as solar, wind, and geothermal—are very promising. They, too, have the potential to reduce the generation of polluting byproducts. In one of two planning scenarios recently developed by Royal Dutch/ Shell, the most profitable oil company in the world, renewable energy provides nearly half the world's energy in four to five decades.[28] In a quiet energy revolution that has received little attention in the press, the costs of renewable power have come down dramatically.[29]

For example, since 1980, research funded by DOE has brought down the cost of photovoltaic (PV) electricity from sunlight by a factor of five to under 20 cents per kilowatt-hour. This price is already competitive for developing countries that haven't yet built an extensive and expensive electricity grid. The sales of PVs have been rising steadily, and reached $300 million last year. With continued research, development, and economies of scale from increased market share, PV electricity will continue to decline in price for decades. PVs may have a market of $300 billion per year in the middle of the next century, if Shell's scenario proves true.

What is exciting about the emergence of renewable energy and fuel cells as major providers of energy is the possibility of realizing the dream of nearly pollution-free energy in the coming decades, at prices competitive with traditional power plants. As is the case with most longer-term research and development efforts, we cannot know for sure today which specific energy technologies will be successful, which is why the Department pursues a variety of paths simultaneously. We can only be sure that there will be a multitrillion-dollar market for advanced power generation technologies in the coming decades and that environmental and public health concerns will increasingly be factored into decisions about what kind of power to use.

Even with increased use of electricity from natural gas and renewable energy technologies in the coming decades, the nation and the world will be faced with significant environmental problems. Each sector of our economy will be challenged to operate more efficiently and cleanly as economic growth fuels increases in the demands for energy.

Cleaner manufacturing. The industrial sector will continue to be the major source of hazardous and toxic waste, and the vast majority of that pollution will come from a handful of very energy-intensive industries, most of which have historically spent far less than the rest of the manufacturing sector in research and development. The half dozen most energy-intensive industries in the country—pulp and paper, chemicals, steel, aluminum, petroleum refining, glass, and metal casting—account for 80% of the energy consumed in U.S. manufacturing, 80% of the toxic waste, and 95% of U.S. hazardous waste. They represent the biggest opportunities to increase energy and resource efficiency while reducing pollution. The public health benefits of reducing toxic and hazardous waste emissions are an added bonus.

That's why DOE began partnering with these industries two years ago to create industry visions and technology road maps: the former lays out the industry's vision for a low-polluting, highly energy-efficient, and very economically competitive factory or industry of the future, and the latter is a research timeline for developing the technologies needed to achieve this vision. This Industries of the Future program has already had startling success.

According to a trade magazine of the pulp and paper industry, the industry's vision, Agenda 2020, is helping to demonstrate to EPA that a prevention-based strategy can be a better way to meet environmental standards.[30] This may result in a final set of EPA standards with substantially reduced compliance costs, from $11.5 billion down to $3-$4 billion. This from a DOE program costing just a few millions of dollars a year.

One government-supported project has helped reduce glassmaking emissions of nitrogen oxides by 90% while cutting furnace energy use 25%; it is now used in manufacturing 15% of all glass made in the United States. Another technology, a process for de-zincing scrap steel, provided the breakthrough that industry needed in order to recycle 10 million tons of scrap metal annually. By the year 2005, electro-chemical de-zincing could reduce the cost of raw materials $160 million per year, save 50 trillion BTUs of energy, and provide 75,000 tons of inexpensive zinc.

The nation with the first businesses to make the shift to pollution prevention will acquire several unique benefits. Its businesses will become more competitive since their costs for purchasing resources and disposing of waste will be lower.[31] That nation will capture the lion's share of an enormous global market for clean technology and environmental services. But most important, it will reap the benefits of improved public health at home.

Cleaner transportation. As much as 80% of urban air pollution is caused by transportation energy use. Energy-efficient transportation and alternative fuel technologies can substantially cut these emissions, improving local environmental quality and cutting health care costs as well.

The DOE's research efforts include advanced transportation technologies to use fuel much more efficiently with far fewer emissions, such as hybrid vehicles that combine an advanced internal combustion engine with an energy storage device. The Department recently developed an advanced natural gas vehicle with a 300-mile range, twice the range of existing natural gas vehicles, and we are working on even more advanced ones, including a gas turbine engine. The Department is developing advanced batteries as well as zero-emission fuel cells for use in transportation. At the same time, the Department is working to advance the infrastructure for alternative fuel vehicles to run on natural gas, electricity, and renewable biofuels.

The technologies will have another benefit, reducing dependence on imported oil. The United States currently imports about half its oil, which adds $50 billion to our trade deficit annually. Without more efficient transportation and alternative fuels, domestic oil consumption is projected to rise steadily, yielding an annual trade deficit in oil in excess of $100 billion a year by 2010.

Cleaner buildings. Buildings account for one-third of all energy use and two-thirds of all electricity use, contributing $200 billion to the nation's energy bill. Developing and deploying energy-efficient technologies could dramatically reduce emissions and improve public health while cutting energy bills by one-third.

The Department's research efforts include developing advanced lighting, window, heating, and cooling technologies as well as integrated design techniques for new building construction that can reduce energy consumption and associated emissions 25% or more with a lower first cost and dramatically reduced construction waste. At the same time, we are working to deploy existing energy-efficient technologies through partnerships with the states, the U.S. Conference of Mayors, and federal energy managers, among others.

Research has shown that these technologies not only reduce energy bills but can also increase worker productivity.[32] For example, one post office that underwent an energy efficiency upgrade found that its productivity in sorting mail jumped 7%, which resulted in additional savings six to eight times greater than the energy savings. In other instances, absenteeism dropped substantially with new energy-efficient building technologies or greater use of natural sunlight.[32]

Another key area of research is in the mitigation of urban heat islands. Most cities have dark surfaces and less vegetation than their surroundings, creating a "heat island" that affects climate, energy use, and habitability. For individual buildings, dark roofs and inadequate shading raise summertime air conditioning demands, which increases the pollution caused by power generation. Heat islands raise the temperature of many cities by five degrees Fahrenheit, which has significant environmental and public health costs as ozone smog is typically created only in hot weather. Finally, the urban heat island exacerbates all heat waves, contributing to the dozens of summer fatalities that cities experience during the summer.

Cooling the city is straightforward. Buildings need shade trees for their southern exposure. Buildings, roads, and parking lots require light-colored surfaces. Cooler roads might have a slightly higher first cost, but probably will last 20% to 50% longer because of reduced thermal wear and reduced ultraviolet damage.

Over a 20-year period, trees can be planted cheaply and roads, roofs, and parking lots replaced by cooler surfaces during the course of normal maintenance. This nominal additional cost would, by the year 2015, save the country $10 billion a year in energy and environmental costs. In Los Angeles alone, this would lower air conditioning bills by $360 million, eliminate as much pollution as is generated by three-quarters of the cars on the road, and reduce the creation of ozone smog by 10% or more.[33]

Clearly, urban heat island mitigation is an important effort. The Department is working to help develop and/or identify the best roofing and paving materials, to use computer models to determine the optimal approach to cooling a city, and to disseminate information around the nation.

Research and development of energy-efficient technologies are among the most cost-effective investments the federal government makes. According to a GAO analysis, just two technologies developed by the DOE—software to help architects design more energy-efficient buildings and an energy-saving compressor for refrigerators—have saved consumers and businesses $8 billion.[34] Three other budding technologies advanced by the Department, energy-efficient windows, lighting, and oil burners, have a net present value of more than $3 billion in energy savings. Yet the entire amount of federal support for energy efficiency research and development from 1978 to 1996 came to only $7 billion. So just five successes among hundreds have paid for all that research. And these five technologies alone have prevented 1,000,000 tons of sulfur dioxide, 300,000 tons of oxides of nitrogen, and 25,000 tons of particulates from being generated and released into the atmosphere.

Conclusion

Air pollution causes severe public health problems, and the vast majority of air pollution is energy related. The nation and the world will be experiencing large increases in energy use in the coming decades. If this increase is achieved through traditional resource- and pollution-intensive methods, environment problems at an urban, regional, and global level will be seriously aggravated, at a terrible cost to human health and quality of life.

Pollution prevention and resource-efficient technologies improve the environment while lowering the energy bills of consumers and businesses. They are the key to sustainable development and offer the hope of minimizing or avoiding the risk of global climate change while saving money.

The choice of whether we move toward pollution prevention or stick with business as usual is being made today. Globally we are investing well over a trillion dollars a decade in new energy technology and infrastructure—and we will live with the consequences of these choices for decades to come. We have two paths. One is sustainable, profitable, and environmentally sound. The other is short term, costly, and potentially devastating from an environmental and human health perspective.

The DOE has the largest set of pollution prevention investments in the world, most in the energy efficiency and renewable energy program. While the Bush and Clinton Administrations supported steady increases in funding for these crucial technologies, Congress cut the budget by one-third last year and is proposing another comparable cut this year, which would undermine U.S. efforts to advance clean technologies at home and retain world leadership in this crucial area. These investments provide cost-effective alternatives to command and control regulation and form a vital part of our nation's environmental and public health strategy. They cannot be abandoned when our nation needs them most.

Groups at Special Risk

Children are at risk. While exposure to air pollution causes adverse health effects in most people, children are especially susceptible. Children spend much more time outdoors (an average of 50% more than adults), particularly in the summertime when ozone levels are the highest. Children spend more time engaged in vigorous activity. Such activity results in more air, and therefore more pollution, being taken deep into the lungs.

Nearly 24 million children under age 13 in the United States live in areas with unhealthy exposure to particulate matter.[35] Researchers with the EPA and the Harvard School of Public Health studied nearly 1,850 school children in six U.S. cities. When ozone (smog) went up, some children coughed more; when ozone and sulfur dioxide levels went up, some children suffered from wheezing, chest pain, coughing, and phlegm. When particulate pollution increased, all children suffered symptoms—even when the pollution was substantially lower than the current national danger standard.[36] Another study found that hospital admissions of children for asthma were consistently higher than average the day following elevated ozone levels.[37]

Air pollution has been linked to asthma, acute respiratory infections, allergies, and other ailments in children. Among chronic diseases, asthma ranks first in the number of children affected, first in making kids miss school, and first in sending them to the hospital. Scientists are concerned that children who experience more frequent lower respirator infections may be at greater risk of lower-than-normal lung function later in life.[18] Inner-city children have twice the national average rate of asthma (8.6% vs. 4.3%).[38]

Minorities are at risk. A disproportionate number of African Americans and Hispanics, because of their concentration in central city areas, are particularly hard hit by ambient air pollution. Thirty-one percent of Hispanics, 20% of African Americans, and only 12% of whites live in the 29 U.S. counties designated as nonattainment areas for three or more key pollutants.[39]

Thus it is not surprising that minorities are disproportionately affected by asthma. In 1993, the prevalence rate of asthma among African Americans was 22.3% higher than among whites. Although African Americans represent 12.4% of the U.S. population (one in eight), they account for 21% (one in five) of deaths due to asthma. And African Americans are four times as likely as whites to be hospitalized for asthma.[40]

The elderly are at risk. Older people often are frailer and weaker and significantly less resistant to infection than they were earlier in life. Some lung function decline appears to be part of the natural aging process. Air pollutants aggravate susceptibilities to influenza and pneumonia, of which older people are the primary victims. Many elders suffer chronic respiratory or heart conditions that may be markedly worsened by the effects of air pollution. A number of epidemiological studies have linked particulate matter with premature death and hospital admissions for cardiovascular and respiratory problems in the elderly.[41-44] Over 11 million elderly people in the United States live in areas with unhealthy exposure to particulate matter.[35]

References

1. Office of Air and Radiation. *National air pollutant emission trends 1900-1994.* Research Triangle Park (NC): Office of Air Quality Planning and Standards, Environmental Protection Agency; 1995. Report No. EPA-454/R-95-011.

2. Pope CA III, Thun MJ, Namboordiri MM, Dockery DW, Evans JS, Speizer FE, Heath Jr. CW. Particulate air pollution as a predictor of mortality in a prospective study of U.S. adults. *Am J Respir Crit Care Med* 1995;151:669-674.

3. *Lung disease data 1995.* New York: American Lung Association 1995.

4. Özkaynak H, Spengler JD, O'Neill M, Xue J, Zhou H, Gilbert K, Ramstrom S. *Ambient ozone exposure and emergency hospital admissions and emergency room visits for respiratory problems in thirteen U.S. cities.* Washington, DC: American Lung Association; 1996:5.

5. *Dollars and cents: the economic and health benefits of potential particulate matter reductions in the United States.* New York: American Lung Association; 1995.

6. Hall JV, Winer AM, Kleinman MT, Lurman FW, Brajer V, Colome SD. Valuing the health benefits of clean air. *Science* 1992;255:812-817.

7. Weiss KS, Gergen PJ, Hodgson TA. An economic evaluation of asthma in the United States. *New Engl J Med* 1992;326:862-866.

8. American Thoracic Society Environmental and Occupational Health Assembly. Health effects of outdoor air pollution. *Am J Respir Crit Care Med* 1996;153:3-50.

9. *Health effects of outdoor air pollution.* Washington DC: American Lung Association; 1996.

10. Dockery DW, Pope CA, Xu X, Spengler JD, Ware JH, Fay ME, et al. An association between air pollution and mortality in six U.S. cities. *New Engl J Med* 1993;329:1753-1759.

11. Sheiman Shprentz D, Bryner GC, Shprentz JS. *Breath-taking: premature mortality due to particulate air pollution in 239 American cities.* Washington DC: Natural Resources Defense Council; 1996.

12. Sheppard D, Wong WS, Uehara CD, Nadel JA, Boushey HA. Lower threshold and greater bronchomotor responsiveness of asthmatic subjects to sulfur dioxide. *Am Rev Respir Dis* 1980;122:873-878.

13. Neas LM, Dockery DW, Ware JH, Spengler JD, Speizer FE, Ferris Jr. BG. Association of indoor nitrogen dioxide with respiratory symptoms and pulmonary function in children. *Am J Epidemiol* 1991;134:204-209.

14. *Out of breath—populations at risk to alternative ozone levels.* Washington DC: American Lung Association; 1995.

15. *Why NO$_x$? The costs, consequences and control of nitrogen oxides in the human and natural environment.* Washington, DC: American Lung Association; 1989.

16. Office of Air and Radiation. *Air quality trends.* Research Triangle Park (NC): Office of Air Quality Planning and Standards, Environmental Protection Agency; 1995. Report No. EPA-454/F95/003.

17. Office of Technology Assessment. *Catching our breath.* Washington DC: Government Printing Office; 1989. Report No. OTA-O-412.

18. First annual report. Washington, DC: Council on Environmental Quality; 1970:67-69.

19. Holguin AH, Buffler PA, Contant Jr. CF, Stock TH, Kotchmar D, Hsi BP, et al. *The effects of ozone on asthmatics in the Houston area; evaluation of the scientific basis for ozone/oxidant standards*. Pittsburgh (PA): Pollution Control Association; 1985.

20. Kinney PL, Özkaynak H. Associations between ozone and daily mortality in Los Angeles and New York City. *Am Rev Respir Dis* 1992;45:A95.

21. Molfino NA, Wright SC, Karz I, Tarlo S, Silverman F, McClean PA, et al. Effect of low concentrations of ozone on inhaled allergen responses in asthmatic subjects. *Lancet* 1991 July; No. 8761:199-203.

22. Abbey DE, Petersen F, Mills K, Beeson WL. Long-term ambient concentrations of total suspended particulates, ozone, and sulfur dioxide and respiratory symptoms in a nonsmoking population. *Arch Environ Health* 1993;48:33-46.

23. National Health Interview Survey, 1982-1993. Hyattsville (MD): National Center for Health Statistics.

24. Roughton FJW, Darling RC. The effect of CO on the oxyhemoglobin dissociation curve, *Am J Physiol* 1944;141:17-31.

25. *Update and revision of the air quality guidelines for Europe: "classical" air pollutants*. Copenhagen: World Health Organization Regional Office for Europe Working Group; 1995.

26. Hazucha MJ, Folinsbee LJ, Seal E, Bromber PA. Lung function response of healthy women after sequential exposures to NO_2 and O_3. *Am J Respir Crit Care Med* 1994;150:642-647

27. National Science and Technology Council. *Technology for a sustainable future*. Washington DC: Office of Science and Technology Policy, Executive Office of the President; 1994.

28. Fay C. *Fossil fuels and beyond—meeting the needs of the 21st century*. Shell Oil Corp., United Kingdom; 1996.

29. Office of Technology Assessment [U.S.]. *Renewing our energy future*. Washington DC: Government Printing Office; 1995. Report No. OTA-ETI-614.

30. Rooks A. A new partnership. [editorial]. *PIMA Magazine* 1995 Dec.;77:6.

31. Porter ME, van der Linde C. Green and competitive: ending the stalemate. *Harvard Business Review* 1995 Sept.-Oct.;73:120-34.

32. Romm J. *Lean and clean management.* New York: Kodansha America Inc.; 1994.

33. Rosenfeld A, Romm J, Akbari H, Pomerantz M. *Heat island mitigation: benefits and implementation strategies. Proceedings, 1996 Summer Study on Energy Efficiency in Buildings.* Washington DC: American Council for an Energy Efficient Economy. In press.

34. *DOE's success stories. Report to the Chairman, House Committee on the Budget.* Washington DC: General Accounting Office; 1996. Report No.: GAO/RCED-96-120R.

35. *The perils of particulates.* New York: American Lung Association; 1994.

36. Schwartz J, Dockery DW, Neas LM, Wypij D, et al. Acute effects of summer air pollution on respiratory symptom reporting in children. *Am J Respir Crit Care Med* 1994; 150:134-142.

37. Bates DV. The strength of the evidence relating air pollutants to adverse health effects. *Carolina Environmental Essay Series.* Chapel Hill (NC): Institute for Environmental Studies, University of North Carolina, 1985.

38. Thurston C, Weiss K. Double the (asthma) risk for inner city children. Paper presented at American Lung Association meeting; 1996 Jan.; New York, NY.

39. Wernett DR, Nieves LA. Breathing polluted air: minorities are disproportionately exposed. *EPA J* 1992 March-April;18:16-17.

40. *Minority lung disease data.* New York: American Lung Association; 1995.

41. Schwartz J. What are people dying of on high air pollution days? *Environ Res* 1994;6:26-35.

42. Schwartz J. PM10, ozone, and hospital admissions for the elderly in Minneapolis, MN. *Arch Environ Health* 1994;40:366-374.

43. Schwartz J. Air pollution and hospital admissions for the elderly in Birmingham, Alabama. *Am J Epidemiol* 1994;139:589-598.

44. Schwartz J. Air pollution and hospital admissions for the elderly in Detroit, Michigan. *Am J Respir Crit Care Med* 1994; 150:618-655.

—by Joseph J. Romm and Christine A. Ervin

Both authors are with the U.S. Department of Energy. Dr. Romm, a physicist, is the Acting Principal Deputy Assistant Secretary for Energy Efficiency and Renewable Energy. Ms. Ervin is the Assistant Secretary. The authors are indebted to David Bassett, David Kovner, and Tina Kaarsberg, Ph.D., for assisting with the research for this article.

Address correspondence to Dr. Romm, Office of Energy Efficiency and Renewable Energy, Department of Energy, 1000 Independence Ave. SW, Washington, DC 20585; tel: (202)586-9220; fax: (202)586-9260; e-mail: <joseph.romm@hq.doe.gov>.

Chapter 30

Noncancer Respiratory Health Effects of Passive Smoking

Background

Tobacco smoking has long been recognized (e.g., U.S. Department of Health, Education, and Welfare [U.S. DHEW], 1964) as a major cause of mortality and morbidity, responsible for an estimated 434,000 deaths per year in the United States (Centers for Disease Control [CDC], 1991a). Tobacco use is known to cause cancer at various sites, in particular the lung (U.S. Department of Health and Human Services [U.S. DHHS], 1982; International Agency for Research on Cancer [IARC], 1986). Smoking can also cause respiratory diseases (U.S. DHHS, 1984, 1989) and is a major risk factor for heart disease (U.S. DHHS, 1983). In recent years, there has been concern that nonsmokers may also be at risk for some of these health effects as a result of their exposure ("passive smoking") to the tobacco smoke that occurs in various environments occupied by smokers. Although this ETS is dilute compared with the mainstream smoke (MS) inhaled by active smokers, it is chemically similar, containing many of the same carcinogenic and toxic agents.

Excerpted from "Respiratory Health Effects of Passive Smoking: Lung Cancer and Other Disorders," December 1992; and "Secondhand Smoke: What You Can Do about Secondhand Smoke as Parents, Decisionmakers, and Building Occupants," [Online] April 2,1997. Available: http://www.epa.gov/iaq/pubs/etsbro.html. Produced by the U.S. Environmental Protection Agency (EPA). For complete contact information, please refer to Chapter 68, "Resources."

In 1986, the National Research Council (NRC) and the Surgeon General of the U.S. Public Health Service independently assessed the health effects of exposure to ETS (NRC, 1986; U.S. DHHS, 1986). Both of the 1986 reports conclude that ETS can cause lung cancer in adult nonsmokers and that children of parents who smoke have increased frequency of respiratory symptoms and acute lower respiratory tract infections, as well as evidence of reduced lung function.

More recent epidemiologic studies of the potential associations between ETS and lung cancer in nonsmoking adults and between ETS and noncancer respiratory effects more than double the size of the database available for analysis from that of the 1986 reports. This EPA report critically reviews the current database on the [noncancer] respiratory health effects of passive smoking; these data are utilized to make quantitative estimates of the public health impacts of ETS for various respiratory diseases.

The weight-of-evidence analyses for the noncancer respiratory effects are based primarily on a review of epidemiologic studies. Most of the endpoints examined are respiratory disorders in children, where parental smoking is used as a surrogate of ETS exposure. For the noncancer respiratory effects in nonsmoking adults, most studies used spousal smoking as an exposure surrogate. A causal association was concluded to exist for a number of respiratory disorders where there was sufficient consistent evidence for a biologically plausible association with ETS that could not be explained by bias, confounding, or chance. The fact that the database consists of human evidence from actual environmental exposure levels gives a high degree of confidence in this conclusion. Where there was suggestive but inconclusive evidence of causality, as was the case for asthma induction in children, ETS was concluded to be a risk factor for that endpoint. Where data were inconsistent or inadequate for evaluation of an association, as for acute upper respiratory tract infections and acute middle ear infections in children, no conclusions were drawn.

Population estimates of ETS health impacts are made for certain noncancer respiratory endpoints in children, specifically lower respiratory tract infections (i.e., pneumonia, bronchitis, and bronchiolitis) and episodes and severity of attacks of asthma. Estimates of ETS-attributable cases of LRI in infants and young children are thought to have a high degree of confidence because of the consistent study findings and the appropriateness of parental smoking as a surrogate measure of exposure in very young children. Estimates of the number of asthmatic children whose condition is aggravated by exposure to ETS are less certain than those for LRIs because of different measures of outcome in various studies and because of increased extraparental exposure to ETS in older children. Estimates of the number of new cases of asthma in previously asymptomatic children also have less confidence because at this time the weight of evidence for asthma induction, while suggestive of a causal association, is not conclusive.

Most of the ETS population impact estimates are presented in terms of ranges, which are thought to reflect reasonable assumptions about the estimates of parameters and variables required for the extrapolation models. The validity of the ranges is also dependent on the appropriateness of the extrapolation models themselves.

Primary Findings

1. Exposure of children to ETS from parental smoking is causally associated with

    - increased prevalence of respiratory symptoms of irritation (cough, sputum, and wheeze),

    - increased prevalence of middle ear effusion (a sign of middle ear disease), and

    - a small but statistically significant reduction in lung function as tested by objective measures of lung capacity.

2. ETS exposure of young children and particularly infants from parental (and especially mothers') smoking is causally associated with an increased risk of LRIs (pneumonia, bronchitis, and bronchiolitis). This report estimates that exposure to ETS contributes 150,000 to 300,000 LRIs annually in infants and children less than 18 months of age, resulting in 7,500 to 15,000 hospitalizations. The confidence in the estimates of LRIs is high. Increased risks for LRIs continue, but are lower in magnitude, for children until about age 3; however, no estimates are derived for children over 18 months.

3. Exposure to ETS is causally associated with additional episodes and increased severity of asthma in children who already have the disease. This report estimates that ETS exposure exacerbates symptoms in approximately 20% of this country's 2 million to 5 million asthmatic children and is a major aggravating factor in approximately 10%.

4. In addition, the epidemiologic evidence is suggestive but not conclusive that ETS exposure increases the number of new

287

cases of asthma in children who have not previously exhibited symptoms. Based on this evidence and the known ETS effects on both the immune system and lungs (e.g., atopy and airway hyperresponsiveness), this report concludes that ETS is a risk factor for the induction of asthma in previously asymptomatic children. Data suggest that relatively high levels of exposure are required to induce new cases of asthma in children. This report calculates that previously asymptomatic children exposed to ETS from mothers who smoke at least 10 cigarettes per day will exhibit an estimated 8,000 to 26,000 new cases of asthma annually. The confidence in this range is medium and is dependent on the conclusion that ETS is a risk factor for asthma induction.

5. Passive smoking has subtle but significant effects on the respiratory health of nonsmoking adults, including coughing, phlegm production, chest discomfort, and reduced lung function.

This report also has reviewed data on the relationship of maternal smoking and sudden infant death syndrome (SIDS), which is thought to involve some unknown respiratory pathogenesis. The report concludes that while there is strong evidence that infants whose mothers smoke are at an increased risk of dying from SIDS, available studies do not allow us to differentiate whether and to what extent this increase is related to in utero versus postnatal exposure to tobacco smoke products. Consequently, this report is unable to assert whether or not ETS exposure by itself is a risk factor for SIDS independent of smoking during pregnancy.

Regarding an association of parental smoking with either upper respiratory tract infections (colds and sore throats) or acute middle ear infections in children, this report finds the evidence inconclusive.

ETS and Noncancer Respiratory Disorders

Exposure to ETS from parental smoking has been previously linked with increased respiratory disorders in children, particularly in infants. Several studies have confirmed the exposure and uptake of ETS in children by assaying saliva, serum, or urine for cotinine. These cotinine concentrations were highly correlated with smoking (especially by the mother) in the child's presence. Nine to twelve million American children under 5 years of age, or one-half to two-thirds of all children in this age group, may be exposed to cigarette smoke in the home (American Academy of Pediatrics, 1986; Overpeck and Moss, 1991).

With regard to the noncancer respiratory effects of passive smoking, this report focuses on epidemiologic evidence appearing since the two major reports of 1986 (NRC and U.S. DHHS) that bears on the potential association of parental smoking with detrimental respiratory effects in their children. These effects include symptoms of respiratory irritation (cough, sputum production, or wheeze); acute diseases of the lower respiratory tract (pneumonia, bronchitis, and bronchiolitis); acute middle ear infections and indications of chronic middle ear infections (predominantly middle ear effusion); reduced lung function (from forced expiratory volume and flow-rate measurements); incidence and prevalence of asthma and exacerbation of symptoms in asthmatics; and acute upper respiratory tract infections (colds and sore throats). The more than 50 recently published studies reviewed here essentially corroborate the previous conclusions of the 1986 reports of the NRC and Surgeon General regarding respiratory symptoms, respiratory illnesses, and pulmonary function, and they strengthen support for those conclusions by the additional weight of evidence. For example, new data on middle ear effusion strengthen previous evidence to warrant the stronger conclusion in this report of a causal association with parental smoking. Furthermore, recent studies establish associations between parental smoking and increased incidence of childhood asthma. Additional research also supports the hypotheses that in utero exposure to mothers' smoke and postnatal exposure to ETS alter lung function and structure, increase bronchial responsiveness, and enhance the process of allergic sensitization, changes that are known to predispose children to early respiratory illness. Early respiratory illness can lead to long-term pulmonary effects (reduced lung function and increased risk of chronic obstructive lung disease).

The 1986 reports of the NRC and Surgeon General conclude that both the prevalence of respiratory symptoms of irritation and the incidence of lower respiratory tract infections are higher in children of smoking parents. In the 18 studies of respiratory symptoms subsequent to the 2 reports, increased symptoms (cough, phlegm production, and wheezing) were observed in a range of ages from birth to midteens, particularly in infants and preschool children. In addition to the studies on symptoms of respiratory irritation, 10 new studies have addressed the topic of parental smoking and acute lower respiratory tract illness in children, and 9 have reported statistically significant associations. The cumulative evidence is conclusive that parental smoking, especially the mother's, causes an increased incidence of respiratory illnesses from birth up to the first 18 months to 3 years of life, particularly for bronchitis, bronchiolitis, and pneumonia.

Overall, the evidence confirms and strengthens the previous conclusions of the NRC and Surgeon General.

Recent studies also solidify the evidence for the conclusion of a causal association between parental smoking and increased middle ear effusion in young children. Middle ear effusion is the most common reason for hospitalization of young children for an operation.

At the time of the Surgeon General's report on passive smoking (U.S. DHHS, 1986), data were sufficient to conclude only that maternal smoking may influence the severity of asthma in children. The recent studies reviewed here strengthen and confirm these exacerbation effects. The new evidence is also conclusive that ETS exposure increases the number of episodes of asthma in children who already have the disease. In addition, the evidence is suggestive that ETS exposure increases the number of new cases of asthma in children who have not previously exhibited symptoms, although the results are statistically significant only with children whose mothers smoke 10 or more cigarettes per day. While the evidence for new cases of asthma itself is not conclusive of a causal association, the consistently strong association of ETS both with increased frequency and severity of the asthmatic symptoms and with the established ETS effects on the immune system and airway hyperresponsiveness lead to the conclusion that ETS is a risk factor for induction of asthma in previously asymptomatic children.

Regarding the effects of passive smoking on lung function in children, the 1986 NRC and Surgeon General reports both conclude that children of parents who smoke have small decreases in tests of pulmonary output function of both the larger and smaller air passages when compared with the children of nonsmokers. As noted in the NRC report, if ETS exposure is the cause of the observed decrease in lung function, this effect could be due to the direct action of agents in ETS or an indirect consequence of increased occurrence of acute respiratory illness related to ETS.

Results from eight studies on ETS and lung function in children that have appeared since those reports add some additional confirmatory evidence suggesting a causal rather than an indirect relationship. For the population as a whole, the reductions are small relative to the interindividual variability of each lung function parameter. However, groups of particularly susceptible or heavily exposed children have shown larger decrements. The studies reviewed suggest that a continuum of exposures to tobacco products starting in fetal life may contribute to the decrements in lung function found in older children. Exposure to tobacco smoke products inhaled by the mother during pregnancy may contribute significantly to these changes, but there is strong evidence indicating that postnatal exposure to ETS is an important part of the causal pathway.

What You Can Do to Reduce the Health Risks of Passive Smoking

In the home:

- Don't smoke in your house or permit others to do so.

- If a family member insists on smoking indoors, increase ventilation in the area where smoking takes place. Open windows or use exhaust fans.

- Do not smoke if children are present, particularly infants and toddlers. They are particularly susceptible to the effects of passive smoking.

- Don't allow babysitters or others who work in your home to smoke in the house or near your children.

Where children spend time:

- EPA recommends that every organization dealing with children have a smoking policy that effectively protects children from exposure to environmental tobacco smoke.

- Find out about the smoking policies of the day care providers, preschools, schools, and other caregivers for your children.

- Help other parents understand the serious health risks to children from secondhand smoke. Work with parent/teacher associations, your school board and school administrators, community leaders, and other concerned citizens to make your child's environment smoke free.

In the workplace:

EPA recommends that every company have a smoking policy that effectively protects nonsmokers from involuntary exposure to tobacco smoke. Many businesses and organizations already have smoking policies in place but these policies vary in their effectiveness.

- If your company does not have a smoking policy that effectively controls secondhand smoke, work with appropriate management and labor organizations to establish one.

291

- Simply separating smokers and nonsmokers within the same area, such as a cafeteria, may reduce exposure, but nonsmokers will still be exposed to recirculated smoke or smoke drifting into nonsmoking areas.

- Prohibiting smoking indoors or limiting smoking to rooms that have been specially designed to prevent smoke from escaping to other area of the building are two options that will effectively protect nonsmokers. The costs associated with establishing properly designated smoking rooms vary from building to building, and are likely to be greater than simply eliminating smoking entirely.

- If smoking is permitted indoors, it should be in a room that meets several conditions:

  1. Air from the smoking room should be directly exhausted to the outside by an exhaust fan. Air from the smoking room should not be recirculated to other parts of the building. More air should be exhausted from the room than is supplied to it to make sure ETS doesn't drift to surrounding spaces.

  2. The ventilation system should provide the smoking room with 60 cubic feet per minute (CFM) of supply air per smoker. This air is often supplied by air transferred from other parts of the building, such as corridors.

  3. Nonsmokers should not have to use the smoking room for any purpose. It should be located in a non-work area where no one, as part of his or her work responsibilities, is required to enter.

- Employer-supported smoking cessation programs are an important part of any smoking policy. Approximately 25 percent of American adults still smoke. Many smokers would like to quit, but cigarette smoking is physically and psychologically addictive, and quitting is not easy. While working in a smoke-free building may encourage some smokers to quit, a goal of any smoking policy should be to actively support smokers who want to kick the habit.

- If there are designated outdoor smoking areas, smoking should not be permitted right outside the doors (or near building ventilation system air intakes) where nonsmokers may have to pass through smoke from smokers congregated near doorways. Some employers have set up outdoor areas equipped with shelters and ashtrays to accommodate smokers.

In restaurants and bars:

- Know the law concerning smoking in your community. Some communities have banned smoking in places such as restaurants entirely. Others require separate smoking areas in restaurants, although most rely on simply separating smokers and nonsmokers within the same space, which may reduce but not eliminate involuntary exposure to ETS.

- If smoking is permitted, placement of smoking areas should be determined with some knowledge of the ventilation characteristics of the space to minimize nonsmoker exposure. For example, nonsmoking areas should be near air supply ducts while smoking areas should be near return registers or exhausts.

- Ask to be seated in nonsmoking areas as far from smokers as possible.

- If your community does not have a smoking control ordinance, urge that one be enacted. If your local ordinances are not sufficiently protective, urge your local government officials to take action.

- Few restrictions have been imposed in bars where drinking and smoking seem to go together. In the absence of state or local laws restricting smoking in bars, encourage the proprietor to consider his or her nonsmoking clientele, and frequent places that do so.

In Other Indoor Spaces

Does your state or community have laws addressing smoking in public spaces? Many states have laws prohibiting smoking in public facilities such as schools, hospitals, airports, bus terminals, and other public buildings. Know the law. Take advantage of laws designed to protect you. Federal laws now prohibit smoking on all airline flights of six hours or less within the U.S. and on all interstate bus travel.

A Special Message for Smokers

This is a difficult time to be a smoker. As the public becomes more aware that smoking is not only a hazard to you but also to others, nonsmokers are becoming more outspoken, and smokers are finding themselves a beleaguered group.

If you choose to smoke, here are some things you can do to help protect the people close to you:

- Don't smoke around children. Their lungs are very susceptible to smoke. If you are expecting a child, quit smoking.

- Take an active role in the development of your company's smoking policy. Encourage the offering of smoking cessation programs for those who want them.

- Keep your home smoke free. Nonsmokers can get lung cancer from exposure to your smoke. Because smoke lingers in the air, people may be exposed even if they are not present while you smoke. If you must smoke inside, limit smoking to a room where you can open windows for cross-ventilation. Be sure the room in which you smoke has a working smoke detector to lessen the risk of fire.

- Test your home for radon. Radon contamination in combination with smoking is a much greater health risk than either one individually.

- Don't smoke in an automobile with the windows closed if passengers are present. The high concentration of smoke in a small, closed compartment substantially increases the exposure of other passengers.

More than two million people quit smoking every year, most of them on their own, without the aid of a program or medication. If you want to quit smoking, assistance is available. Smoking cessation programs can help. Your employer may offer programs, or ask your doctor for advice.

For More Information

Indoor Air Quality Information Clearinghouse (IAQ INFO)
P.O. Box 37133, Washington, DC 20013-7133
(800)438-4318, (703)356-4020
fax: (703)356-5386
Website: www.epa.gov/iaq

Office on Smoking and Health
Centers for Disease Control and Prevention, Mail Stop K-50
4770 Buford Highway, N.E.
Atlanta, GA 30341-3724
(770) 488-5493

National Cancer Institute
Building 31, Room 10A24
9000 Rockville Pike
Bethesda, MD 20892
(800)4-CANCER

National Heart, Lung, and Blood Institute
Information Center
P.O. Box 30105
Bethesda, MD 20824-0105
(301)592-8573

National Institute for Occupational Safety and Health
4676 Columbia Parkway
Cincinnati, OH 45226-1998
(800)35-NIOSH

Chapter 31

Fragrances and Health

The health effects of fragrances are a general health issue, an indoor air quality issue, an access issue, and an environmental issue. Unfortunately, the only issue the fragrance industry has addressed is that of skin safety for the user of the products. This leaves many areas of concern.

Allergic disease affects 20% of the population and is the sixth leading cause of chronic disease. There are an estimated 17 million asthmatics, and migraine headaches affect as many as 25 million people in the United States. Individuals with nonallergic rhinitis, chronic respiratory disease, and chemical sensitivities should also be included in these numbers. Fragrances are known to trigger and exacerbate all of these conditions. The impact of fragrances on health is a general health issue.

Fragrance chemicals are volatile by nature. This means some of each fragranced product used ends up in the air. The result is [a] complex mixture of chemicals that is constantly changing. Fragrance chemicals are often air, heat, and light sensitive. Very often the compounds that result from the reactions and breakdown that occurs in the air are more irritating than the original compounds. In indoor

Excerpted from "Fragrances and Health," by Betty Bridges, in *Environmental Health Perspectives* (Correspondence), Vol. 107, No. 7 [Online] July 1999. Available: http://ehpnet1.niehs.nih.gov/docs/1999/107-7/correspondence.html. Produced by the National Institute of Environmental Health Sciences (NIEHS), P.O. Box 12233, Research Triangle Park, NC 27709. For complete contact information, please refer to Chapter 68, "Resources."

environments where air exchange is poor, the problems are compounded.

Fragrance chemicals are not removed from wastewater by present sewage treatment methods. Synthetic musk compounds are being found in waterways and in aquatic wildlife. The implications are not known because so little research has been done in the area of fragrance chemical safety. These materials are now in the food chain.

The main focus of safety testing in the fragrance industry has been adverse skin effects. Fragrance materials penetrate the skin, are absorbed into the bloodstream, and are distributed to other organs. Other routes of exposure, such as respiratory and neurologic exposure via olfactory pathways, have been ignored. Ingestion is another route of exposure because many of the same materials are used as flavors in foods.

There are legitimate concerns about the scope and effectiveness of safety testing by the fragrance industry. In the late 1970s it was found that acetylethyltetramethyltetralin (AETT) caused the internal organs of laboratory animals to turn blue. This substance was also severely neurotoxic. Testing by the industry had not pinpointed these side effects, which were discovered by accident after the material had been used in products for over 20 years[1,2].

Musk ambrette was also used in fragrances for years. Testing by the Research Institute for Fragrance Materials indicated that it was safe for use. It was later determined that musk ambrette caused photosensitivity reactions and had neurotoxic properties[3]. The International Fragrance Association recommended in 1985 that musk ambrette not be used in products with skin contact. In 1991, musk ambrette was still being found in products tested by the Food and Drug Administration (FDA).

More recent concerns are being focused on musk xylol, which was used to replace musk ambrette. Safety testing by the industry indicated that musk xylol was safe for use. Later studies outside the industry found musk xylol to be carcinogenic when fed to mice. Musk xylol has been used since the turn of the century. It accumulates in human tissue and has been found in human adipose tissue and breast milk.

Some fragrance materials are known to act as haptens in the skin. Although there is significant respiratory exposure to these materials, the possibility of respiratory sensitization has not been addressed. In some individuals with asthma, fragrances are primary triggers, whereas other irritants do not initiate a response. This suggests that there may be respiratory sensitization involved. If fragrance materials have the ability to sensitize the respiratory system in the same manner as the skin, the implications are serious and could be one factor in the unexplained increase in asthma rates.

The fragrance industry asserts that adequate safety testing is done, there is adequate monitoring of problems, and no increase in complaints concerning fragranced products has been noted. The present system of monitoring complaints is totally inadequate. The FDA's system of logging complaints is set up for users of the products, and not for those made ill by others' use. Someone who calls the general FDA complaint line may not be given instructions on whom to contact. Any complaints on "secondhand" fragrance should be addressed specifically to Lark Lambert, HFS-106, Office of Cosmetics and Colors, Cosmetic Adverse Reaction Monitoring Program, 200C Street SW, Washington, DC 20204 USA. Telephone: (202)205-4706; Fax: (202)205-5098.

Even with the limited method of collecting data, there was an increase in records of complaints from 1995 to 1997. These complaints included respiratory and neurologic effects. The FDA suspended the Voluntary Cosmetic Registration Program in March 1998 because of budget cuts; it was reinstated 1 January 1999. This program is totally voluntary, and the industry is not required to participate.

The FDA only addresses the safety of materials in cosmetics. Fragrances in household products come under the jurisdiction of the Consumer Product Safety Commission. Once the products volatilize, air quality falls under U.S. Environmental Protection Agency jurisdiction. The fragrance industry does not have a centralized data collection program in place. This means that there is no method in place for accurately collecting data on the negative impact of fragrances.

The "trade-secret" status of fragrances makes it difficult, if not impossible, to pinpoint substances that cause problems. Present labeling is misleading, as "fragrance-free" and "unscented" products often contain fragrance chemicals. Avoidance is not possible when labeling does not reflect the contents.

It seems to be the industry's position to discount complaints concerning fragrances as reactionary and psychological responses to odors. Fragrances do enhance our lives, just as music does. But taste in music varies—what is music to one may be noise to another. Also, when there is too much noise or noise is too loud, real health problems occur.

When types of substances used by the fragrance industry are used in other industries, they are heavily regulated because of their known health effects. Whereas these substances are generally used at low levels in fragrance materials, the sheer numbers of fragranced products used and the constant exposure causes concern, especially in children. In addition, many of the materials have synergistic effects that cannot be ignored. A much more prudent course of action would be to gather reliable data, do further safety testing, pinpoint the substances causing problems, and eliminate them from use. Further information can be found at the web site of the Fragranced Products Information Network (http://www.ameliaww.com/fpin).

References

1. Spencer PS, Sterman AB, Horoupian DS, Foulds MM. Neurotoxic fragrance produces ceroid and myelin disease. *Science* 204:633-635 (1979).

2. Troy WR. Toxicity of Versalide [letter]. *Food Chem Toxicol* 20:629 (1982).

3. Wisneski HS, Havery DC. Nitro musks in fragrance products: an update of FDA findings. *Cosmetics and Toiletries* 3(6):73-74 (1996).

—by Betty Bridges, R.N.

Betty Bridges heads the Fragranced Products Information Network, Amelia, Virginia; E-mail: bcb56@ix.netcom.com

Chapter 32

Cockroach Antigens

Cockroach antigens are proteins found in the insects' feces, saliva, eggs, and shed cuticles that can trigger allergic reactions (and the corresponding formation of antibodies) when they become airborne and are inhaled by humans. Cockroach antigens produce allergic effects particularly in children, including respiratory symptoms and especially asthma. A recent study concluded that exposure to cockroach antigens may play an important role in asthma-related health problems among inner-city children. Skin tests to detect reactions to cockroach antigens produce positive results at rates second only to house dust mites.

Researchers at the United States Department of Agriculture's Agricultural Research Service (ARS), the Arkansas Children's Hospital Research Institute in Little Rock, Arkansas, and the FDA have teamed up to identify cockroach antigens associated with triggering asthma. Their goal is to reduce asthma symptoms by finding and removing cockroach antigens from dwellings. A key milestone of their work is the development of a home test kit that uses polyclonal antibodies to detect cockroach antigens, which can then be eliminated with common household cleaners.

From "Working the Bugs Out of Asthma," by Carol Potera, in *Environmental Health Perspectives,* Vol. 105, No. 11 [Online] November 1997. Available: http://ehpnet1.niehs.nih.gov/qa/105-11/innovations.html. Produced by the National Institute of Environmental Health Sciences (NIEHS), P.O. Box 12233, Research Triangle Park, NC 27709. For complete contact information, please refer to Chapter 68, "Resources."

Controlling cockroach-induced asthma is difficult. Immunotherapy with injections of cockroach extracts brings little relief. And killing cockroaches by fumigating homes with pesticides fails to significantly reduce allergic symptoms. During their search for better ways to prevent cockroach-induced asthma, the ARS researchers and their colleagues discovered that cockroach antigens persist in buildings for at least five years, even in the absence of cockroaches.

Tracking Cockroaches

Richard Brenner, a medical entomologist and research leader in the imported fire ants and household insects research unit of the ARS in Gainesville, Florida, set out to demonstrate the tenacity of cockroach antigens. In August 1990, Brenner and his colleagues infested a 1,040-square-foot building with 600 German cockroaches (*Blattella germanica*) captured at a Miami housing project. The facility was furnished with wall cabinets, countertops, a sink, refrigerator, electric stove, waste basket, and table. The activity of the cockroaches and their antigen distribution was monitored for five months while moving food and water sources.

Because insect pests redistribute themselves to optimize their survival in any environment, "all infestations are spatial in nature," says Brenner. However, research procedures and statistics traditionally used by entomologists fail to address these spatial relationships fully. So Brenner adapted spatial analysis, a statistical method developed by mining engineers to precisely target the subsurface distribution of minerals, to study the cockroaches.

Unlike traditional statistical methods that assume random sampling and independent observations, spatial analysis recognizes "spatial continuity," which is the phenomenon that samples taken close to each other will appear similar. This parallels ecological systems— trees tend to grow together in groves, grass occurs in continuous patches, and German cockroaches aggregate.

Spatial analysis is modeled by computer programs that generate a contour map showing areas of varying density, similar to topographic maps. Within a data set, sample locations are defined by X and Y spatial coordinates. Spatial analysis pairs each observation with each of the other observations, calculates the distance between the members of each pair, then determines how similar the values are in each pair. The information is then used to estimate values at unsampled locations within the study site.

In Brenner's German cockroach experiment, about 100 live traps, baited with bread soaked in beer, were placed overnight in a grid that covered the scope of ecological diversity in the test building. The next morning, trapped cockroaches were counted. Using these counts and spatial analysis, the researchers estimated the number of cockroaches at one-foot intervals, which added up to 1,040 locations within the facility.

Through spatial analysis Brenner learned that the cockroaches, which are very adaptable creatures, redistributed themselves rapidly after their food and water were relocated. This meant that allergens associated with them were probably broadly distributed as well. The next step was to devise a detection system that could determine the allergen distribution and how long the allergens persisted.

After five months of monitoring the cockroaches, Brenner's crew removed all the insects, closed the building without cleaning it, and set out to build a detection system. In December 1996, they returned with a prototype of the cockroach antigen test kit to determine whether these potential cockroach allergens persisted years later in the absence of cockroaches, and, if so, where they were distributed. Because German cockroaches only live where there are people, Brenner was certain no new ones had taken up residence in the closed building.

A 16-square-inch surface was swabbed at 110 locations, and the swabs were shipped to the laboratory of standards and testing at the FDA's Center for Biologics Evaluation and Research in Bethesda, Maryland, where they were analyzed with an enzyme-linked immuno-adsorbent assay (ELISA) using polyclonal antibodies to detect cock-roach antigens. When the results were returned to Brenner and plugged into the spatial analysis computer program, the distribution of cockroach antigens matched to a remarkable degree the cumulative distribution of cockroaches found five years earlier. The research-ers concluded that the allergen load, expressed by a newly created index called "cockroach hour equivalents," measured as high as 4,100 units five years after all cockroaches were removed. "The allergen load was still enormous. You can see why even when cockroaches are re-moved, asthma does not get better," says Brenner.

Next, the ARS researchers cleaned the facility with a common household cleaner. They took test swabs of the surfaces after clean-ing and sent the samples to the FDA for ELISA testing. Spatial analy-sis showed that cleaning removed 90% of the cockroach antigens and highlighted where the rest remained. The researchers cleaned again, swabbed again, and tested with ELISA. This second cleaning reduced the allergen load to zero cockroach hour equivalents, and confirmed that common cleaners adequately eliminate cockroach antigens.

Perfecting a Home Test Kit

Testing for potential cockroach allergens in homes requires a detection probe that is both highly specific and environmentally sensitive. A monoclonal antibody to a single cockroach antigen fails to detect many others, because 15-20 proteins from several types of cockroaches, including German, American, and Asian varieties, are suspected of causing human allergic reactions, says microbiologist Chris Anderson, chief of the FDA's laboratory of standards and testing. To be environmentally sensitive to cockroach allergens in homes, a probe must be polyclonal, or capable of detecting all major cockroach antigens.

Perfecting the laboratory-based ELISA devised by Anderson's team into a simple, home-based test kit is the next challenge facing the cockroach researchers. The polyclonal ELISA includes two major cockroach antigens characterized and cloned by immunologist Ricki Helm, an associate professor of pediatrics at the Arkansas Children's Hospital Research Institute. Using physicochemical methods such as isoelectric focusing and gel electrophoresis, Helm identified a 36-kilodalton (kd) and a 90-kd antigen, both of which recognize IgE antibodies in serum from people with known cockroach allergies. The 90-kd allergen bound IgE in 77% (17 of 22) of patient sera tested. By definition, a major allergen produces an IgE response in more than 50% of allergic patients.

Other known cockroach antigens range in size from 6 to 100 kd. "Some people react to only one, others to 15 allergens," says Anderson. At this point, the researchers do not know the final combination of cockroach antigens that will be included in a home test kit, but the final mixture has to cover a practical, broad base, says Anderson.

In addition, the team needs to verify that cockroach antigens recovered from swabbed floors that test positive in the ELISA are allergens that trigger asthma. Work is underway to correlate the relationship between these antigens and asthma allergens. "This needs to be done before a test kit can be successful," says Anderson.

Preventing Cockroach-Induced Asthma

A study published in the 8 May 1997 issue of the *New England Journal of Medicine* highlighted the need to detect cockroach allergens in homes. Dust samples from the bedrooms of 476 inner-city asthmatic children were analyzed for dust mite, cat, and cockroach allergens. Multivariate analysis revealed that cockroaches were the most common cause of the children's asthma. In the children's bedrooms, 50.2% had cockroach allergen levels that exceeded the disease-induction threshold, compared with 9.7% for dust mite allergen levels and 12.6% for cat allergen levels. The rate of hospitalization for asthma was 3.4 times higher among children whose skin tested positive to cockroach allergens and whose bedrooms had high cockroach-allergen levels. The same group also had 78% more visits to health care providers, experienced significantly more wheezing, and missed more school because of asthma.

Brenner proposes that a cockroach allergen home test kit can help relieve asthmatic symptoms by precisely targeting the allergens and directing cleaning efforts. "We can have a positive impact on human health by eliminating the pests and their attendant allergens," he says. By analogy, he compares cockroach allergen contamination to having a nuclear waste spill in a home. Both are extremely dangerous even in small quantities—a picogram of cockroach allergen can kill a sensitive asthmatic—and both require clean-up procedures that find and remove all of the contamination. For example, he says, in the case of allergens, removing 95% clearly is good. But the remaining 5% could conceivably be entirely concentrated in one small location—for example, the corner of a child's playroom. Consequently, the remaining 5% is potentially a concentration that could be life-threatening to a severely cockroach-sensitive asthmatic. Brenner says, "That is the essence of our spatial analysis. It tells you exactly where the problem is, not just the magnitude."

Brenner foresees the test kit including many probes to check many sites in a home before and after cleaning with household cleansers. The cockroach allergen test kit could also be adapted by the pest control industry to assess, target, clean, resample, and verify that all cockroach allergens are eliminated. The technology is also helping to develop and test new cockroach repellents that are environmentally friendly.

The exact design of a commercial home test kit will be determined once partners from private industry are selected and patents are obtained. This novel approach of combining polyclonal antibodies for cockroach antigens with spatial analysis "allows us to take a holistic view of indoor environmental quality by examining surface contaminants," says Brenner, "and goes beyond simply testing indoor air quality."

Suggested Reading

Brenner RJ. Preparing for the 21st century: research methods in developing management strategies for arthropods and allergens in the structural environment. In: *Proceedings of the 1st International Conference on Insect Pests in the Urban Environment* (Wildey KB, Robinson WH, eds.). Exeter:BPCC Wheatons Ltd.,1993;57-69.

Rosenstreich DL, Eggleston P, Kattan M, et al. The role of cockroach allergy and exposure to cockroach allergen in causing morbidity among inner-city children with asthma. *N Engl J Med* 336:1356-1363 (1997).

Helm R, Cockrell G, Stanley JS, et al. Isolation and characterization of a clone encoding a major allergen (Bla g Bd90K) involved in IgE-mediated cockroach hypersensitivity. *J Allergy Clin Immunol* 98:172-180 (1996).

—by Carol Potera

Chapter 33

Occupational Asthma

As much as 15% of adult-onset asthma may arise from exposures on the job. A careful history and evaluation of respiratory symptoms can help [the physician] determine whether a patient's asthma is truly occupational.

Asthma far exceeds other causes of occupational pulmonary disease in the industrialized world. An estimated 2-15% of all adult asthma cases are workplace-related, and some 250 triggering agents have been implicated. In comparison to many other job-related illnesses and injuries, asthma often produces more persistent—even permanent—effects.

The public health impact is also considerable. Occupational asthma may result in social and economic disruption for the worker and substantial cost to employers and the state.

The definitive diagnosis of occupational asthma requires meticulous—even arduous—assessments of the patient and workplace. But these assessments must be performed expeditiously—the longer the exposure is allowed to continue, the more serious and persistent asthma is likely to be. Furthermore, because both medicolegal and compensation issues may be involved, the diagnosis and the linkage to the workplace must be as specific as possible.

Excerpted from "Occupational Asthma: Breathing Easier on the Job," by Emil J. Bardana Jr., Philip Harber, and James E. Lockey, in *Patient Care*, Vol. 30, No. 3, February 15, 1996, pp. 100-9. © 1996 by Medical Economics Publishing Co., Five Paragon Dr., Montvale, NJ 07645-1742. Reprinted with permission.

As the first person the patient is likely to consult about the possibility of occupational asthma, [the physician's] primary care role is crucial. While [he] may not wish to undertake all the allergy and pulmonary function testing that eventually may be needed, [he is] the person who can ensure that rapid action is taken.

In 1993, guidelines for assessing the degree of disability and impairment in asthma were established by the American Thoracic Society.[1] These include spirometric measurements of forced expiratory volume in one second (FEV_1) and forced vital capacity, and assessment of symptom reversibility following administration of a bronchodilator. Depending on the severity of impairment, a trial of oral or inhaled corticosteroids also may be performed to document airway hypersensitivity. For less severe symptoms, a histamine or methacholine chloride (Provocholine) challenge also may be done. As [he considers] the diagnosis of occupational asthma, [he should] keep in mind that the first and crucial step is providing objective documentation of reversible airway obstruction.

Exposure and Effects

The clinical effects of workplace exposure depend on a number of factors, including the nature of the substance and the person's predisposition to allergy. Different types of pathologic processes—both immunologic and nonimmunologic—are also involved.

Immunologic Asthma

The most common forms of occupational asthma involve an IgE-mediated response to a high-molecular-weight antigen such as flour or latex, or an inflammatory, non-IgE-mediated response to a low-molecular-weight agent such as a diisocyanate compound (see Table 33.1.). Immunologic asthma can be characterized by an early-phase, late-phase, or biphasic response in FEV_1 or peak-flow values.

Immunologic asthma develops after a latent period of exposure to one or more antigens and tends to develop slowly—over a period of months or even years—usually as a response to low-level, chronic exposure. Immunologic occupational asthma may develop de novo or after sensitization to new antigens at the workplace in a patient with preexistent asthma.

Symptoms initially include nasal congestion and eye and throat irritation that are worse during the workweek and improve somewhat on weekends or during vacations. With continued exposure, lower

Table 33.1. Causes of Occupational Asthma

High-Molecular-Weight-Allergens

Animal proteins	Plant proteins	Foods and enzymes
Danders	Castor bean dust	Bromelain
Feathers	Exotic wood dusts	Crab
Pelts	Grains, flours	Egg powder
Urine	Green coffee bean dust	Garlic powder
Saliva	Gum acacia	Mushrooms
Animal proteins derived from any mammalian species	Gum arabic	Pancreatic extracts
Insect proteins	Latex	Papain
Bee moths	Plant components	Pepsin
Lake flies	Pollens	Prawns
Locusts	Tragacanth	Sea squirt
Mealworms	Pharmaceuticals	Trypsin
Midges	Ipecacuanha	—
Mites	Psyllium	—
Screwworms	—	—
Sewer flies	—	—

Low-Molecular-Weight-Allergens

Organic chemicals	Metallic salts/ Inorganic compounds	Pharmaceuticals
Acid anhydrates	Aluminum	Cephalosporins
—Himic anhydrate	Ammonium persulfate	Isoniazid
—Phthalic anhydrate	—	Macrolide antibiotics
—Tetrachlorophthalic anhydrate	Hard metal and cobalt	Penicillins
—Trimellitic anhydrate	Nickel	Sulfonamides
Colophony	Platinum salts	Tetracycline
—Abietic acid	—Ammonium chloroplatinate	—
—Primaric acid	—Potassium hexachloroplatinate	—
Diisocyanates	—Sodium chloroplatinate	—
—Diphenylmethane diisocyanate	Stainless steel	—
—Hexamethylene diisocyanate	Uranium hexafluoride	—
—Naphthalene diisocyanate	Vanadium	—
—Toluene diisocyanate	—	—
Epoxy resins	—	—
—Diethylenetriamine	—	—
—Ethylenediamine	—	—
—Piperazine (diethylenediamine)	—	—
Western red cedar	—	—
—Plicatic acid	—	—

Adapted from Bardana EJ Jr: Occupational asthma and related respiratory disorders. *Dis Mort* 1995;41(3):143-199.

respiratory symptoms develop, such as nocturnal cough, shortness of breath, and wheezing. Initially these symptoms will improve during weekends and vacations. With continued exposure, however, symptoms can progress and persist even when the person is not at work.

In cases of occupational asthma associated with exposure to low-molecular-weight substances, there is no association with previous smoking, and there is no predisposition because of a history of atopy. The classic presentation of occupational asthma from such exposures is the late or biphasic response. The most common offending agents are diisocyanates, which are used in many manufacturing processes and spray paints. An estimated 5-10% of workers in these environments eventually are affected.

Nonimmunologic Asthma

Breathlessness and wheezing may be sudden and severe after a high-level exposure to a toxic agent such as sulfur dioxide, chloride, chlorine, or anhydrous ammonia. This is known as nonimmunologic asthma.[2] A precipitating event—such as an industrial accident that involves a respiratory irritant—is usually obvious, and asthmalike symptoms soon develop.

Also referred to as reactive airway dysfunction syndrome (RADS), this condition is unrelated to prior atopy. Symptoms show less reversibility following administration of a bronchodilator. The inflammatory response is marked by an absence of eosinophilia and some degree of lymphocytic infiltration. The exact mechanism of persistent airway hyperreactivity is unclear but involves the alteration and disruption of the epithelial lining with subsequent inflammatory and fibrotic changes.

Clues in History

Once the diagnosis of asthma has been established, the more difficult problem of linking the symptoms to the workplace arises. This can require extensive, detailed questioning about the medical history, symptom patterns, present work conditions, and work history.

[The physician should be] as specific as possible. Asking for the person's job title isn't enough. [He needs] to find out exactly what the person does at work, what the environment is like, what materials are present, and if coworkers have had similar difficulties. Many patients have little knowledge of the materials around them and will not make the connection between symptoms and workplace exposure unless asked directly. Others erroneously blame the workplace, referring vaguely to fumes or dust, when the source of the problem may lie elsewhere—such as at home.

As with any occupational illness, the most obvious tip-off is the appearance or worsening of symptoms at the workplace and improvement on weekends and vacations. Unlike some other occupational conditions, however, the symptom pattern is not always so straightforward. The bronchial hyperreactivity typical of asthma tends to be self-perpetuating, especially if exposure continues, and symptoms can persist long after the person leaves the job site. Approximately half of all workers who develop occupational asthma caused by low-molecular-weight compounds never experience complete symptom resolution.

A detailed evaluation of the patient's job history and workplace exposures, home environment, and hobbies is essential. The history must investigate job tasks and potential exposures, the use of protective equipment, types of upper and/or lower respiratory tract symptoms, the relationship of symptoms to home and work environments, and the type and intensity of symptoms when away from both home and work. Here are some of the questions occupational medicine experts always ask:

- Where were you and what were you doing when your symptoms began?

- Have you ever had similar symptoms before, even in childhood?

- Are you allergic to any foods or medicines? Do you have seasonal hay fever? Does anyone in your family have allergies?

- Do you smoke? Have you ever smoked? If so, how much and for how long? Does anyone in your household or workplace smoke?

- What type of dwelling do you live in, and what types of heating and cooling systems are in your home?

- Have you recently had a viral respiratory illness or "sinus trouble"?

- Do you take any prescription medications?

- What nonprescription drugs do you use?

- Do you have pets at home?

- Do you engage in activities such as photography, woodworking, or gardening?

Of course, many more questions are necessary based on the exposure history (see Table 33.2.). It's also important to inquire about the work site, especially about the ventilation system and the type of respirator used. But [the physician needs] to go beyond the worker and the workplace in tracing historical clues. Making an accurate diagnosis requires recognition of the multifactorial nature of asthma and an understanding of the role of predisposing factors, such as a family history of atopic disorders or a recent severe lower respiratory tract infection.

Finding the Link

In attempting to link the symptoms with the workplace, it's important to know as specifically as possible what the patient may have been exposed to and in what circumstances. Doing a walk-through of

Table 33.2. Taking an Exposure History (continued on next page)

Tobacco Smoke
Current cigarette smoking status
Lifetime smoking history, translated to cumulative pack-years
Cigar or pipe smoking history
History of environmental tobacco smoke exposure, especially domestic

Occupational History
List all full-time and part-time jobs in chronological order, including the following:
—Dates of employment
—Name and location of employer
—Title of job
—General description of workplace, including processes
—Description of work performed
—List of any potentially hazardous exposures

Any routine incidents (e.g., pipe breaks) or nonroutine incidents (e.g., explosions) associated with exposures.
—Describe health symptoms, evaluation, and care following such incidents
—Nature of respiratory protection, if any
—Any perceived adverse health effects at the time of exposure
—Any health surveillance (e.g., workplace pulmonary function tests)
—Reason job ended

the site can be extremely helpful. Companies are required by law to keep Material Safety Data Sheets on all possibly toxic agents on their premises, and they must make these available to the employee and physician on request.

Peak-flow monitoring is the first step in relating the person's pattern of respiratory symptoms to workplace exposures. At two-hour intervals throughout the day, the patient [should] record the peak expiratory flow rate (PEFR) and keep a diary of activities and workplace events. This monitoring is done for two weeks on the job, followed by similar monitoring for two weeks away from the workplace. This approach is limited, however, by its reliance on the patient's cooperation, conscientiousness, and flexibility. Reliability improves if a

Table 33.2. (continued) Taking an Exposure History

History of Hobbies

List hobbies, their frequency, and intensity

List types of processes, materials used, location, and ventilation

List any adverse reactions

History of Environment

List residences (judgment may be used as to whether all residences or only current residence should be assessed)

Type of residence (e.g., apartment, single-family dwelling)

Age and location

Basic structure (number of stories, basement, crawl space, cement slab)

Construction materials, including type of insulation

Heating and air conditioning systems (both permanent and portable), including their age, presence of filters or humidification system, maintenance schedule

Floor coverings (especially carpets), curtains, and furnishings

Pets, especially cats, dogs, and birds

Rodents or cockroach infestation

Nearby structures (e.g., factories, gasoline stations)

Other Respiratory Exposures

Marijuana and other nontobacco cigarettes

Freebasing cocaine

Adapted from Bascom R: Occupational and environmental respiratory diseases: A medicolegal primer for physicians. *Occup Med: State of the Art Reviews* 1992;7:331-345.

Asthma Sourcebook, First Edition

health care worker such as a company nurse is present to supervise the monitoring. Consistent decrease in PEFR of 25% or more suggests occupational asthma.

If peak-flow findings support the diagnosis, a workplace challenge is sometimes considered. This requires effort and organization because a technician must accompany the person to the work site to perform spirometric measurements at regular intervals and record the findings. A workplace challenge is reliable and accurate but often impractical. Spirometric measurements performed in the physician's office before and after the work shift may provide sufficient evidence of a consistent pattern of decline in pulmonary function on the job.

Some authorities conduct additional tests such as bronchoprovocation with a subirritant concentration to associate symptoms more firmly with a specific agent, depending on clinical circumstances. These tests can be helpful if the patient strongly desires to remain on the job, because confirmation of the exact immunogen might permit adjustments at the workplace to remove or minimize the exposure.

Bronchoprovocation requires carefully controlled conditions—often including hospitalization—and is performed only by experienced occupational pulmonary medicine specialists. In many cases, however, it's not possible to pin down exactly what substance causes the symptoms because of the multiplicity of chemicals present in many modern workplaces.

Long-Term Concerns

The principles of managing symptomatic occupational asthma are the same as for nonoccupational asthma. Corticosteroids and cromolyn sodium (Intal) are used to alleviate inflammation, and bronchodilators are used for acute attacks. But it's important to keep in mind that continued exposure to the offending agent is very likely to worsen the condition. Once the patient has developed asthma, the level of exposure needed to produce symptoms can drop far below levels that are legally acceptable in the workplace. Providing a bronchodilator won't solve the problem.

The best treatment for occupational asthma is, of course, removal of the person from the job site as promptly as possible. Experts agree that the single most significant determinant of prognosis is the length of exposure before diagnosis. Leaving work altogether isn't necessarily the answer, however. Adjustments can be made to the workplace. Ventilation can be improved, or the person might be relocated to an area protected from exposure.

314

The Americans with Disabilities Act of 1990 requires employers to attempt to adapt the workplace to special needs of employees—and that includes the ability to breathe without impairment. Some asthmatics learn to function with respirators, although some workers find them cumbersome and unpleasant. Others retrain and take positions elsewhere in the company. Those with very severe symptoms, however, may have no choice but to find employment elsewhere.

The patient with occupational asthma needs vocational guidance and, possibly, advice on administrative matters such as workers' compensation. Once the patient's symptoms have stabilized—which can take up to two years—an evaluation of impairment is performed and a long-term impairment rating made for purposes of establishing disability status.[1] This rating should be reevaluated as clinical status warrants because the condition can improve or worsen with time.

References

1. American Thoracic Society: Guidelines for the evaluation of impairment/disability in patients with asthma. *Am Rev Respir Dis* 1993;147:1056-1061.

2. Bardana EJ Jr: Occupational asthma and related respiratory disorders. *Dis Mort* 1995;41(3):143-199.

—by Emil J. Bardana, Jr., Philip Harber, and James E. Lockey

Emil J. Bardana, Jr., M.D., is Professor of Medicine and Chief of the Division of Allergy and Clinical Immunology, Oregon Health Sciences University School of Medicine, Portland.

Philip Harber, M.D., M.P.H., is Professor of Medicine and Director, Occupational and Environmental Medicine, UCLA School of Medicine. He is a former Chairman of the Occupational Lung Disorder Committee of the American College of Occupational and Environmental Medicine.

James E. Lockey, M.D., is Professor and Director, Division of Occupational and Environmental Medicine, Department of Environmental Health, University of Cincinnati College of Medicine. He is Chairman of the Occupational Lung Disorder Committee of the American College of Occupational and Environmental Medicine.

Chapter 34

Agricultural Allergens and Irritants

In contrast to widely held images of urban pollution and blight, the persistence of an "agrarian myth" that associates life on the farm with healthful, bucolic joys ignores a fundamental reality: agriculture can be a dangerous occupation. In agriculture, a large proportion of acute traumatic injury and death comes from accidents involving farm machinery. Farm equipment also inflicts chronic injuries upon workers including noise-induced hearing loss and vibration-associated diseases of the back. Agrichemicals pose a risk for direct toxicity and possibly cancer. Dermatologic diseases, including cancers, among farmers and farm workers are often linked to ultraviolet light exposure, contact dermatitis, and zoonosis. But the most prevalent agricultural hazard involves the respiratory tract. Says Marc B. Schenker, medical epidemiologist and director of the Center for Occupational and Environmental Health at the University of California, Davis, "Despite this litany of significant occupational health problems, respiratory disease remains one of the most common and important issues for those working in the agricultural field." Indeed, occupational mortality studies from the United States, England, and Scandinavia

From "Focus: Danger in the Dust," by Leslie Lang, in *Environmental Health Perspectives,* Vol. 104, No. 1, [Online] January 1996. Available: http://ehpnet1.niehs.nih.gov/docs/1996/104-1/focusdust.html. Produced by the National Institute of Environmental Health Sciences (NIEHS), P.O. Box 12233, Research Triangle Park, NC 27709. For complete contact information, please refer to Chapter 68, "Resources."

reveal higher respiratory disease mortality rates among farmers than the general population.

The farming population in the United States includes approximately 3 million Americans fully engaged in agricultural production and as many as 9 million more who are seasonal and migrant workers, part-time farmers, and farm family members, the latter often considerably active in farm work.

Schenker points out that agriculture is different from many occupations that give rise to respiratory disease. "You have a whole range of respiratory hazards. This isn't like asbestos where you're looking for those fibers, or sandblasting when you're just measuring quartz." Schenker's list of potential respiratory hazards includes gases at potentially lethal concentrations (chlorine, hydrogen sulfide, ammonia), diesel exhaust, solvents, welding fumes, infectious agents and viral diseases from animals, and organic and inorganic dusts, "which can exacerbate any of the others," Schenker says.

Written in the Dust

"It is organic dust that accounts for the most common exposure leading to agricultural respiratory disease," says James Merchant, director of Iowa University's Environmental Health Sciences Research Center. "Virtually everybody who works in agriculture gets exposed to some organic dust."

Indeed, studies indicate that the risk associated with developing respiratory disease appears to be more than threefold greater among those who are heavily exposed to inhalable dust generated in the agricultural environment. According to pulmonologist David A. Schwartz of the University of Iowa College of Medicine, asthma and bronchitis are the main diseases. "Between five and twenty percent of individuals in aggregate will develop some airway disease as a result of agricultural dust exposures," he says.

"The major health effect is airway inflammation, and that extends from the nose to the terminal bronchiole," says Merchant. These dusts and their components are highly respirable, under 10 microns in aerodynamic diameters, so they can penetrate to the terminal bronchiole. "We see an effect in all levels of the airway, but the basic mechanism is airway inflammation, which is manifested clinically as rhinitis, either allergic or irritant; bronchitis, asthma, which can be allergic or irritant; and hypersensitivity pneumonitis."

Agricultural workers encounter a variety of airborne organic dusts generally containing 30-40% of particles in the respirable range. These include molds, pollens, and dusts generated in silos, barns, and grain elevators. Organic dusts measured in enclosed settings such as dairy, poultry, and swine buildings are particularly biologically active. Along with suspended inorganic matter (primarily silicates), they contain plant material (feed and bedding), animal-derived particles (skin, hair, feathers, droppings, urine), bacteria and fungi, mites and other arthropods, insects and insect fragments, feed additives (including antibiotics), pesticides, and microbial toxins (including glucans from molds, fungal mycotoxins, and endotoxin, the lipopolysaccharide fraction of certain bacterial cell walls).

"One thing that's really important is that farmers in general have a relatively low prevalence of cigarette smoking in comparison to the general population," says Schwartz. "And given that, it's really striking that they have such major problems with airway disease. So even if it turns out not to be endotoxin or grain dust, there's something in the environment that's causing them to have major problems with airway disease in comparison with other groups."

By Any Other Name

In the early 18th century, the Italian physician Bernardo Ramazzini recorded his observations associating respiratory disorders with worker exposure to dusts from vegetable fibers and grain. Only in the 20th century has careful study of these phenomena occurred. Among the factors that may have accounted for this lack of study was the rise of manufacturing. Victorian-era social concerns were focused on factories with their concentrations of workers and related issues of workplace conditions, safety, and child labor. Agriculture was still individual in nature in that people worked for themselves, on their own farms, and in small groups. The art and literature of the day painted a healthy and wholesome picture of agrarian life in contrast to highly publicized industrial disasters such as mine cave-ins, factory explosions, and sweatshop fires. "Occupational health, since its inception, has largely ignored agriculture, even though agriculture was the source of some of the earliest recognized occupational diseases," Schenker observes.

Still, the Industrial Revolution did help draw some attention to adverse health effects of exposure to agricultural dusts. As NIOSH Senior Medical Epidemiologist Robert M. Castellan points out, "The increasingly regular work schedule associated with the Industrial Revolution and its concentrations of workers in manufacturing facilities led to the recognition of a peculiar 'Monday phenomenon' among cotton textile workers. This was characterized by symptoms of chest tightness and other breathing difficulties occurring predominately on the first day back to work after Sunday break." In 1877, the term "byssinosis," derived from the Latin byssus, meaning "a fine cotton or linen," first entered the scientific literature.

Since then, adverse health effects arising from exposures to many other agricultural dusts have been described and documented, but myriad syndromes such as silo unloader's syndrome, bark stripper's disease, farmer's lung, and grain fever have caused confusion among clinicians and epidemiologists. "People thought they were looking at many diseases, all of which needed to be attacked separately. But essentially they're the same, except one was diagnosed, say, in mushroom growers, the other in British pigeon handlers," says NIOSH physiologist Vincent Castranova. "The most recent understanding of the situation is that there are acute and chronic forms of agricultural dust disease in general, or responses to either isolated or multiple exposures to organic dust." For example, Castranova explains that the flulike mill fever among cotton workers that follows initial, intense exposures to cotton dust is not present after repeated exposures, though chronic exposures can result in byssinosis, with its symptoms of chest tightness, decline in lung function, and bronchitis.

Acute responses to isolated exposures have been lumped under the term organic dust toxic syndrome (ODTS). ODTS typically occurs in the presence of large amounts of airborne, organic dust. The syndrome often occurs in small clusters and is characterized by fever occurring 4-12 hours after exposure and flulike symptoms such as general weakness, headache, chills, body aches, and cough. Chest tightness and shortness of breath may also occur.

Chest examination usually reveals normal breathing sounds, although lung crackles and wheezing may be present. Chest X-rays are usually normal. Pulmonary function may be impaired, and an increase in the number of white blood cells (leukocytosis) is common. Circulating blood antibodies to the specific dust are usually not present. ODTS usually disappears within 24 hours to a few days following removal from the exposure. However, repeated ODTS episodes can occur after reexposure to the organic dust. An estimated 30-40% of workers exposed to organic dusts will develop ODTS. Grain fever, pulmonary mycotoxicosis, silo unloader's syndrome, inhalation fever, and mill fever in cotton textile workers are all included under ODTS.

A 1988 case reported by NIOSH researchers exemplifies a typical cluster of ODTS. Eleven male workers, aged 15-60, moved 800 bushels of oats from a poorly ventilated storage bin. The oats were reported to contain pockets of powdery, white dust. Work conditions were described as extremely dusty, and all workers wore disposable masks while inside the bin. The workers shoveled oats for 8 hours in groups of two or three in shifts of 20-30 minutes. Within 4-12 hours, all 9 men who worked inside the bin became ill with fever and chills, chest discomfort, weakness, and fatigue. Eight reported shortness of breath, six had nonproductive coughs, five complained of body aches, and four developed headaches. Upon medical examination, crackle sounds in the lungs were found in two workers, wheezing in one. No symptoms developed in the two workers who remained outside the storage bin. Symptoms in all affected workers disappeared within 2-12 days.

"As to the chronic response," Castranova explains, "symptoms would be similar. But you would have a history of prior exposure, presence of serum antibodies to that dust, and the response in the lung is lymphocytic [an accumulation of specific white blood cells that participate in cell-mediated immune responses]."

Farmer's lung disease (an immunologic lung response involving antibodies to the fungi found in moldy hay), mushroom worker's lung, bark stripper's disease, and allergic alveolitis are examples of chronic responses and are synonymous with hypersensitivity pneumonitis. Symptoms often become progressively worse with increasing exposure and may lead to chronic bronchitis, shortness of breath, loss of appetite, and severe reductions in lung volume and diffusing capacity (the volume of gases that move through lung tissue membranes). Five to eight percent of workers exposed to organic dusts develop hypersensitivity pneumonitis. Although it has been studied for more than 25 years, the precise pathological mechanism of hypersensitivity pneumonitis remains unknown.

The conceptual road from acute to chronic responses to organic dusts may not be so clear. According to Castranova, if dust exposure levels are high enough, an affected worker may have neutrophils and lymphocytes in the lungs typical of both acute inflammatory and immunologic reactions. "It's never quite as simple as we'd like to make it," he says.

From Acute to Chronic

In his five-year longitudinal study of 611 workers employed at six cotton mills, biomedical engineer Henry Glindmeyer of Tulane University Medical Center's environmental medicine section reported a significant association between the acute and chronic effects of cotton dust exposure. Cotton dust exposure levels and acute pulmonary function changes measured across workshifts were predictive of annual declines in lung function. Moreover, an inverse exposure-response relationship was found. Yarn production workers in the initial manufacturing process were exposed to lower dust levels (below OSHA permissible exposure limits of 200 micrograms/ cubic meter of air [g/m3]) than workers exposed to the higher permissible levels (750 g/m3) in their slashing and weaving jobs in the later production process. Yet yarn production workers showed a greater annual decline in lung function, a finding which Glindmeyer and his colleagues interpreted as a dust potency effect, possibly due to endotoxin.

Early processing includes bringing the cotton into the warehouse, opening the bales, then manufacturing the cotton into long yarn. "Slashing and weaving is, number one, generally less dusty, but more importantly, tends to have a less potent dust," Glindmeyer explains. "Whatever might be in the dust is generally scrubbed out in the early process."

He adds, "In yarn manufacturing we were able to pick up a dose-response relationship at the 200 g/m3 level. But we were not able to find one in the slashing and weaving area." The slashing and weaving area of the mill, he points out, does not necessarily have cleaner air. "In fact, it can have more dust, but it's less potent."

In this study, smoking proved also to be a significant determinant of decline in lung function. The Tulane researchers say their findings support lowering cotton dust exposures and excluding smokers from working in yarn manufacturing.

The implications of this and other recent longitudinal studies were summarized by McGill University epidemiologist Margaret Becklake. "There is some uncertainty as to whether the acute responses are always in the causal pathway for chronic responses or are independently related to exposure, or whether both mechanisms operate," she said. However, she points to similar findings for exposure to grain dust among grain elevator workers in Vancouver, British Columbia. These studies, she says, indicate a much broader role for occupational exposures in the development of chronic obstructive pulmonary disease than has been previously assumed.

In Keokuk County, Iowa, Merchant is directing a large-scale longitudinal rural health study. Begun just four years ago, this study comparing farm families, rural nonfarm families, and urban families is still in the first round of data collection. It involves children and adults and focuses particularly on effects on the elderly and women. "We are taking a hard look at not only symptoms, but pulmonary function, airway responsiveness, and immunological factors in terms of lung disease risk, " he says. The study is aimed at assessing and quantitating the risk to a variety of rural, agricultural, and other environmental exposures ranging from farm equipment to pesticides and agricultural dusts.

Endotoxin: A Critical Component

Endotoxins are a combination of lipid (lipid A) and polysaccharide side chains and are integral components of the outer membrane of gram negative bacteria. Endotoxins are released into the surrounding environment during active cell growth or breakdown (lysis), or when bacterial cells are engulfed by immune cells called phagocytes.

In the 1930s and early 1940s, widespread outbreaks were reported of an acute, self-limited respiratory illness that appears to have been clinically identical to mill fever, but that also included chest tightness and cough much like symptoms of byssinosis. But rather than textile mill workers, those affected were poor rural families making mattresses for personal use from surplus, low-grade, stained cotton provided by a federally sponsored program.

"With our current knowledge, staining would be indicative of microbial growth on that cotton," says Castellan. "And on subsequent investigation, it was found that this cotton was highly contaminated, much more than it normally is, with an enterobacter species, a gram negative bacteria." The U.S. Public Health Service investigation of this outbreak resulted in the first scientific evidence suggesting that gram negative bacteria or its products are a likely cause of mill fever and possibly also a contributing factor in the etiology of acute and chronic pulmonary effects associated with byssinosis.

Endotoxins have been known to cause profound inflammation of any tissue exposed to them, including lung tissue. "Exposure to endotoxins causes an influx of inflammatory cells into the lungs," says NIOSH immunologist Stephen A. Olenchock. "They bring with them and they release various agents called cytokines, which cause swelling, exudate, or seepage, from blood vessels. These are very potent inflammatory agents."

Initially, the response to endotoxin may seem to be allergic. But unlike allergy, the active component is lipid A, and not an antigenic protein. "This is not an allergy at all," Olenchock explains. "Allergy involves a type of antibody associated with a specific antigen. Here, there is an absence of antibody. Endotoxins activate the complement system, which causes inflammation and then removal of foreign agents."

Occupational inhalation of endotoxins induces fever and constriction of airways. According to Castranova, endotoxins tend to upregulate the activity of lung phagocytes, encouraging pulmonary inflammation. "Many studies seem to show that if you put lung phagocytes in a test tube and add endotoxin, not much happens," he explains. "But if you add endotoxin and then add a second stimulus, the [phagocytic] response to that second stimulus is greater than if the endotoxin weren't there. The second stimulus could be the dust, the particulate matter."

In vitro studies of animal lung phagocytes reveal that endotoxins may initiate this response following a single dose, but decline in ability to do so after multiple doses. Castranova says this may explain the Monday phenomenon in cotton textile workers with byssinosis. "The cells are more responsive to endotoxin given once. After that they downregulate. Their receptors are internalized with the cell wall and are not available to respond again. After a weekend period of no exposure, those receptors are externalized on the cell surface and are ready to respond to endotoxin again."

In the 1980s, controlled experimental exposures of human volunteers to cotton dusts contaminated with endotoxins provided insight into the roles of endotoxins in eliciting acute respiratory responses. Castellan and his colleagues reported a highly correlated relationship between acute changes in pulmonary function and endotoxin concentrations.

Experimental human exposure studies have been aimed at closely mimicking dust conditions experienced by mill workers. These results show decreases in lung function, such as forced expiratory volume (FEV), to be associated more strongly with endotoxin content than with mass exposures of dust. Moreover, studies involving cotton that was washed to lower its endotoxin content showed such cotton dust to be a less potent inducer of airway obstruction.

In one experiment, Castellan and colleagues investigated acute respiratory responses (FEV) to a wide range of cotton dust types— cotton raised in different parts of the country and of differing grades. "We note there is a much stronger dose-response relationship using endotoxin as the index of exposure, and in fact, no dose-response relationship [for] gravimetric dust." Gravimetric dust is measured by a device called a vertical elutriator designed to collect lint-free samples of aerodynamic size corresponding to inhaled dust particles deposited at or below an individual's trachea.

Signs and symptoms of respiratory exposures to dusts contaminated with endotoxins have also been reported for grain workers and those involved in animal production, including swine and poultry.

Attempting to identify the role of endotoxin in grain dust-induced lung disease, Schwartz and his colleagues conducted a population-based, cross-sectional investigation comparing a cohort of grain handlers and postal workers in eastern Iowa. After controlling for age, gender, and cigarette-smoking status, the researchers found that occupational exposure to grain dust was associated with acute and chronic respiratory symptoms, objective measures of diminished airflow, and enhanced bronchial reactivity (hyperresponsiveness). While it wasn't shown that endotoxin causes airway disease in grain handlers, airway disease appeared to be more pronounced in those exposed to higher concentrations of airborne endotoxin in the work setting.

"Other exposures associated with microbial contamination of grain dust may be involved here," Schwartz says. "Endotoxin may serve as a good surrogate marker for the more pathogenic components. We don't know whether it's the cause, but it seems to be."

In studying workers in swine confinement buildings, which are minimally ventilated, Schwartz found decreases in lung function that were independently associated with greater cross-shift changes (a measure of a worker's respiratory function over a specific workshift) in FEV and higher concentrations of airborne endotoxins. Moreover, acute declines in lung airflow across the workshift and higher concentrations of endotoxin were linked to accelerated declines in airflow during the period of observation, about two years. According to Schwartz, this indicates that acute airway responses are predictive of chronic changes in airflow.

Animal models have been developed that mimic the fever and acute pulmonary response reactions to organic dust inhalation. These studies have also exhibited a strong correlation between endotoxin levels and lung responses to organic dusts, including grain and cotton dusts. Schwartz used genetic strains of endotoxin-sensitive and endotoxin-resistant mice to perform corn dust inhalation studies. Endotoxin-sensitive mice showed a more profound inflammatory response in the lower respiratory tract to inhaled corn dust than the endotoxin-resistant mice. Endotoxin-sensitive mice that were made tolerant to endotoxins showed a significantly diminished inflammatory response to inhaled corn dust.

In experiments with guinea pigs, in which airway reactivity to organic dust closely mimics that of humans, Castranova demonstrated that changes in breathing pattern—the "Monday accentuation" response—depended on the endotoxin content of cellulose, which when untreated with endotoxin did not alter respiratory responses in the animals.

"In general, more work needs to be done with animal models," Castranova says. "The importance of various mediators has been brought out, including tumor necrosis factor, a product of lung phagocytes. If one gives the animal antibody to that, so that it's no longer active, the animal's acute pulmonary response to organic dust is mitigated."

Beyond the Tip of the Iceberg

The interaction between environmental and physiological factors may play a significant role in exposure to organic dusts, but the specifics remain to be clarified. As Schenker observes, "The determinants of the hypersensitivity pneumonitis response remain poorly understood. Initiation [of this response] in farmers who may have had similar exposures for years without pulmonary problems is unexplained."

Cigarette smoking is associated with diminished lung function responses to cotton and grain dusts, but the prevalence of hypersensitivity pneumonitis is higher in nonsmokers than in smokers. Some investigators point to cigarette-mediated immune alterations such as reduced cytokine production by lung macrophages. Others suggest that smokers are generally less susceptible to irritants, which may be a factor in why they smoke.

Clarification of environment and host interactions is often complicated by another element: "the healthy worker effect." Rates of long-term ill effects may be reduced because of early departure of sensitized workers from an industry. In grain workers, for example, smoking, mite allergy, and nonspecific bronchial hyperreactivity may increase departure rates.

Studies in the cotton industry have shown that mill workers may still have accelerated declines in lung function related to cotton dust in the absence of symptoms characteristic of the Monday syndrome. "To many of us, that's not surprising," says Castellan. "The more we study the phenomena of occupational respiratory disease, the more we realize that the gross symptoms and gross findings are the tip of the iceberg. There's much more going on in terms of very subtle effects."

Minimizing Health Risks

Prevention, ventilation, and avoidance of exposures appear to be key recommendations for workers facing occupational health risks from agricultural dusts. According to some authorities, primary prevention through dust control, though more readily applicable in some agricultural industries such as cotton, is difficult elsewhere. "Dust presents a challenge because of its ubiquity," says Schenker.

In many situations there are steps that can effectively prevent dust generation," he said. Some of the steps he outlines for specific work practices include reducing levels of microorganisms in cut grasses to be used for feed or bedding via adequate drying in the field before baling, adding fat to the diet of animals in confinement facilities and using covered feed troughs filled through enclosed spouts to reduce ambient dust levels, capping silage materials to reduce spoilage, and pouring a quart of water on the cut surface of a hay bale prior to use in a bedding chopper, which can reduce dust levels by 85%.

In terms of ventilation, NIOSH recommends local exhaust ventilation for barns and confinement houses. *NIOSH Alert,* an agency publication, advises agricultural workers and employers on a number of practices aimed at minimizing risk of exposure to dusts, including wearing respirators with the highest assigned protection factor. In accordance with the OSHA respiratory protection standard, employers must train and monitor personnel in the use of respiratory protection equipment, as well as how to maintain, inspect, store, and clean it.

Cotton dust is the only specific agricultural dust that currently has an OSHA standard, although the main regulatory requirements apply only to regulated cotton industries and processes. Growing, harvesting, ginning, classing, warehousing, and knitting of cotton are not currently regulated. Handling and processing of woven or knitted cotton fabrics are also not regulated. Several different exposure limits ranging from 200 g/m3 to 750 g/m3 apply in textile mill operations. The cotton dust standard also requires medical examinations for new employees as well as periodic monitoring for all workers exposed to cotton dust. OSHA also has a standard for nonspecific dusts: 15 g/m3 for total dust and 5 g/m3 for respirable dust.

Future Needs

The extent of risks associated with dust exposures needs to be refined. Specific agents within agricultural dusts that are responsible for toxic and immunologic responses remain in question, as do methods for quantifying these components. Research is also needed to elucidate susceptibilities to these exposures. And more work is needed in the area of education and intervention to develop sound strategies aimed at preventing acute and chronic respiratory symptoms for a widespread and varied population of agricultural workers.

—by Leslie Lang

Chapter 35

Latex Allergy

"Latex is the allergen of the '90s. We simply can't afford to sensitize and potentially lose a large segment of our highly trained, well-paid health care professionals," says Kevin J. Kelly, M.D., Director of Pediatric Allergy and Immunology at Children's Hospital of Wisconsin in Milwaukee. "I've seen physicians, surgeons, nurses, laboratory technicians, and researchers develop such severe occupational asthma that they become totally disabled professionally."

Latex allergy is an unexpected result of the adoption of universal precautions against infectious diseases in recent years. Because products manufactured from the milky sap of *Hevea brasiliensis* are impermeable to transmissible viruses—especially HIV and hepatitis—the demand for them has increased exponentially. Latex now is ubiquitous in the health care environment and is used in dressings, catheters,

Excerpted from "Latex Allergy: Potentially Disabling," by Nancy Walsh D'Epiro, in *Patient Care,* Vol. 30, No. 3, February 15, 1996, pp.32-4. © 1996 by Medical Economics Publishing Co., Five Paragon Dr., Montvale, NJ 07645-1742. Reprinted with permission. Excerpted from "Latex Allergies Stretch beyond Rubber Gloves," in *Environmental Health Perspectives,* Vol. 104, No. 9 [Online] September 1996. Available: http://ehpnet1.niehs.nih.gov/docs/1996/104-9/forum.html. Produced by the National Institute of Environmental Health Science (NIEHS), National Institutes of Health (NIH). Excerpted from "NIOSH Alert: Preventing Allergic Reactions to Natural Rubber Latex in the Workplace," Publication No. 97-135 [Online] June 1997. Available: http://www.cdc.gov/niosh/latexalt.html. Produced by the U.S. Department of Health and Human Services (HHS). For complete contact information, please refer to Chapter 68, "Resources."

tapes, and, most notably, protective gloves. Before the adoption of universal precautions, an estimated 300 million gloves were used annually. This figure has grown to 9.6 billion per year.

The initial manifestation of latex allergy is an urticarial condition that develops on the hands, often after an initial contact dermatitis that may break down the skin barrier. In up to 50% of exposed persons, however, the condition also affects the respiratory tract. This occurs because high concentrations of powder on latex gloves become airborne and are inhaled by workers in hospitals and clinics. The result can be severe rhinoconjunctivitis, asthma, and anaphylaxis. Fatalities have occurred.

Approximately 15-17% of health care workers are now thought to be sensitized to latex, and many of them manifesting occupational asthma may have permanent respiratory sequelae that force them to leave their jobs. Anaphylaxis may occur in 5-10% of allergic persons.

Gloves causing asthma? Some unusual operating room events in the early 1990s helped researchers make the connection.

Wisconsin, 1991: Anaphylaxis during Surgery

The first report of contact urticaria involving rubber products appeared in 1979, and a scattering of further cases was seen throughout Europe in the 1980s. Then, in 1991, some unexpected events occurred. One was at Children's Hospital of Wisconsin, where an unexplained epidemic of anaphylactic reactions occurred during surgery.[1] Another took place at Henry Ford Hospital in Detroit, where a number of allergic reactions—including fatalities—were associated with barium enemas. Other children's hospitals were reporting similar unexplained incidents.

Dr. Kelly, who is also Associate Professor of Pediatrics at the Medical College of Wisconsin, Milwaukee, explains what happened at his hospital: "During a 6-7-month period in 1991, there were 12 episodes of anaphylaxis in our operating room. The likelihood of anaphylaxis during surgery ranges from 1 in 5,000 to 1 in 15,000. In a hospital such as ours, where we do about 7,500 operations each year, you might expect one case. In fact, the previous year, we had none."

Specialists from the Centers for Disease Control and Prevention (CDC) went to Milwaukee to help determine the cause of the epidemic. They reviewed the types of surgical procedures and the patient populations involved. This analysis revealed that 11 of the 12 reactions occurred in patients with spina bifida—yet only 152 operations out of the 7,500 involved this patient group. Because of the extremely high statistical connection between spina bifida and anaphylaxis during surgery, the CDC and FDA ordered a moratorium on elective surgery for children with spina bifida until the cause of the problem could be identified. It was a year before the latex connection was found.

Two years earlier there had been a report of two cases of latex allergy in children with spina bifida at Children's National Medical Center in Washington, D.C.[2] This prompted Dr. Kelly and his colleagues to consider the possibility of latex sensitization occurring during surgery. They found that 68% of all spina bifida patients in southeast Wisconsin were indeed sensitized to latex. "These children were being sensitized to latex very early in life, in numerous procedures exposing mucosal surfaces to the antigen," Dr. Kelly explains.

Young children with spina bifida typically undergo surgery at least twice a year because of the numerous genitourinary, neurologic, and orthopedic problems associated with the condition. Born with myelomeningocele [protrusion of the membranes of the brain or spinal cord through a defect in the skull or spinal column], most of these children undergo two surgical procedures during the first week of life, one to repair the spinal abnormality and the second to insert a shunt for hydrocephalus. This early and repeated exposure to latex during surgery resulted in an extremely high incidence of sensitization.

Diagnosis: Clues and Hazards

Identifying the patient with latex allergy, particularly with symptoms of asthma, requires an awareness of the magnitude of the problem in the health care environment affecting both patients and workers. It's quite likely that patient groups other than children with spina bifida also are at risk if they undergo multiple procedures that allow contact with latex. Anyone who exhibits any allergic symptoms during surgery should be tested for latex hypersensitivity. So should any health care worker who complains of symptoms ranging from urticaria on the hands to severe and worsening asthma that appears to have a temporal relation to the workplace.

Serologic testing can be done easily in the primary care office, with results available in about a week. Several tests are available, and one has recently been approved by the FDA (Alastat Latex-Specific IgE Allergen Test Kit, Diagnostic Products Corp., Los Angeles). The sensitivity of these tests is limited, however—10-20% of positive results may be missed. More specific tests are available through reference laboratories, and a negative result in light of a strong history and clinical suspicion may warrant further investigation and referral to an allergist.

331

A standardized skin test extract has not yet been made commercially available, and improvised in-office challenge testing is highly undesirable. Because the antigen is water-soluble and easily washes out of the gloves, some clinicians have attempted skin testing with a saline solution into which a latex glove has been immersed. Others have tested by having the patient actually try on a wet glove. These practices are potentially dangerous and have led to systemic reactions. Any challenge testing for latex allergy should be done by specialists under carefully controlled conditions.

A curious but important diagnostic clue involves the phenomenon of cross-reactivity. Some persons with latex allergy also experience a positive response to several food substances, most notably bananas and other tropical fruits such as kiwi and passion fruit. Chestnuts and pitted fruits such as peaches and cherries also have been implicated. It is not yet known if some unidentified proteins in these foods that are similar to those present in latex are responsible.

Investigators have suggested that certain chemicals and enzymes sprayed on rubber trees to preserve the sap until it can be processed may be involved. Others also suggest that chemicals used as antioxidants and accelerants in rubber processing may contribute to the initial development of dermatitis.[3] In vitro reactivity doesn't necessarily translate into clinical reactivity, however, and immunologists are still investigating the nature and variability of the cross-reactivity seen with latex and certain foods. Until the connection is clarified, Dr. Kelly advises presuming a latex allergy in anyone who is exposed frequently to latex and exhibits an allergic reaction to one of these fruits, because true allergy to them is uncommon.

Looking for a Solution

Some have suggested that the burgeoning demand for latex gloves spurred by the AIDS epidemic was accompanied by changes in manufacturing practices intended to meet the increased demand but which inadvertently resulted in increased antigenicity. The manufacturers deny substantial changes in practice, however, according to Dr. Kelly. "And unfortunately," he says, "the question probably won't be solved in a scientific forum, but in a court of law." A number of individual and class-action product-liability suits have been filed against latex manufacturers, similar to those involving silicone breast implants.

While no one doubts the benefits of latex in protecting against infectious diseases, the magnitude of the latex allergy problem now is forcing some hard questions to be asked. Should the universal use of latex gloves be rethought? Dr. Kelly suggests that consideration be given to man-made alternatives with less antigenic potential, such as vinyl. He acknowledges that vinyl is more permeable than latex and is therefore a less effective barrier against HIV and hepatitis, but he points out that permeability does not necessarily translate into infection. Wearing gloves is imperfect protection: Latex won't stop needlesticks. "We have no proof that health care workers wearing other types of gloves would actually become infected at a greater rate than those wearing latex gloves," he observes.

Low-allergen gloves and alternatives for some other products are now available, and a Compendium of Non-Latex Gloves was published by the Medical Devices Bureau, Health Protection Branch, Health Canada, in July 1994 [See below, "Latex in the Air"]. Until a broad solution to the problem is found, however, the American Academy of Allergy, Asthma and Immunology recommends the following guidelines for preventing latex sensitization:[4]

- Patients in high-risk groups should be identified.

- All patients, regardless of risk group status, should be questioned about a history of latex allergy.

- All high-risk patients should be offered testing for latex allergy.

- Procedures on all patients with spina bifida should be performed in an environment free of latex—one in which no latex gloves are used by any personnel. In addition, there should be no latex accessories (catheters, adhesives, tourniquets, anesthesia equipment) that come into direct contact with the patient.

- Procedures on all patients with a positive history, regardless of risk group status, should be performed in an environment free of latex.

- Low-risk patients with no history of latex allergy are extremely unlikely to react to latex. At this time, routine testing is not recommended for such persons.

- Patients identified as latex-allergic by history or testing should be advised to obtain a Medic Alert bracelet and self-injectable epinephrine.

Latex in the Air

With the number of latex allergies jumping from a single case report in 1979 to 6.5% of Americans in 1994, it would seem that latex is dropping from the sky. A report in the January 1995 issue of the *Journal of Allergy and Clinical Immunology* and a followup article in the March 1996 issue of *Chest* find that urban air does contain latex particles, shed into the environment by normal tire wear.

Along a four-lane road in Denver, Colorado, a team from the Allergy Respiratory Institute of Colorado led by immunologist Brock Williams collected particulate air pollution. Their samples included black fragments containing latex proteins, which were recognized in tests by human antibodies to latex. More than half (58%) of the airborne debris was small enough to be inhaled into the lungs. Airborne latex could partially explain the rise in latex sensitization. "Until we know more about it," says Williams, "it's difficult to weigh the importance of airborne latex to the overall problem. But it's probably in every city in the world with cars."

Because 57 latex proteins are known allergens, removing them is impractical. So is avoiding rubber, which is found in 40,000 items, including 300 medical products [See below, "Products Containing Latex"]. To circumvent latex allergies, USDA researchers at the Western Regional Research Center in Albany, California, have developed hypoallergenic rubber from guayule (Parthenium argentatum), a shrub native to the southwestern United States. In clinical trials to be published in the *Journal of Allergy and Immunology*, people allergic to Hevea latex do not react to guayule.

The USDA team, headed by plant physiologist Katrina Cornish, created processing methods to extract guayule and manufacture rubber products with superior resilience, strength, and elasticity. The USDA granted an exclusive license for the patented technology to American Medical Products in Burlingame, California. The first guayule products will be medical supplies for latex-sensitive patients and medical workers. Cornish is continuing genetic studies to improve latex yields and adapt guayule for growth in diverse climates.

Products Containing Latex

A wide variety of products contain latex: medical supplies, personal protective equipment, and numerous household objects. Most people who encounter latex products only through their general use in society have no health problems from the use of these products. Workers who repeatedly use latex products are the focus of this Alert. The following are examples of products that may contain latex:

Emergency Equipment

Blood pressure cuffs
Stethoscopes
Disposable gloves
Oral and nasal airways
Endotracheal tubes

Tourniquets
Intravenous tubing
Syringes
Electrode pads

Personal Protective Equipment

Gloves
Surgical masks
Goggles

Respirators
Rubber aprons

Office Supplies

Rubber bands

Erasers

Hospital Supplies

Anesthesia masks
Catheters
Wound drains

Injection ports
Rubber tops of multidose vials
Dental dams

Household Objects

Automobile tires
Motorcycle and bicycle handgrips
Carpeting
Swimming goggles
Racquet handles
Shoe soles
Expandable fabric (waistbands)

Dishwashing gloves
Hot water bottles
Condoms
Diaphragms
Balloons
Pacifiers
Baby bottle nipples

Individuals who already have latex allergy should be aware of latex-containing products that may trigger an allergic reaction. Some of the listed products are available in latex-free forms.

References

1. Kelly K, Sitlock M, Davis JP: Anaphylactic reactions during general anesthesia among pediatric patients—United States, January 1990-January 1991. *MMWR* 1991;40:437-443.

2. Slater JE: Rubber anaphylaxis. *N Engl J Med* 1989;320:1126-1130.

3. Sussman GL, Beezhold DH: Allergy to latex rubber. *Ann Intern Med* 1995;122:43-46.

4. Task Force on Allergic Reactions to Latex: Committee report. *J Allergy Clin Immunol* 1993;92:16-18.

Chapter 36

Food and Asthma

While allergy to pollen or other outdoor sources typically causes a lot of discomfort during spring, summer, and fall, food allergy is one condition that knows no season. Surveys show that approximately one in three adults believe they have a food allergy. The reality is that true food allergy actually affects less than two percent of adults, or approximately 5 million Americans, according to the National Institutes of Health.

People tend to diagnose themselves, believing they have allergic reactions to certain foods or food ingredients. Unfortunately, self-diagnosis of food allergy often leads to unnecessary food restrictions. In some cases, it can be life-threatening because some symptoms that occur after eating may be caused by medical conditions other than food allergy. Therefore, experts urge people to see a board-certified allergist for proper diagnosis of food allergy.

What Is a Food Allergy?

A food allergy is an adverse reaction to a food or food component that involves the body's immune system. There are some adverse reactions to foods that involve the body's metabolism but not the immune

Excerpted from "Backgrounder—Food Allergy/Asthma," and "Everything You Need to Know about Asthma and Food," [Online] 1997, 1998. Available: http://ificinfo.health.org. Produced by the International Food Information Council Foundation, 1100 Connecticut Ave. NW, Ste. 430, Washington, DC 20036. Reprinted with permission. For complete contact information, please refer to Chapter 68, "Resources."

system. These reactions are known as food intolerance. Examples of food intolerance are food poisoning or the inability to properly digest certain food components such as lactose, or milk sugar.

A true allergic reaction to a food involves three primary components:

1. contact with food allergens (reaction-provoking substance, usually protein);

2. immunoglobulin E (IgE—antibody in the immune system that reacts with allergens); and

3. mast cells (tissue cells) and basophils (blood cells), which when connected to IgE antibodies release histamine or other substances causing allergic symptoms.

The body's immune system recognizes an allergen in the food as foreign and produces antibodies to halt the "invasion." As the battle rages, symptoms appear throughout the body. The most common sites are the mouth (swelling of the lips), digestive tract (stomach cramps, vomiting, diarrhea), skin (hives, rashes, or eczema), and the airways (wheezing or breathing problems).

Allergic reactions to food are rare and can be caused by any food. However, the most common food allergens are fish, shellfish, milk, egg, soy, wheat, peanuts, and tree nuts such as walnuts. Symptoms of a food allergy are highly individual and usually begin within minutes to a few hours after eating the offending food. People with food allergies must avoid the offending food altogether.

There are some misconceptions regarding allergy to food additives and preservatives. Although some additives and preservatives have been shown to trigger asthma or hives in certain people, these reactions are not the same as those reactions observed with food. These reactions do not involve the immune system and therefore are examples of food intolerance rather than food allergy. Most Americans consume a wide variety of food additives daily, with only a small number having been associated with adverse reactions.

What Are Major Triggers of Asthma?

There are many factors that can trigger an asthma attack:

- Upper respiratory infections
- Weather changes
- Allergens from dust, molds, pollen, animals, and occasionally food

- Exercise
- Environmental irritants such as cigarette smoke, auto exhaust, smog, or cleaners
- Emotions
- Early morning
- Certain medications
- Sulfites and sulfiting agents—sulfur dioxide, sodium bisulfite, potassium bisulfite, sodium metabisulfite, potassium metabisulfite, and sodium sulfite.

Where Are Sulfites Found?

Sulfites or sulfiting agents, both occurring naturally or used in food processing, have been found to trigger asthma. If sulfites are used in food preparation or processing as a preservative agent, you will find them listed on the food label. Common food sources of sulfites include:

- dried fruits or vegetables
- potatoes (some packaged and prepared)
- wine, beer
- bottled lemon or lime juice
- shrimp (fresh, frozen, or prepared)
- pickled foods, such as pickles, relishes, peppers, or sauerkraut (some)

Do Other Food Ingredients Trigger Asthma?

Other food ingredients have been previously suspected to trigger asthma. However, scientific evaluation has not been able to conclusively link these food components to asthma. They include tartrazine (and other food dyes or colorings); benzoates (food and drug preservative); BHA and BHT (food preservatives); monosodium glutamate (MSG, flavor enhancer); aspartame (NutraSweet™, intense sweetener); and nitrate and nitrite (food preservatives).

Life-Threatening Reactions

Most allergic reactions to food are relatively mild. However, a small percentage of food-allergic individuals have severe reactions, called anaphylaxis, that can be life-threatening. Anaphylaxis is a rare but potentially fatal condition in which several different parts of the body experience food-allergic reactions simultaneously, causing hives, swelling of the throat, and difficulty breathing. It is the most severe allergic reaction to an allergen.

Symptoms usually appear rapidly, sometimes within minutes of exposure to the allergen. Because they can be life-threatening, immediate medical attention is necessary when an anaphylactic reaction occurs. Standard emergency treatment often includes an injection of epinephrine (adrenaline) to open up the airway and blood vessels.

Diagnosing Food Allergy

Diagnosis usually begins with a thorough medical history, a complete physical examination, and selected tests to rule out underlying medical conditions not related to food allergy. Patients may also have to keep a food diary and record symptoms over a period of time.

Several tests are available to determine if a person is allergic to a certain food. In skin-prick testing, a diluted extract of the suspected food is placed on the skin, which is scratched or punctured. A blood test can provide similar information as that obtained by skin testing. The "gold" standard for food allergy testing is the double-blind, placebo-controlled food challenge (DBPCFC). This test is performed by a board-certified allergist. The suspected allergen (e.g., milk, fish, soy) is placed in a capsule or hidden in food, and fed to the patient under strict supervision. Neither the allergist, nor the patient, is aware of which capsule, or food, contains the suspected allergen-hence the name "double-blind." For the test to be effective, the patient must also be fed capsules or food which do not contain the allergen to make sure the observed reaction, if any, is to the allergen and not to some other factor—hence the name "placebo-controlled." These tests have enabled allergists to identify the most common allergens, and also to determine what foods and additives do not cause allergic reactions.

What Can You Do to Prevent Asthma Triggered by Foods?

The best way to avoid food-induced or aggravated asthma is by avoiding or eliminating the food or food ingredient from your diet or the environment. Remember that these substances can be both released into the air or consumed when eating or drinking.

Reading ingredient labels on food packages and knowing where food triggers are found in foods are your best protections against an asthma attack. By working with your physician on a care plan and proper use of medications, you will be prepared to act in case of an asthma attack.

Other Resources

Asthma and Allergy Foundation of America
1233 20th Street, NW, Suite 402
Washington, DC 20036
1-800-7-ASTHMA

Food Allergy Network
10400 Eaton Pl., Ste. 107
Fairfax, VA 22030-2208
1-800-929-4040
http://www.foodallergy.org

Chapter 37

Risk Factors Associated with Fatal Asthma Attacks in Children

The number of children dying from their asthma is increasing. The death rate for asthmatics 5-24 years old nearly doubled, from 1980 to 1993. The still unanswered question is "Why?" With all the new medicines available and our greater understanding of the disease process, the death rate should be falling.

Children who die from asthma fall into two scenarios. The most common scenario is the child who arrives for care too late. The symptoms have been present for hours or even days, getting progressively worse. Yet treatment is delayed. Prompter treatment would have saved their lives.

In the second scenario, children have a sudden and severe attack without any warning. Sometimes even the quickest of treatments doesn't make any difference.

Doctors at the Washington University School of Medicine, St. Louis, MO, investigated the possible causes of the delay in seeking treatment. What happens all too often is that the parents don't pay attention to their children who have severe asthma. Family discord or conflict interferes with good care and recognizing when symptoms are worsening.

From "Asthma Deaths," produced by the Immunology and Allergy Clinics of North America (June 1998), in *Pediatrics for Parents,* January 1999, p.1. © 1999 by Pediatrics for Parents Inc., 747 S. 3rd St., Philadelphia, PA 19147-3324. Reprinted with permission.

There are a number of family problems that may interfere with good asthma care including recent loss of a loved one, alcoholism, unemployment, spousal abuse, etc.

Certain factors increase the risk a child will have a fatal asthma attack:

- Poor family support for ongoing and acute care
- A history of a near fatal attack
- Recent hospitalization despite proper medications
- Denial by the child of the severity of his/her disease
- Poor understanding of the disease
- Difficulty in accessing immediate medical care
- Depression over how the asthma interferes with his/her life
- Poor control of their asthma

The study found three basic steps that can help reduce the risk of death.

1. Educate both the family and the child about the disease and its potentially serious consequences

2. Establish a medical regime that controls the asthma

3. Determine if the child is at high risk for dying from asthma

It's important to determine how effective the asthma treatment is. Pulmonary function tests are one way to monitor a child's respiratory status. Also important are the degree the child participates in school activities and how many absences are due to the asthma.

Chapter 38

Access to Asthma Health Care by African American Families

Today there is much discussion about access to health care for vulnerable populations such as children or members of at-risk ethnic groups. Aday stated, "Access implies that people have a place to go and the financial and other means of obtaining care. The way services are organized and the methods that exist to pay for them may not always facilitate either entry or continuity, however." (p.180)[1] Families in a pilot study reported in this article shared their experiences regarding access to health care.

This article focuses on a vulnerable group of African American families who have children with a chronic illness. Families' perspectives of access to health care for asthma are described. Asthma is "the most common chronic illness affecting children in the U.S. . . . The prevalence increased 33% between 1981 and 1988 . . . for all children younger than 18 years of age." (p.56)[2] Despite increasing mortality rates among white children, African American children still had a higher prevalence of asthma in 1988.[3] Betz[4] analyzed ethnic representation in pediatric nursing research and found a lack of diversity among populations studied. In most studies the sample size of African Americans was small and therefore statistically insignificant so that findings are contextualized in the dominant culture.

From "Access to Health Care: Perspectives of African American Families with Chronically Ill Children," (Vulnerable Population, part 1), by Jane W. Peterson, Yvonne M. Sterling, and DeLois P. Weekes, in *Family and Community Health,* January 1997, Vol. 19, No. 4, pp. 64-75. © 1997 by Aspen Publishers, Inc., 200 Orchard Ridge Dr., Gaithersburg, MD 20878. Reprinted with permission.

This article discusses African Americans within their own families and communities. The discussion centers around general beliefs and behaviors of the family that affect and are affected by the chronic illness of a child. The intent is to give voice to their viewpoint and advocate inclusion of their perspective as an integral part of a health assessment. This should lead to greater collaboration in the selection of interventions by health care providers and clients. Increased utilization of health care at appropriate primary, secondary, and tertiary levels is more likely with this more collaborative approach leading to positive health outcomes for the population. Advocacy is a strategy for enhancing health care. Families would feel they "had a place to go." (p.180)[1]

Literature Review

National and international attention has recently been drawn to the plight of African American children in the United States. The United Nations Development Programme (UNDP) introduced a human development index (HDI) to assess, compare, and provide choices on human development in any country. This index "combines indicators of real purchasing power, education, and health [which offer] a measure of development much more comprehensive than GNP [gross national product] alone." (p.10)[5] According to this index, black (African American) children in the United States are disadvantaged from birth and rank 31st in the world, while the white population in the United States ranks first. One factor that contributes to this disparity, according to Thomas,[6] is lack of access to health services. Davidson and associates,[7] in their study on access to care for 170 asthma patients ages 2 to 17, found that black and Hispanic patients and patients on Medicaid used the emergency room more, without first calling their doctor or clinic, than did white patients. Shields and associates[8] tried a specific education program at a Chicago health maintenance organization (HMO) to reduce this pattern of emergency room utilization among 253 primarily low-income black children with asthma but failed to change their pattern. The researchers attributed this to their failure to target the education program to the specific population and their not increasing knowledge about behavior change while increasing knowledge about asthma.

Evans[9] summarized the lack of access to health care among minority children with asthma. He found the following reasons for problems with access:

- no hospital in the area, poor transportation system,

- lack of care for well children while caring for the ill child,
- long clinic and hospital waiting times,
- inconvenient hours of service,
- problems understanding the language, and
- lack of money to pay for service or treatment.

Bosco and associates found that even if access problems were eliminated, in the treatment of childhood asthma "the black urban patient continued to receive less effective therapy with fixed-combination products well after these products had been abandoned in other groups of Medicaid patients." (p.1,731)[10] Thus, access to health care might result in different patterns of service and less effective therapy received by this population.

Asthma is a leading cause of disability in people younger than 17 years of age.[10] It "is frequently misdiagnosed or undertreated and causes more hospital admissions, more visits to hospital emergency rooms and more school absences than any other chronic disease in childhood." (p.1)[11] Hospitalization, morbidity, and mortality rates have all increased for asthma patients. The population most affected appears to be nonwhite children living in urban areas and the poor.[2, 12] Death rates among children 5 to 14 years are 0.7 per 100,000 population for black children and 0.1 per 100,000 for white children.[9] In 1987, black males 5 to 34 years old had a mortality rate five times higher than white patients of both sexes.[12] The prevalence of asthma was 150 times greater for black children than for others during the period 1965 to 1984.[13] A review of hospital admissions for children with status asthmaticus revealed most patients to be young black males.[14] Between 1981 and 1988, the incidence rate for asthma increased more in white than black children, and black children still had a higher prevalence rate in 1988.[3]

What emerges from the literature are high asthma rates for hospitalization, morbidity, and mortality among black children. However, the underlying causes for these findings are not precisely understood. It is not clear whether race or socioeconomic status or an interaction among multiple factors is responsible for the high morbidity and mortality rates.[15, 16] It may be that a complex interaction among socioeconomic status, inner-city problems, family adaptive patterns, social support, cultural beliefs, physical environment, and the health care delivery system has unique and combined effects on the vulnerability of black children.[12, 17] Newacheck[18] concluded that chronic health problems in children from poor families are not adequately addressed by the existing health care system. He found that these children were more likely than children from nonpoor families to not report chronic illnesses, have a higher risk of severe chronic conditions, experience lack of access to care, be uninsured, and lack a usual source of care. Black children have differential vulnerability[1] reflected by their multiple cumulative risk factors, indicating that a disease such as asthma will hurt them more than others.

It appears that black children perceive illness through their cultural lens and are influenced by multiple factors. Health care providers view illness through their professional lens and focus mainly on the disease process and health restoration. A mediator could bridge these two views. Cultural brokering or mediating[19-22] between family and health care provider would help clarify the perspectives of both and the impact of low socioeconomic status and cultural beliefs on a family's access to health care. A cultural broker can "interpret expectations based on beliefs, values, and traditions, clarify issues, and provide a common understanding between two groups." (p.71)[19] Cultural brokering is an outcome of this study, which asked the question, what are the experiences of black families with a chronically ill child? The ethnographic study design allowed families to share their views as they relate to access to health care services, or "gettin' help" as one mother put it.

Method

This study used an ethnographic design. Ethnography "is the work of describing culture" (p.3)[23] and makes explicit the meaning of events and actions of the people being studied. Participant observation and interviews were carried out by three African American nurse researchers living in the cities in which the study was conducted. This ensured that the language used by African Americans was faithfully recorded and interpreted within their cultural context. Purposeful sampling was done by obtaining families who had experience with children with asthma and were of African American ethnicity. Families were obtained through outpatient or community health clinics in Seattle, New Orleans, and the San Francisco Bay Area.

Seven families with a child diagnosed with asthma are discussed in this article. Three were from Seattle and two each from the other cities. A total of 11 contacts occurred. Four families were contacted twice and three families only once due to cancelled appointments. Most visits were held in the family's home, with a few in a clinic or an office. The mean age of the children was 11.3 years; the youngest was 5 and the oldest 17. There were four girls and three boys. The seven key informants, all adult women, were the primary caregivers. Six of the caregivers were the mothers (including one foster mother) and one was a paternal grandmother. These women ranged from 31 to 46 years of age, with a mean age of 37. Four women were married and lived with their spouses, while three were single mothers. Two women worked full time, two worked part time, and three were not employed outside the home. One of the women, not employed, had taken what she termed an early "medical retirement" due to her own problems with asthma. Although interviews were conducted mainly with the caregivers, three of the children and one maternal grandmother who was not a primary caregiver participated in the interviews. Each family had a history of asthma. Two of the key informants reported that they had never been responsible for the care of a person with asthma before caring for the child in this study.

All interviews were audiotaped and notes were made. Interview material was transcribed and identifying material removed. Families were referred to by codes, and informants, health care facilities, and health care providers were given pseudonyms to maintain confidentiality. All informants signed consent forms. The researchers met face to face prior to, during, and after data collection to plan, review, and analyze data as a team. Second interviews with four of the families allowed the researcher to validate impressions with the family and receive feedback from them. Families commented on how much they appreciated this and sought to clarify points they thought the researcher misunderstood.

Analysis

All families studied were concerned about the health of their children. Parents or health care providers reported that all children had been diagnosed with asthma by a physician. From the family's perspective, "gettin' help" meant getting the health care they wanted and found acceptable from the health care system. Despite spending time, energy, and family resources the results were not always successful.

The families' perspectives comprised four distinct categories:

1. getting health care that is wanted—three families;

2. getting health care that is unwanted—two families;

3. not getting health care that is wanted—one family; and

4. not getting health care that is unwanted—one family.

Getting Health Care That Is Wanted

The three families who were able to get the health care they wanted did so by negotiating with the system, using the system on their own terms, or joining the system.

Case 1. Eddy is a 10-year-old boy who was diagnosed with asthma at 3 months. He lives with his mother, father, and younger sister. Both parents work. However, his mother lost her full-time job and thus her family health benefits due to her many absences from work to care for her son. She now has a part-time job in food services, but no health benefits. This family has been able to negotiate with the health care system to obtain care for Eddy. The mother recounts that when she felt that she was not being heard, and therefore unable to negotiate for health care, she switched health care facilities.

> At Mercy Hospital . . . From the time they diagnosed him with the asthma, he's been going every Monday for approximately 4 years, taking two shots, and that's to determine, to try to slow the asthma down. At their determining that his condition looked like it wasn't going to get no better at Mercy Hospital, I switched him to Children's Hospital under the care of Dr. Thomas. Since going to Children's he's improved, he don't go every Monday, he go every 3 months now. The medication has increased, they put him on Provental, and they put him on a steroid tablet at night so he has to take that every night.

This mother considered moving closer to the hospital. "We were constantly going to Mercy, it was like every other day, it was like let's move closer to Mercy, 'cause the child just couldn't make it." The family has strong support from family members and friends who help them decide what actions to take. These people also sanctioned health care decisions. This is evident when Eddy's mother states, "Until one day a friend of mine told me to contact respiratory. I did. I got the machine for him, it prevented me from having to go to the hospital as much, now I only go to the hospital with him if for some reason that he's having an attack . . . where the machine don't do him no good."

This mother was able to advocate for her child and herself. After losing her health benefits, she applied for a medical card for her son, but was told that he was too old to qualify. She pursued this issue on her son's behalf:

I went through social welfare, through CHAMPUS, they denied it. . . . So one day I was . . . trying to call the clinic and I wound up getting the governor's office. So I spoke to the people at the governor's office, I told them that the child is an asthmatic patient and I was depending on getting the [medical] card for him for his medicine, because I could not afford to pay for his medicine, it's hard. So I went on and talked to somebody in the office and the next month they reinstated his card and I wound up getting his card back for him, that was luck, pure luck.

Thus, this case illustrates how a family obtained the care they wanted by negotiating the system.

Case 2. Derek is a 13-year-old boy diagnosed with asthma at age 3. He lives with his mother who is a secretary at a local university and a younger sister. His older sister is married. His mother's large extended family lives in the area and offers their help when needed. This family uses the health care system on their own terms. For them, the health care delivery system is only one strategy used to maintain Derek's health. His mother views an active life as an essential part of keeping healthy: "What I have done with him is I've kept him real active in sports, push him real hard about running. . . . I'd say maybe once a year he'll have a chiropractic adjustment, but hardly [have] any problems with Derek."

Her feeling toward doctors is clear when she says, "it's just like doctors aren't all that necessary." Her own sense of control and faith keeps her centered, "it is mind over matter, but it's a matter, . . . my children think more on the lines of they know the Lord will heal them." This belief was talked about in terms of an active belief, one that was incorporated into everyday life, the way they lived, the choices they made. "Faith plays a big part in our life now. . . . There is a lot more peace in my life . . . it's just like l don't allow chaos in my house, you know, no matter what form it comes in.

However, this mother readily takes her child to the hospital when she feels he needs to go. She had certain expectations of the health care system and created ways to have these met.

. . . in terms of interacting with hospitals and clinics . . . they are there when you need them. And there's 2,000 people in emergency [room] or something like that—and I'm going to stay there all day? And I just go to the emergency [room] and tell them something fantastic. "My daughter has a snake on her leg. I want somebody to look at it." And of course when children are

351

having problems with asthma, nobody's going to sit in the waiting room. Because I've never had any body make me wait in a waiting room for any length of time for my children if they ever have problems with asthma. Never.

This mother often calls a sister who has a master's degree in nursing for advice when she does not understand health care providers' instructions. "And they [doctors] told me, 'Give him this thing tonight and in the morning give him this other.' And then I called [my sister] and she said, 'Well, go on. You give him the medication, the whole thing and call me in an hour or so.' And then I called her back and she said, 'Well how is he doing'?"

With the support of a relative, this mother was able to care for her child successfully through an illness episode. For the most part, Derek goes to his regular clinic appointments by himself. He has an inhaler, and he has medications that he manages on his own. The case exemplifies a family effectively using the system on their own terms.

Case 3. Arthur is 10 years old. He was diagnosed with asthma at 10 months, "since he got here practically," says his paternal grandmother, who is his primary caregiver. He lives with his grandparents. His mother lives in a different part of the state with her husband and children. His father, who is also married and has children, lives in the same city. The strategy this family uses for getting wanted health care is joining the system. Arthur's grandmother became a respiratory therapist. Talking about herself she says, "I don't work as a respiratory therapist now. . . . I had to retire medically from the post office. . . . See, I worked there for 11 years, and I couldn't take it any more, so then I retired and I was in and out of the hospital all the time, and I just happened to be scanning my hospital bill, and I noticed every time the respiratory therapist came it was $50, right? . . . And I said well, hey, I can do this!"

She worked for a while as a respiratory therapist. She finds that experience "really helpful" in taking care of Arthur. "I have trained Arthur. He can do his own breathing treatments. . . . He knows that when his chest gets tight, what he has to do, and he knows that when there's a cat or something in the house, he knows he shouldn't be there, so he's taking care of himself."

Because of her knowledge, she is able to talk to health care providers using their language:

One particular time we went to the emergency room. He was having a terrible, terrible asthma attack at this particular time, as a matter of fact he wasn't getting any oxygen, OK? . . . What blew me out was I had to tell the doctors, "Look he is not getting any oxygen, you know. He can't breathe. . ." When I let them know that I know what's going on, they sometimes talk to me a little bit different. Because I do know what's going on, they can tell me certain things in medical terms, so I can really understand it. They don't have to use layman language; they can just say what they have to say, and I'll understand it right away.

Her satisfaction with health care is summarized when she says, "Well, the last clinic visit was a very good clinic visit . . . they determine everything and then they make suggestions. They ask me what do I think, and I tell them what I think. Then they tell me what they think, and then we meet somewhere on common ground, and everything, so it works out pretty well."

Getting Health Care That Is Unwanted

Two families expressed concern that the health care they received was not the care they wanted. For one family, health care did not fit what Kleinman[24] called the family's explanatory model of the illness. Explanatory models "offer explanations of sickness and treatment to guide choices among available therapies and therapists and to cast personal and social meaning on the experience of sickness." (p.105)[24] The other family felt so indebted to the health care system that they accepted whatever was suggested even when opposed to the suggestions.

Case 4. Ramona, a 17-year-old girl, has an infant son. They live with Ramona's mother and three younger sisters. Ramona and her husband are separated but he comes to the apartment frequently to help with the baby. Ramona was diagnosed with asthma at age 5. Her dislike of the health care system started at the time of diagnosis and persists to the present. Her dissatisfaction with her health care is closely associated with the family's explanatory model of asthma. Ramona's mother describes asthma in the following way: "When I hear asthma, I picture an old man . . . walking down the street with pee stain hat and pee stain pants real dirty and dandruff collar maybe grease on his pants, maybe a bug or two stuck on it, panhandler with his hand out. This is what asthma reminds me of . . . it is the noise, just the noise. I can handle anything . . . puky old stuff from this old man, but the wheeze. The noise I can't [take]."

Ramona's mother's view of asthma is triggered by the wheezing sound and very much associated with aging.

Even when she was little when she first started wheezing. She was that little old man even then. . . . I didn't see her getting any better, I didn't see any progress whatsoever. The only thing I saw was that she is getting old. And then I saw her heart getting old, her inside parts getting old. So, l figure those are getting old, how could she be getting better? . . . She wouldn't take [her pills] because they would make her heart beat fast. . . . I really did not want her on the pills anyway. Because I felt that if your heart beats . . . twice as fast all the time, that is like speeding up the aging process. I figure her heart is getting really old and by the time she hits 25 or such she'd have a heart attack. This is in the back of my mind, okay? And I figured they just didn't give her good care.

The family's explanatory model also accounted for the fact that Ramona had not grown out of the disease, and to them it did not seem that she was ever going to grow out of it.

The doctor said I should relax and she would grow out of it. I didn't think it was anything permanent. If they had told me it would only last 2 months I could handle that. But years! She may be a teenager, God, I'd be dead. So, this is like sentencing somebody to death row to me, that's torture. They said she could outgrow it anytime, but definitely by the time she is a teenager. . . . I only held onto that [outgrowing asthma] until she was 11 or 12. By that time I knew she was going to have it for life. . . . l didn't see her getting any better. I didn't see any progress whatsoever. The only thing I saw was that she is getting old.

Ramona internalized her mother's explanatory model of asthma. "I feel like an old man. That's how I feel. . . . When you are the oldest child, like me, you have pressure to be doing better than you should be doing. . . . You're suppose to set examples and therefore you can't get sick. . . . Asthma means I am sick. It means you can't be the best you can be because you have a sickness. It means you are different from everybody else. 'Cause you can't do any of the things they can do. And when I think of asthma, I think of medicine."

Ramona's view of asthma impacts decisions she makes in her life. She feels that she has little control and there is little predictability in what happens to her. This case illustrates the explanatory model of asthma as a condition of the aged who cannot care for themselves and of medication hastening that process.

Case 5. Tameka is 13 years old and was diagnosed with asthma at 5 months. Two of her four siblings have asthma. The children live with their mother and maternal grandmother. The mother's sister and only sibling gave her a car to transport the children to and from the doctor. The overall view of this family toward the health care system is indebtedness for having saved Tameka's life. Because of this they accept most suggestions made by health care providers, even those they do not like. "I love City Hospital. [Tameka] likes to go to City, but Mercy Hospital is the one—before they transferred her to City they [Mercy Hospital staff] really, I think, saved her life; 'cause my baby had stopped breathing, twice."

Mercy Hospital in many ways has become an extension of the family referred to as Tameka's "second home." Her mother says, "She's been there [to the hospital] so many times and they know her—I feel comfortable when I'm home [and she is in the hospital]. I know they know her and she know them. . . . "

Despite this strong positive feeling for Mercy Hospital, Tameka's mother no longer takes her there. She says, "I don't bring her back to Mercy Hospital. City Hospital doctors get mad. So now I start bringing her to City. . . . Tameka likes City. . . . " This family also puts its trust in God. They are willing to accept whatever happens to them in the belief that God will take care of them.

It bothers me now when she gets sick but I know it's the Man up above who's gonna take care of us. He wouldn't have let her been here this long, 'cause He could have took her when she was small, how sick she was . . . day after day you wonder if she gonna make it this day or if she gonna pass that day and it just help you wondering, keep you praying a lot. The first year of her life was the real hard year of her life.

At first the family refused to consider surgery for Tameka. Her mother prayed, "I ask the Lord that she doesn't have to have the surgery. But if she do, I'll hesitate, stop what I'm doing and put myself in His hands." Tameka's mother's belief that the Lord would do what was right was unshakable. She was willing to live with the consequences no matter how painful for her. She said that doctors did procedures and treatments that she told them she did not want for

Tameka. However, she felt there was no use pursuing these differences as she was told that the treatment was to help her daughter. This family passively accepted care given that was not wanted. They felt God was the ultimate decision maker and He would do the right thing; they could live with that.

Not Getting Health Care That Is Wanted

One family fell into this category. This was a family whose socio-economic status had decreased. The family felt they were not treated as well as they had been in the past by health care providers.

Case 6. Daria, now 5 years old, was diagnosed with asthma when almost 3. She lives with both parents and an 11-year-old brother. Her father is starting a new business with his brother, and her mother can no longer hold a steady job because "it's no telling when she's gonna go into a asthma attack . . . it's back and forth . . . you can't keep somebody who's never at work."

Daria's illness adds to the strain on the family finances and in the marital relationship. The family's desire for wanted health care for their daughter is hindered by the family finances.

> When we have to get medical [coverage] then it is a big fight. Well, of course I don't feel good when I have to go down to the welfare office for any reason. And then I take that out on him [husband] and he take it out on me 'cause he's mad 'cause he doesn't have a job that has medical and we go round and round like that. . . . I tell him, he can't afford to work there because we need medical. . . . So, it's a real strain when you don't have medical and don't have resources to take care of it. And we're still paying bills from way back. . . . [This last time] I swallowed my pride and went down to the welfare and I, actually I made him [husband] go. . . . I said, "Well, if you can't get a job doing things and get medical, you have to go down there and feel what I feel when I have to go down to the welfare to do this." So he went down there and signed us all up for medical and now we have medical. But it is so hard when you have a fluctuating income.

Balancing the budget is a constant source of strain in this household. They don't eat properly because they prefer to use their money to pay medical bills. As the mother says, "You get to know the doctors and you don't want to cheat anybody of their money." However, they felt their ability to pay affected the health care they received. "I come down here and beg from you guys to get my bills taken care of. And then you go to the doctor and sometimes they don't treat you right, you know, sometimes they look at you kind a like, 'well you know, if you would just get off your behind and take care of your business this wouldn't be' . . . it's rough everywhere you go." The family was also upset because no one told them that a different but equally effective medication was covered by welfare.

Not Getting Health Care That Is Unwanted

One family fell in this category. They ignored asthma as a disease. Asthma was normalized by referring to the symptoms as common problems of all children—cough, common cold, and sneezing. Health care was not sought and not wanted, which preserved the notion that the child was "normal, just like her friends."

Case 7. Nicole is 11 years and 11 months. She was diagnosed with asthma shortly after her 11th birthday. She lives in a foster home in which both parents work and their two children attend school with Nicole. Nicole's foster mother has a large extended family with a familial history of asthma. Other than the initial diagnosis, Nicole has not had health care for her asthma. When asked about the recent move into their new home and how Nicole had managed, she and her mother replied in unison, "Fine." Nicole continued, "I helped unpack the kitchen. That was OK. . . I sneeze . . . " Her mother interjected, "when I noticed that the painting was bothering her, I just restricted her from that area until it was dry. See, we painted everything in here, she was fine."

Nicole has very limited knowledge about asthma. When asked what asthma means to her, she says, "I haven't even had an asthma attack. I don't know what asthma is like. . . . They say I have asthma because I keep on breathing harder." Her treatment for asthma is an "asthma pump," which she had left at school the day of the interview. Her mother said she had gone camping overnight and had forgotten to taken her pump. She takes no other medication for asthma. On the one hand her mother tries to manage the asthma; "I told her yesterday to go get her breather. . . . I know she was coughing a lot, I told her to use her inhaler." On the other hand the family leaves it up to Nicole to manage care of her health. However, her focus is not on the day-to-day problems of the asthma symptoms, which have been normalized, but on the potential "asthma attacks." She says, "I don't get it. People with asthma have asthma attacks and I don't have any." Yet Nicole has an unusual fear of having an asthma attack. She says, "If I have an asthma attack . . . They might keep me in the hospital for the rest of my life. . . . I have never been in the hospital." When asked about Children's Hospital she was frankly surprised that there was a hospital exclusively for children and wanted to know if there were lots of children there. "If I be at the hospital until I get to be 21, then will they admit me to a big hospital [hospital for adults]?" she asked. Nicole's model for a hospital was that of a jail with juvenile and adult prisoners and the potential for life sentences. She had no concept of hospital, chronic disease, or treatment regimen.

Discussion and Findings

All families in this study said they were "dealin' with the asthma." Family reports of access to health care and obtaining the health care they wanted fell into four categories. Each category presents different implications for advocating for an African American family with a child who has asthma. There are also different and quite promising research implications.

Three of the seven families in this pilot study obtained the health care they wanted. These families were able to negotiate with health care providers, had strong support systems that sanctioned their health care requests, used the health care system on their terms, and understood and spoke health care language. This group does not need an advocate to help them access or utilize the health care system. However, a strong partnership model would enhance an already successful health care system for these families.

Two families obtained health care they did not want. One had an explanatory model for asthma that differed from those of the health care providers. For this family, the treatment at times seemed worse than the illness. The expectation that the child would outgrow the disease by a certain age gave them hope. When this did not happen, the family felt that the health care they were getting was "bad," and their unmet expectation was their evidence. The second family in this category felt indebted to the nurses and doctors for saving their child's life but were unable to question health care practices. Faith in God and the belief that "everything will turn out for the best" was another concept that deterred this family from challenging health care practices that they questioned. An advocate can play a useful role in situations such as these. An advocate, somewhat like the mediators[19] or cultural brokers,[22] can help family and health care providers articulate and understand the others' perspective and explanatory model. Advocates can also help the two parties operate in an arena of balanced reciprocity where the family's participation in their health care is rewarded and the health care providers' sensitivity to the family's explanatory model is acknowledged.

The third category included only one family who did not get the health care they wanted. This family's income decreased. They had to "swallow their pride and sign up for welfare." Their perception of themselves diminished, and they reported doctors not treating them as well. An advocate in this situation can help the family assert their right to health care they find acceptable. Specific areas in which this needs to be done are gaining a sense of control over one's own health, knowing the options available, and feeling comfortable making a request. Advocates can also help health care providers understand the effect they have on families with ill children and discuss alternatives so families can make informed health care decisions.

The last category, not getting health care and not wanting health care, contained one family. This family normalized illness symptoms of the child diagnosed with asthma. The mother had experience with and information about asthma but minimized the condition to such an extent that the child had limited opportunity to develop understanding of her illness and its treatment. Treatment regimens for asthma were not followed in this family. This is a family in which an advocate could be of great help making information about asthma relevant to the family and the child in a way that does not directly challenge their beliefs and that fits their lifestyle. Such an advocate would seek opportunities to supplement the family's understanding and their health care activities and help this child to manage her own asthma condition. Advocates for families who have negative feelings toward the health care system and who do not want health care face an immense challenge. Finding and contacting these families must become a legitimate activity for health care advocates. For families who will not acknowledge their illness, advocates should respond to issues families present. When health care is seen as one factor among multiple complex interrelationships, indirect information on health issues can be provided as other factors are addressed.

Vulnerable populations are those "in a position of being hurt or ignored, as well as being helped, by [others]." (p.1)[1] Access to health care is an issue for vulnerable populations. Understanding access from a sociocultural perspective deepens the health care provider's appreciation of these people's vulnerability. In order for African American families to have access to health care, "a place to go,"[1] they need to believe that they have some say in their care. Families in this study describe when they thought they had access to health care and when they thought they did not. The use of an advocate is a strategy that can enhance access. Advocates can make an immense contribution to helping families and health care professionals design collaborative health care interventions to "meet somewhere on common ground . . . so it all works out," as Arthur's mother says.

Much remains to be learned about African American families and how they understand asthma in their children. Studying explanatory models of health and illness can provide answers to how the chronically ill child is managed and why and when the health care system is accessed. Research on the role of cultural brokers could also provide strategies to enhance access to wanted health care for families. Health researchers need to investigate how to work with vulnerable families who are unwilling or unable to acknowledge their illness. Only when such research is done will more answers be provided about who the key players are in African American families and their participation in health care.

References

1. Aday LA. *At Risk in America: The Health and Health Care Needs of Vulnerable Populations*. San Francisco, Calif: Jossey Bass; 1993.

2. Halfon N, Newacheck PW. Childhood asthma and poverty: differential impact and utilization of health services. *Pediatrics*. 1993;91(1):56-61.

3. Weitzman M, Gortmaker SL, Sobol AM, Perrin JM. Recent trends in the prevalence and severity of childhood asthma. *JAMA*. 1992;268(19):2,673-2,677.

4. Betz CL. A culturally biased perspective. *J Pediatr Nurs*. 1992;7:229.

5. United Nations Development Programme. *Human Development Report*. New York, NY: Oxford University Press; 1993.

6. Thomas S. The health of the black community in the twenty-first century: a futuristic perspective. In: Braithwait RL, Taylor SE, eds. *Health Issues in the Black Community*. San Francisco, Calif: Jossey-Bass; 1992.

7. Davidson AK, Klein DE, Settipane GA, Alario AJ. Access to care among children visiting the emergency room with acute exacerbations of asthma. *Ann Allergy.* 1994;72(5):469-473.

8. Shields MC, Griffin KW, McNabb WL. The effect of a patient education program on emergency room use for inner-city children with asthma. *Am J Public Health.* 1990;80(1):36-38.

9. Evans R. Asthma among minority children. *Chest.* 1992;101(6, suppl):368S-371S.

10. Bosco LA, Gerstman BB, Tomita DK. Variations in the use of medication for the treatment of childhood asthma in the Michigan Medicaid population, 1980 to 1986. *Chest.* 1993;104(6):1,727-1,732.

11. Plaut TF. *Children with Asthma: A Manual for Parents.* 2nd ed. Amherst, Mass: Pedipress, 1990.

12. Weiss KB, Gergen PJ, Crain EF. Inner-city asthma. *Chest.* 1992;101(6, suppl):362S-367S.

13. Evans R, Mullally DI, Wilson RW, et al. National trends in the morbidity and mortality of asthma in the US. Prevalence, hospitalization and death from asthma over two decades: 1965-1984. *Chest.* 1987;91(6, suppl):65S-74S.

14. Richards W. Hospitalization of children with status asthmaticus: a review. *Pediatrics.* 1989;84(1):111-118.

15. Gergen PJ, Mullally Dl, Evans R. National survey of prevalence of asthma among children in the United States, 1976-1980. *Pediatrics.* 1988;81(1):1-7.

16. Wissow LS, Gittelsohn AM, Szklo M, Starfield B, Mussman M. Poverty, race, and hospitalization for childhood asthma. *Am J Public Health.* 1988;78(7):777-782.

17. Weitzman M, Gortmaker SL, Sobol AM. Racial, social and environmental risks for childhood asthma. *Am J Dis Children.* 1990;144(11):1,189-1,194.

18. Newacheck PW. Poverty and childhood chronic illness. *Arch Pediatr Adolesc Med.* 1994;148(11):1,143-1,149.

19. LaFargue JP. Mediating between two views of illness. *Topics Clin Nurs.* 1985;7(3):70-77.

20. Leininger MM. *Culture Care Diversity and Universality: A Theory of Nursing*. New York, NY: National League for Nursing Press; 1991.

21. Jackson LE. Understanding, eliciting, and negotiating clients' multicultural beliefs. *Nurse Practitioner*. 1993;18(4):30-43.

22. Jezewski MA. Cultural brokering as a model for advocacy. *Nurs Health Care*. 1993,14(2):78-85.

23. Spradely JP. *Participant Observation*. New York, NY: Holt, Rinehart & Winston; 1980.

24. Kleinman A. *Patients and Healers in the Context of Culture*. Berkeley, Calif: University of California Press; 1980.

—by Jane W. Peterson, Yvonee M. Sterling, and DeLois P. Weekes

Jane W. Peterson, R.N., Ph.D., is a professor and anthropologist, Seattle University School of Nursing, Seattle, Washington.

Yvonne M. Sterling, R.N, D.N.Sc., is a professor and coordinator, Louisiana State University Medical Center School of Nursing, Graduate Program, New Orleans, Louisiana.

DeLois P. Weekes, R.N., D.N.S., is an associate professor and associate dean, Boston College School of Nursing, Chestnut Hill, Massachusetts.

Part Five

Diagnosis and Treatments

Chapter 39

Asthma Assessment and Diagnosis

Diagnosis of Asthma in Adults and Children over 5 Years of Age

Recurrent episodes of coughing or wheezing are almost always due to asthma in both children and adults. Cough can be the sole symptom. Findings that increase the probability of asthma include:

- Medical history
  1. Episodic wheeze, chest tightness, shortness of breath, or cough
  2. Symptoms worsen in presence of aeroallergens, irritants, or exercise
  3. Symptoms occur or worsen at night, awakening the patient
  4. Patient has allergic rhinitis or atopic dermatitis
  5. Close relatives have asthma, allergy, sinusitis, or rhinitis

- Physical examination of the upper respiratory tract, chest, and skin
  1. Hyperexpansion of the thorax

Excerpted from "Initial Assessment and Diagnosis of Asthma," in *Practical Guide for the Diagnosis and Management of Asthma,* based on the *Expert Panel Report 2: Guidelines for the Diagnosis and Management of Asthma.* Produced by U.S. Department of Health and Human Services, National Heart, Lung, and Blood Institute (NHLBI), NIH Publication No. 97-4053, October 1997. For complete contact information, please refer to Chapter 68, "Resources."

2. Sounds of wheezing during normal breathing or a prolonged phase of forced exhalation

3   Increased nasal secretions, mucosal swelling, sinusitis, rhinitis, or nasal polyps

4. Atopic dermatitis/eczema or other signs of allergic skin problems

To establish an asthma diagnosis, determine the following.

History or presence of episodic symptoms of airflow obstruction (i.e., wheeze, shortness of breath, tightness in the chest, or cough). Asthma symptoms vary throughout the day; absence of symptoms at the time of the examination does not exclude the diagnosis of asthma.

Airflow obstruction is at least partially reversible. Use spirometry to:

• Establish airflow obstruction: FEV_1 [forced expiratory volume in 1 second] <80 percent predicted; FEV_1 /FVC [forced vital capacity] <65 percent or below the lower limit of normal. (If obstruction is absent, see Table 39.1., below.)

• Establish reversibility: FEV_1 increases ≥12 percent and at least 200 mL after using a short-acting inhaled beta$_2$-agonist (e.g., albuterol, terbutaline).

• Alternative diagnoses are excluded (e.g., vocal cord dysfunction, vascular rings, foreign bodies, or other pulmonary diseases). See Table 39.1. for additional tests that may be needed.

NOTE: Older adults may need to take oral steroids for 2 to 3 weeks and then take the spirometry test to measure the degree of reversibility achieved. Chronic bronchitis and emphysema may coexist with asthma in adults. The degree of reversibility indicates the degree to which asthma therapy may be beneficial.

In general, FEV_1 predicted norms or reference values used for children should also be used for adolescents.

Diagnosis in Infants and Children Younger than 5 Years of Age

Because children with asthma are often mislabeled as having bronchiolitis, bronchitis, or pneumonia, many do not receive adequate therapy.

- The diagnostic steps listed previously are the same for this age group except that spirometry is not possible. A trial of asthma medications may aid in the eventual diagnosis.

- Diagnosis is not needed to begin to treat wheezing associated with an upper respiratory viral infection, which is the most common precipitant of wheezing in this age group. Patients should be monitored carefully.

- There are two general patterns of illness in infants and children who have wheezing with acute viral upper respiratory infections: a remission of symptoms in the preschool years and persistence of asthma throughout childhood. The factors associated with continuing asthma are allergies, a family history of asthma, and perinatal exposure to aeroallergens and passive smoke.

Patient Education After Diagnosis

Identify the concerns the patient has about being diagnosed with asthma by asking: "What worries you most about having asthma? What concerns do you have about your asthma?"

Address the patient's concerns and make at least these key points:

- **Asthma can be managed and the patient can live a normal life.**

- **Asthma can be controlled when the patient works together with the medical staff.** The patient plays a big role in monitoring asthma, taking medications, and avoiding things that can cause asthma episodes.

- **Asthma is a chronic lung disease characterized by inflammation of the airways.** There may be periods when there are no symptoms, but the airways are swollen and sensitive to some degree all of the time. Long-term anti-inflammatory medications are important to control airway inflammation.

- **Many things in the home, school, work, or elsewhere can cause asthma attacks** (e.g., secondhand tobacco smoke, allergens, irritants). An asthma attack (also called episodes, flareups, or exacerbations) occurs when airways narrow, making it harder to breathe.

367

- **Asthma requires long-term care and monitoring.** Asthma cannot be cured, but it can be controlled. Asthma can get better or worse over time and requires treatment changes.

Patient education should begin at the time of diagnosis and continue at every visit.

Table 39.1. Additional Tests for Adults and Children. Additional tests may be needed when asthma is suspected but spirometry is normal, when coexisting conditions are suspected, or for other reasons. These tests can aid diagnosis or confirm suspected contributors to asthma morbidity (e.g., allergens and irritants).

Reasons for Additional Tests	The Tests
• Patient has symptoms but spirometry is normal or near normal	• Assess diurnal variation of peak flow over 1 to 2 weeks • Refer to a specialist for bronchoprovocation with methacholine, histamine, or exercise; negatite test may help rule out asthma
• Suspect infection, large airway lesions, heart disease, or obstruction by foreign object	• Chest x-ray
• Suspect coexisting chronic obstructive pulmonary disease, restrictive defect, or central airway obstruction	• Additional pulmonary function studies • Diffusing capacity test
• Suspect other factors contribute to asthma (These are not diagnostic tests for asthma.)	• Allergy tests—skin or in vitro • Nasal examination • Gastroesophageal reflux assessment

Assessment of Asthma Severity

[See Chapter 47, Table 47.1. Clinical Features before Treatment to Classify Severity] to estimate the severity of chronic asthma in patients of all age groups. These levels of severity correspond to the "steps" of pharmacologic therapy discussed later.

General Guidelines for Referral to an Asthma Specialist

Based on the opinion of the Expert Panel, referral for consultation or care to a specialist in asthma care is recommended if assistance is needed for:

- **Diagnosis and assessment** (e.g., differential diagnosis is problematic, other conditions aggravate asthma, or confirmation is needed on the contribution of occupational or environmental exposures)

- **Specialized treatment and education** (e.g., considering patient for immunotherapy or providing additional education for allergen avoidance)

- **Other cases:**

  1. Patient is not meeting the goals of asthma therapy (defined in next section) after 3 to 6 months. An earlier referral or consultation is appropriate if the physician concludes that the patient is unresponsive to therapy.

  2. Life-threatening asthma exacerbation occurred.

  3. Patient requires step 4 care [see Chapter 47, Table 47.2.] or has used more than two bursts of oral steroids in 1 year. (Referral may be considered for patients requiring step 3 care.)

  4. Patient is younger than age 3 and requires step 3 or 4 care. Referral should be considered for patients under age 3 who require step 2 care [see Chapter 47, Table 47.3.].

An asthma specialist is usually a fellowship-trained allergist or pulmonologist or, occasionally, a physician with expertise in asthma management developed through additional training and experience.

Patients with significant psychiatric, psychosocial, or family problems that interfere with their asthma therapy should be referred to an appropriate mental health professional for counseling or treatment.

Establish the Goals of Asthma Therapy with the Patient

The goals of asthma therapy provide the criteria that the clinician and patient will use to evaluate the patient's response to therapy. The goals will provide the focus for all subsequent interactions with the patient.

First, determine the patient's personal goals of therapy by asking a few questions, such as: "What would you like to be able to do that you can't do now or can't do well because of your asthma?" "What would you like to accomplish with your asthma treatment?"

Then, share the general goals of asthma therapy with the patient and the family.

Finally, agree on the goals you and the patient will set as the foundation for the patient's treatment plan.

General Goals of Asthma Therapy

- Prevent chronic asthma symptoms and asthma exacerbations during the day and night. (Indicators: No sleep disruption by asthma. No missed school or work due to asthma. No or minimal need for emergency department visits or hospitalizations.)

- Maintain normal activity levels—including exercise and other physical activities.

- Have normal or near-normal lung function.

- Be satisfied with the asthma care received.

- Have no or minimal side effects while receiving optimal medications.

Chapter 40

Asthma Medications

Asthma Medications: Long-Term Control and Quick Relief

Long-term-control asthma medications are taken daily to achieve and maintain control of persistent asthma. The most effective long-term-control medications for asthma are those that reduce inflammation. Inhaled steroids are the most potent inhaled anti-inflammatory medication currently available.

Inhaled Steroids

The daily use of inhaled steroids results in the following:[1,2,3-9]

- Asthma symptoms will diminish. Improvement will continue gradually.

- Occurrence of severe exacerbations is greatly reduced.

- Use of quick-relief medication decreases.

- Lung function improves significantly, as measured by peak flow, FEV_1, and airway hyperresponsiveness.

Excerpted from "Pharmacologic Therapy: Managing Asthma Long Term," in *Practical Guide for the Diagnosis and Management of Asthma*, based on the *Expert Panel Report 2: Guidelines for the Diagnosis and Management of Asthma*. Produced by U.S. Department of Health and Human Services, National Heart, Lung, and Blood Institute (NHLBI), NIH Publication No. 97-4053, October 1997. For complete contact information, please refer to Chapter 68, "Resources."

Table 40.1. Estimated Comparative Daily Dosages for Inhaled Steroids

Adults

Inhaled steroid	Low dose	Medium dose	High dose
Beclomethasone dipropionate 42 mcg/puff 84 mcg/puff	4-12 puffs—42 mcg 2-6 puffs—84 mcg	12-20 puffs—42 mcg 6-10 puffs—84 mcg	>20 puffs—42 mcg >10 puffs—84 mcg
Budesonide DPI 200 mcg/dose	200-400 mcg 1-2 inhalations	400-600 mcg 2-3 inhalations	>600 mcg >3 inhalations
Flunisolide 250 mcg/puff	500-1,000 mcg 2-4 puffs	1,000-2,000 mcg 4-8 puffs	>2,000 mcg >8 puffs
Fluticasone MDI: 44, 110, 220 mcg/puff	88-264 mcg 2-6 puffs—44 mcg or 2 puffs—110 mcg	264-660 mcg 2-6 puffs—110 mcg	>660 mcg >6 puffs—110 mcg or >3 puffs—220 mcg
DPI: 50, 100, 250 mcg/dose	2-6 inhalations—50 mcg	3-6 inhalations—100 mcg	>6 inhalations—100 mcg or >2 inhalations—250 mcg
Triamcinolone acetonide 100 mcg/puff	400-1,000 mcg 4-10 puffs	1,000-2,000 mcg 10-20 puffs	>2,000 mcg >20 puffs

Children ≤12 years

Inhaled steroid	Low dose	Medium dose	High dose
Beclomethasone dipropionate 42 mcg/puff 84 mcg/puff	84-336 mcg 2-8 puffs—42 mcg 1-4 puffs—84 mcg	336-672 mcg 8-16 puffs—42 mcg 4-8 puffs—84 mcg	>672 mcg >16 puffs—42 mcg >8 puffs—84 mcg

	Low dose	Medium dose	High dose
Budesonide DPI 200 mcg/dose	100-200 mcg	200-400 mcg 1-2 inhalations—200 mcg	>400 mcg >2 inhalations—200 mcg
Flunisolide 250 mcg/puff	500-750 mcg **2-3 puffs**	1,000-1,250 mcg **4-5 puffs**	>1,250 mcg **>5 puffs**
Fluticasone **MDI:** 44, 110, 220 mcg/puff	88-176 mcg **2-4 puffs—44 mcg**	176-440 mcg **4-10 puffs—44 mcg** or **2-4 puffs—110 mcg**	>440 mcg **>4 puffs—110 mcg** or **>2 puffs—220 mcg**
DPI: 50, 100, 250 mcg/dose	2-4 inhalations—50 mcg	2-4 inhalations—100 mcg	>4 inhalations—100 mcg or >2 inhalations—250 mcg
Triamcinolone acetonide 100 mcg/puff	400-800 mcg **4-8 puffs**	800-1,200 mcg **8-12 puffs**	>1,200 mcg **>12 puffs**

Clinician judgment of patient response is essential to appropriate dosing. Once asthma is controlled, medication doses should be carefully titrated to the minimum dose required to maintain control, thus reducing the potential for adverse effect.

Data from in vitro and clinical trials suggest that different inhaled corticosteroid preparations are not equivalent on a per puff or microgram basis. However, few data directly compare the preparations. The Expert Panel developed recommended dose ranges for different preparations based on available data.

Inhaled corticosteroid safety data suggest dose ranges for children equivalent to beclomethasone dipropionate 200-400 mcg/day (low dose), 400-800 mcg/day (medium dose), and >800 mcg/day (high dose).

Table 40.2. Usual Dosages for Long-Term Control Medications

Medication	Dosage form	Adult dose	Child dose
Oral steroids			
Methylprednisolone	2, 4, 8, 16, 32 mg tabs	7.5-60 mg daily in a single dose or qod as needed for control;	0.25-2 mg/kg day in single dose or qod as needed for control;
		short course "burst": 40-60 mg/day as single or 2 divided doses for 3-10 days	short course "burst": 1-2 mg/kg/day, max 60 mg/day for 3-10 days
Prednisolone	5 mg tabs, 5 mg/5 cc, 15 mg/5cc		
Prednisone	1, 2.5, 5, 10, 20, 25 mg tabs; 5 mg/cc, 5 mg/5 cc		
Cromolyn and nedocromil			
Cromolyn	MDI 1 mg/puff (200 sprays/canister); nebulizer sol. 20 mg/ampule	2-4 puffs tid-qid; 1 ampule tid-qid	1-2 puffs tid-qid; 1 ampule tid-qid
Nedocromil	MDI 1.75 mg/puff (104 sprays/canister)	2-4 puffs bid-qid	1-2 puffs bid-qid

Long-Acting bronchodilators

Salmeterol

Inhaled:
MDI 21 mcg/puff,
60 or 120 puffs
(120 sprays/canister);
DPI 50 mcg/blister

2 puffs q 12 hrs;
1 blister q 12 hrs

1-2 puffs q 12 hrs;
1 blister q 12 hrs

Sustained-release albuterol

Tablet:
4 mg tab

4 mg q 12 hrs

Theophylline

Liquids,
sustained-release tabs
and caps

Starting dose 10 mg/kg/day
up to 300 mg max; usual max
800 mg/day

0.3-0.6 mg/kg/day,
not to exceed 8 mg/day

Starting dose 10 mg/kg/day;
usual max:
≥1 yr of age: 16 mg/kg/day;
<1 yr of age: 0.2 (age in
weeks) + 5 = mg/kg/day

Leukotriene modifiers

Zafirlukast

20 mg tab

40 mg/day (1 tab bid)

Zileuton

300 mg tab; 600 mg tab

2,400 mg/day (two 300-mg tabs
or one 600-mg tab, qid)

All chlorofluorocarbon (CFC)-propelled inhalers are being phased out. The new non-CFC products should have similar effectiveness and safety levels as the original product.

375

Table 40.3. Asthma Quick-Relief Medications

Medication	Adult dose	Child dose
Inhaled short-acting beta₂-agonists		
Albuterol		
—nebulizer sol (5 mg/mL)	2.5-5 mg every 20 min for 3 doses, then 2.5-10 mg every 1-4 hrs as needed, or 10-15 mg/hr continuously	0.15 mg/kg (min dose 2.5 mg) every 20 min for 3 doses, then 0.15-0.3 mg/kg up to 10 mg every 1-4 hrs as needed, or 0.5 mg/kg/hr by continuous nebulation
—MDI (90 mcg/puff)	4-8 puffs every 20 min up to 4 hrs, then every 1-4 hrs as needed	4-8 puffs every 20 min for 3 doses, then every 1-4 hrs as needed
Systemic (injected) beta₂-agonists		
Epinephrine 1:1000 (1 mg/mL)	0.3-0.5 mg every 20 min for 3 doses SQ	0.01 mg/kg up to 0.3-0.5 mg every 20 min for 3 doses SQ
Terbutaline (1mg/mL)	0.25 mg every 20 min for 3 doses SQ	0.01 mg/kg every 20 min for 3 doses, then every 2-6 hrs as needed SQ
Anticholinergics		
Ipratropium bromide		
—nebulizer sol (0.25 mg/mL)	0.5 mg every 30 min for 3 doses, then every 2-4 hrs as needed	0.25 mg every 20 min for 3 doses, then every 2-4 hrs as needed
—MDI (18 mcg/puff)	4-8 puffs as needed	4-8 puffs as needed
Steroids		
Prednisone, methylprednisolone, prednisolone	120-180 mg/day in 3 or 4 divided doses for 48 hrs, then 60-80 mg/day until PEF reaches 70% of predicted or personal best	1 mg/kg every 6 hrs for 48 hrs, then 1-2 mg/kg/day (max = 60 mg/day) in 2 divided doses until PEF 70% of predicted or personal best

Problems due to asthma may return if patients stop taking inhaled steroids.

Inhaled steroids are generally well tolerated and safe at recommended doses. To reduce the potential for adverse effects, patients taking inhaled steroids should:

- Use a spacer/holding chamber.

- Rinse and spit following inhalation.

- Use the lowest possible dose to maintain control. Consider adding a long-acting inhaled beta$_2$-agonist to a low-to-medium dose of inhaled steroid rather than using a higher dose of inhaled steroid.[10,11]

Quick-Relief Medications

Quick-relief medications are used to provide prompt treatment of acute airflow obstruction and its accompanying symptoms such as cough, chest tightness, shortness of breath, and wheezing. These medications include short-acting inhaled beta$_2$-agonists and oral steroids. Anticholinergics are included in special circumstances.

References

1. Van Essen-Zandvliet EE, Hughes MD, Waalkens HJ, Duiverman EJ, Pocock SJ, Kerrebijn KF. Effects of 22 months of treatment with inhaled steroids and/or beta$_2$-agonists on lung function, airway responsiveness, and symptoms in children with asthma. *Am Rev Respir Dis* 1992;146:547-54.

2. Haahtela T, Jarvinen M, Kava T, et al. Comparison of a beta$_2$-agonist, terbutaline, with an inhaled corticosteroid, budesonide, in newly detected asthma. *N Engl J Med* 1991;325:388-92.

3. Haahtela T, Jarvinen M, Kava T, et al. Effects of reducing or discontinuing inhaled budesonide in patients with mild asthma. *N Engl J Med* 1994;331:700-5.

4. Waalkens HJ, Van Essen-Zandvliet EE, Hughes MD, et al. Cessation of long-term treatment with inhaled corticosteroid (budesonide) in children with asthma results in deterioration. *Am Rev Respir Dis* 1993;148:1252-7.

5. Dahl R, Lundback E, Malo JL, et al. A dose-ranging study of fluticasone propionate in adult patients with moderate asthma. *Chest* 1993;104:1352-8.

6. Fabbri L, Burge PS, Croonenborgh L, et al. On behalf of an International Study Group. Comparison of fluticasone propionate with beclomethasone dipropionate in moderate to severe asthma treated for one year. *Thorax* 1993;48:817-23.

7. Gustafsson P, Tsanakas J, Gold M, Primhak R, Radford M, Gillies E. Comparison of the efficacy and safety of inhaled fluticasone 200 mcg/day with inhaled beclomethasone dipropionate 400 mcg/day in mild and moderate asthma. *Arch Dis Child* 1993;69:206-11.

8. Jeffery PK, Godfrey RW, Adelroth E, Nelson F, Rogers A, Johansson SA. Effects of treatment on airway inflammation and thickening of basement membrane reticular collagen in asthma. *Am Rev Respir Dis* 1992;145:890-9.

9. Rafferty P, Tucker LG, Frame MH, Fergusson RJ, Biggs BA, Crompton GK. Comparison of budesonide and beclomethasone dipropionate in patients with severe chronic asthma: assessment of relative prednisolone-sparing effects. *Br J Dis Chest* 1985;79:244-50.

10. Greening AP, Wind P, Northfield M, Shaw G. Added salmeterol versus higher-dose steroid in asthma patients with symptoms on existing inhaled steroid. *Lancet* 1994;344:219-24.

11. Woolcock A, Lundback B, Ringdal N, Jacques LA. Comparison of addition of salmeterol to inhaled steroids with doubling of the dose of inhaled steroid. *Am J Respir Crit Care Med* 1996;153:1481-8.

Chapter 41

Pediatric and Geriatric Drug Safety

Despite seven days, "about 26 hours a day," spent preparing to testify about the labeling of drugs for children's use, Wendy Goldberg told Food and Drug Administration experts at a 1997 hearing, "I have become neither a scientist nor a doctor. Not even close." But, she said, "I do know one thing—I use a lot of medicines on Abby that are not approved by the FDA for use on children her age."

Of the nine-item laundry list of medicines Goldberg's 6-year-old daughter Abby was taking for her severe asthma, not a single one was tested or approved in the United States for children under 12. "I feel as though I am testing drugs on my own child, every day, and it isn't helping anyone," Goldberg said.

While some drugs do come with pediatric use information (notably, vaccines and antibiotics), asthma medications by no means stand alone in their lack of labeling for kids' treatment. Other types of drugs that often lack pediatric labeling include those for depression, epilepsy, severe pain, gastrointestinal problems, allergic reactions, and high blood pressure.

Overall, more than half of the drugs approved every year that are likely to be used in children are not adequately tested or labeled for treating youngsters, according to FDA estimates. Safety and effectiveness

From "Pediatric Drug Studies: Protecting Pint-Sized Patients," by Tamar Nordenberg, in *FDA Consumer* magazine, May-June 1999 [Online] April 1999. Available: http://www.fda.gov. Produced by the U.S. Food and Drug Administration (FDA). For complete contact information, please refer to Chapter 68, "Resources."

information is especially sparse for the over 7 million children under age 2.

A recent survey by the agency identified the 10 drugs that were prescribed most often to children in 1994 that lacked pediatric labeling. Together, they were prescribed for kids more than 5 million times. (See below "Top 10 Drugs Prescribed to Kids without Pediatric Labeling.")

"At times, children have been harmed and maybe even killed because of a lack of knowledge of how drugs would affect them," says Robert M. Ward, M.D., chair of the American Academy of Pediatrics' Committee on Drugs. Among Ward's historical examples: the deaths of a number of newborn babies in the 1960s when their immature livers were unable to break down the antibiotic chloramphenicol. "Those types of therapeutic misadventures are certainly part of pediatric medicine, and we'd rather they didn't repeat," he says.

To help prevent future chloramphenicol-type disasters, FDA finalized a rule last December requiring manufacturers of many drugs to provide information about how their drugs can safely and effectively be used in children (from newborns to adolescents), including information on the proper doses for kids.

A Healthy Dose of Regulation

The pediatric studies rule, published in the Dec. 2, 1998, *Federal Register*, requires that new drugs (generally prescription drugs, including biologics, or drugs derived from living organisms) that are important in the medical treatment of children or will be commonly used in children include labeling information on safe pediatric use.

The information would usually be required when a drug is approved. For drugs already on the market, FDA can require children's studies in certain compelling circumstances—when pediatric labeling could avoid significant risks to kids, for example.

The rule expands on a 1994 regulation that simplified the information needed for a manufacturer to label its drugs for children's use. That rule required drug makers to look at existing data and determine if they could support safe and effective use in children.

"That was the voluntary effort, and we weren't making much headway," says Rosemary Roberts, M.D., chair of the pediatric subcommittee in FDA's Center for Drug Evaluation and Research. "Most manufacturers just went back to saying that safety and effectiveness had not been established for children."

Without pediatric data about a drug, Roberts says, doctors are sometimes reluctant to treat a child with it. "Some physicians won't even try a drug in a child if they don't have enough information," she says. It is legal, however, to prescribe a drug for use in children despite its approval only for adults (termed "off-label" use).

If doctors decide against using adult drugs in their young patients because the appropriate dose is unknown, children may be deprived of useful treatments, especially some AIDS drugs and other breakthrough therapies that carry considerable risks.

Doctors can be faced with quite a dilemma, says Timothy Westmoreland of the Elizabeth Glaser Pediatric AIDS Foundation. "Do you choose to withhold a potentially effective drug that is useful in adults or expose a child to a drug you don't know is safe?"

Because of their immature organs and different metabolic and immune systems, children react unlike adults to many drugs. Treating children with adult drugs, then, can carry the risk of unforeseen adverse reactions.

Besides the chloramphenicol tragedy, other serious adverse reactions in children have included:

- jaundice in newborns from sulfa drugs

- seizures and cardiac arrest from the local anesthetic bupivacaine

- withdrawal symptoms from prolonged use of the painkiller fentanyl

- staining of teeth from the antibiotic tetracycline

"It can be a real guessing game as to whether we're treating a child effectively," Roberts says. "Sometimes a child's body will handle the drug very much like an adult's," she explains, "while other times a child's body will react quite differently. There may be no way of knowing in advance."

While dosing information sometimes becomes available to physicians through references such as journal articles and pediatric handbooks, it may take years for this information to appear. Even then, the information may not be based on adequate testing and may contain gaps, about its use in certain age groups, for example.

Even if the correct dose is known, the medicine will do no good, of course, if a child can't ingest it. So the 1998 rule in some cases requires manufacturers to make a special formulation of a drug product— liquid or chewable tablet instead of a tablet that must be swallowed whole, for example—to enable kids to take the drug.

Wendy Goldberg knows first-hand the frustrations of treating her child with drugs made in tablet form for adults. "I need to cut two of

381

them in half," she told the panelists at the hearing preceding the rule. One, she said, is "like a little stone. I got a gadget from my pharmacist that is supposed to cut it in half, but it doesn't work exactly right. Do I give her the big 'half' or the small 'half'? I usually give her the big piece in the morning, on the theory that if something bad happens, at least she'll be awake."

Controlled Risk

To those who point out that bad things can happen during drug studies, too, the American Academy of Pediatrics has responded that treating children with untested drugs may place more kids at risk than including them in controlled studies of the drugs in the first place.

Children enrolled in drug studies "are sick children that stand to benefit from getting new drugs sooner," says AAP's Ward. "Yes, they will be at risk, just like adults are at risk, if the drug is later found to have problems. But because we're treating children with illnesses, that risk is justified."

Under the rule, the timing of studies in children will depend on the seriousness of the disease, the availability of other treatments, the amount of safety and effectiveness information already available, and the types of studies that are needed.

FDA will not delay the approval of a drug for adults to await completion of children's studies. Instead, the agency could approve the drug for adults on the condition that the company completes pediatric studies in a timely way.

The pediatric study requirement may be waived entirely if a drug is not medically important for children and will not be commonly used in children or if:

- there is strong evidence that the drug product would be ineffective or unsafe in all pediatric patients or

- children's studies are impossible or highly impractical because, for example, the number of patients is too small or geographically spread-out or

- attempts to develop a pediatric formulation have failed.

The Pediatric AIDS Foundation's Westmoreland is confident that "virtually all" drugs with significance to children will be studied because of the new FDA rule, as well as the complementary financial incentives under the FDA Modernization Act of 1997, which gives an extra six months of exclusive marketing or patent protection for studying certain drugs in children.

"We see the rule as a real victory," says Janis Stire, executive director of the foundation. "For too long, children have been seen as an afterthought, with so many drugs not available to them. A child is not just half an adult to be given half the adult dose."

Top 10 Drugs Prescribed to Kids without Pediatric Labeling

(Based on 1994 data from research firm IMS America, Ltd.)

These 10 drugs were prescribed more than 5 million times in a single year to children in age groups for which the drugs were not adequately labeled.

1. Drug: **Albuterol inhalation solution for nebulization**
   Condition: Asthma
   Prescribed: 1,626,000 times to children under 12

2. Drug: **Phenergan**
   Condition: Allergic reactions
   Prescribed: 663,000 times to children under 2

3. Drug: **Ampicillin injections**
   Condition: Infection
   Prescribed: 639,000 times to children under 12

4. Drug: **Auralgan otic solution**
   Condition: Ear pain
   Prescribed: 600,000 times to children under 16

5. Drug: **Lotrisone cream**
   Condition: Topical infections
   Prescribed: 325,000 times to children under 12

6. Drug: **Prozac**
   Condition: Depression, obsessive-compulsive disorder
   Prescribed: 349,000 times to children under 16, including 3,000 times to infants under 1

7. Drug: **Intal**
   Condition: Asthma
   Prescribed: Solution prescribed 109,000 times to children under 2; aerosol prescribed 399,000 times to children under 5

8. Drug: **Zoloft**
    Condition: Depression
    Prescribed: 248,000 times to children under 16

9. Drug: **Ritalin**
    Condition: Attention deficit disorder, narcolepsy
    Prescribed: 226,000 times to children under 6

10. Drug: **Alupent syrup**
    Condition: Asthma
    Prescribed: 184,000 times to children under 6

Protecting Older Patients

To help ensure the safe and effective use of prescription drugs in older people (specifically, aged 65 and older), a rule finalized by FDA in August 1997 requires drug companies to include a separate "Geriatric use" section in their drugs' labeling. Drug companies do not have to perform additional studies like the pediatric rule requires, but must include available information in a specific format and location.

"If the information is dispersed throughout the whole label, it doesn't make for a user-friendly information source," says Robert Michocki, a clinical pharmacist and professor at the University of Maryland's school of pharmacy. "People are busy. Physicians don't sit down and read the whole drug label. They try to read the important sections that answer questions like 'what's the dose?' or 'what are the side effects?'"

While drugs for everything from heart problems and high blood pressure to pneumonia and the flu can be lifesavers for older people, the dangers of medicine can be magnified in this population, too.

One reason for the increased risk is people's changing physiology as they get older, says Charles Ganley, M.D., FDA's medical team leader for cardiorenal drug products. For example, he says, certain drugs that are eliminated from the body by the kidneys could cause problems in the elderly because kidney function can decline with age.

Also, the elderly take more medicines than any other age group— around 30 percent of the prescription drugs sold in the United States, according to FDA, although they make up only about 12 percent of the country's population. The use of multiple drugs can increase the risk of dangerous drug interactions.

Michocki says, "start low and go slow" is an adage that applies to giving older people medicines. "For the most part, with older people you're using medications to try and manage their chronic diseases like diabetes or arthritis. There's no reason to go in there and try to fix something overnight."

The rule will prove beneficial, Michocki thinks, because "after reading the special section on geriatrics, a physician who is not familiar with the drug may start out giving half the dose he was going to give in the first place."

New labels are appearing gradually, first on those drugs that FDA has determined are most likely to create problems for geriatric patients. These include psychotropic drugs such as antidepressants and antipsychotics, as well as some heart medications and nonsteroidal anti-inflammatory drugs (NSAIDs).

—by Tamar Nordenberg

Tamar Nordenberg is a staff writer for FDA Consumer.

Chapter 42

Corticosteroids:
Benefits and Risks

Corticosteroids

Frequently people have concerns about taking corticosteroid ("steroid") medications because they are not well-informed about their benefits, indications, and risks. Please discuss concerns that you have about steroid use with your health care provider.

Corticosteroids are anti-inflammatory medications for the treatment of allergic conditions, asthma, and other diseases. They are NOT the same as anabolic steroids, used by athletes to increase muscle tissue.

Corticosteroids are related to cortisol, a hormone produced by the adrenal glands and one of the body's own natural steroids. Cortisol is essential for life and well-being. During stress, our bodies produce additional cortisol to keep us from becoming seriously ill.

Normally the adrenal glands release cortisol into the blood stream every morning. The brain monitors this amount and regulates the adrenal function accordingly. It cannot, however, tell the difference between its own natural cortisone and that of steroid medicines. Therefore, when a person takes high doses of steroids over a prolonged period of time, the brain may decrease or stop cortisol production. Health care providers generally decrease a steroid dosage slowly to allow the adrenal gland to recover and produce cortisol at a normal level again.

Excerpted from "Med Facts: Corticosteroids,"[Online] 1994; and "Med Facts: Use of the Chickenpox Vaccine in Children," [Online] 1995. Available: http://www.njc.org/MFhtml/. © 1994-1995 by the National Jewish Medical and Research Center, 1400 Jackson St., Denver, CO 80206. Reprinted with permission. For complete contact information, please refer to Chapter 68, "Resources."

How Do Corticosteroids Work?

No one knows exactly how corticosteroids work. Studies show that their effectiveness in asthma may relate to their ability to:

1. Decrease inflammation and swelling in the airways, lessening airway hyperreactivity;

2. Reduce the release of body chemicals from certain inflammatory cells;

3. Increase the effect of bronchodilator medications.

Corticosteroid Preparations

Corticosteroid medications are available as nasal sprays, metered-dose-inhalers (inhaled steroids), oral forms (pills or syrups), and injections and intravenous (IV) solutions. Health care providers at National Jewish rarely use corticosteroid injections for the treatment of chronic respiratory disorders. With severe episodes or emergencies, high-dose steroids are generally given in an IV. As the patient stabilizes, the medication is changed from IV to oral forms and then gradually decreased.

The two most commonly prescribed forms of corticosteroids for most people with a chronic lung condition are inhaled steroids and oral steroids.

Inhaled Corticosteroids

For many people with asthma, an inhaled steroid is the primary medication that is used to prevent symptoms. When taken on a regular schedule, an inhaled steroid reduces inflammation in the airways, making them less sensitive. Also, an inhaled steroid may help reduce symptoms associated with chronic bronchitis or chronic obstructive pulmonary disease (COPD).

An inhaled steroid is generally prescribed as a preventive medication. This means that you need to take it on a daily basis whether you have symptoms or not. Also, it will not provide immediate relief for breathing difficulty. Most people with asthma benefit from using an inhaled steroid year round, but those with seasonal asthma may need to use it for only certain months of the year.

Your clinician may adjust the dosage of your inhaled steroid based on your symptoms, how often you use your bronchodilator to control asthma symptoms, and your peak flow results. You may continue to need an occasional short-term burst of oral steroids when you experience more severe episodes.

Available inhaled steroids include:

- beclomethasone: Beclovent®, Vanceril®
- flunisolide: AeroBid®
- triamcinolone: Azmacort®

An inhaled steroid has a low risk of side effects when used at recommended doses. Studies show that the medication is usually broken down by the liver and very little circulates in the blood stream, thereby decreasing the risk of significant side effects. When a dosage is prescribed that is higher than recommended in the package insert, some systemic side effects could occur. Keep in mind, however, that an inhaled steroid has much less potential for side effects than oral (tablet or syrup) steroids. The most common side effects with inhaled steroids are cough, hoarseness, or a yeast infection of the mouth or throat (thrush). Using a spacer device with an inhaled steroid and rinsing your mouth with water (spitting after use) can help lessen these side effects.

Steroid Tablets

Oral steroids are given as a short-term burst or as routine maintenance therapy. Although there are several corticosteroid tablets available, we recommend either prednisone or methylprednisolone because they are short-acting and reliably well-absorbed and available to the lungs.

A short-term burst is generally used for severe episodes of your condition. A burst may last three to seven days and not require a gradually decreasing dosage. Rarely, a burst may need to continue for several weeks with a gradually decreasing dosage (taper). Your health care provider should closely monitor bursts and tapers. Side effects that may be associated with a burst include mood swings, swelling, increased appetite, flushing of the face, and high blood pressure. These side effects usually disappear when the medication is stopped.

Long-Term Oral Corticosteroid Use

A small percentage of persons with chronic disease require the use of oral steroids for prolonged periods, possibly weeks, months, or longer. In several lung diseases, the primary treatment is high-dose oral steroids for several months or longer. If you have a lung condition

389

such as asthma or COPD, the treatment program should include a combination of several medications rather than oral steroids alone. If you have asthma, it is especially important that your treatment include an inhaled steroid with an adequate dosage before beginning maintenance oral steroids. National Jewish physicians recommend that you see a specialist (pulmonologist or allergist) if your condition requires long-term oral steroids.

Steroid side effects usually occur after prolonged use with high doses. It is important to note that some people who take long-term oral corticosteroids experience only minimal side effects. Side effects which may occur in some persons taking high-dose oral steroids include:

- Thinning of bones (osteoporosis) which may lead to fractures or compressions, especially of the vertebral bones (backbone) and the hip;

- Loss of blood supply to bones (aseptic necrosis) which may cause severe bone pain and may require surgical correction;

- High blood pressure (hypertension);

- Increased pressure in the eye (glaucoma);

- Permanent clouding of vision in one or both eyes (cataracts);

- Weight gain with increased appetite, fluid retention, and stretch marks;

- Facial fullness;

- Increase in body hair and acne;

- A tendency to easy bruising and thinning of the skin, along with poor wound healing;

- Interference with growth in children (remember that an untreated chronic illness can impair growth as well);

- Muscle weakness or cramps, and joint pain;

- Changes in menstrual cycle;

- Elevations in blood sugar (diabetes);

- Suppression of the body's adrenal gland which makes the necessary amount of cortisol at times of stress (adrenal insufficiency). The adrenal gland function usually resumes when steroids are stopped or when they are taken in a single AM dose or a single PM dose every other day;

- Irritation of stomach and esophagus with possible ulcer symptoms and, rarely, bleeding;

- Emotional disturbances such as irritability, depression, euphoria, or hallucinations.

- Steroids may also suppress your body's response to certain viral infections, for example varicella (chickenpox). If you or your child are exposed and susceptible to chickenpox while receiving oral steroids or high dose inhaled steroids, notify your health care provider immediately to determine if any special treatment is needed.

Some precautions can lessen your risk of side effects with long-term oral corticosteroids:

- Take the steroid dose as a single dose in the morning, as this is closer to how the body produces its own natural steroid. (Some individuals receive greater benefit from a mid afternoon, evening, or split dose.)

- If prescribed by your physician, take the steroid every other day to minimize side effects.

- Take your steroid dose with food to lessen irritation of the stomach lining.

- Take the full dosage (complete number of puffs) of your inhaled steroid as prescribed to allow the lowest possible dosage of oral steroids.

- If you notice a deterioration in peak flows or increased symptoms, notify your health care provider. A short course of oral steroids given early may help alleviate the need for longer courses if treated later.

It is extremely important to follow your health care provider's directions. Don't make any changes without this approval!

Diet Recommendations

Make sure you get proper nutrition when taking oral corticosteroids. Oral steroid use can cause you to lose calcium and potassium, important minerals for bone strength and good muscle function. An imbalance of these minerals may cause muscle cramping or heart irregularities. Don't take a potassium supplement unless prescribed by

391

your clinician. To make sure that you are getting enough calcium, increase your intake of dairy products to 4-5 servings per day. If you experience swelling, your clinician may recommend a diet low in sodium. This may include limited use of salt or sodium-rich condiments and processed foods. Eat a well-balanced diet including citrus fruits and fruit juices. Remember that corticosteroids can increase your appetite, so if you are eating more food, be sure you choose low-fat, low sugar items to control calories. Your health care provider or dietitian can help you with a specific diet plan.

Osteoporosis

Long-term oral corticosteroid use depletes the bones of calcium which can lead to osteoporosis. Osteoporosis, or brittle bones, places you at greater risk of fractures. Even low-dose corticosteroid therapy can cause this calcium loss; post-menopausal women are at particular risk. If you have osteoporosis or a family history of it, inform your physician.

Several tests can determine the extent of bone loss. These include laboratory calcium tests to measure the amount of calcium in the blood or urine, CT scans, and bone densitometry. Bone densitometry is much more sensitive than routine X-ray of the bone. After a baseline measurement of bone density is determined, your clinician may want to repeat this test every 6-12 months for children and 12-18 months for adults to monitor possible mineral loss.

Regular weight-bearing exercise and supplemental calcium can reduce the risk of osteoporosis. Weight-bearing activities include walking, running, and bicycling. Supplements of calcium and vitamin D may be recommended if your diet doesn't supply the required amount. Discuss your particular needs with your health care provider.

Newer treatments to prevent steroid-induced bone loss include the injections thyrocalcitonin and etidronate. The majority of post-menopausal women on corticosteroid therapy benefit from estrogen replacement to prevent or lessen osteoporosis.

Chickenpox and the New Vaccine

Chickenpox (varicella) is one of the most common childhood viral diseases. Chickenpox is highly contagious and can now be prevented with a safe and effective vaccine. Although chickenpox is usually mild, vaccinating children can prevent complications of severe chickenpox and reduce costs associated with children missing school and adults missing work. The chickenpox vaccine is very effective in preventing chickenpox. If children who are vaccinated do get chickenpox, they will generally have a much milder form of the illness.

Special Considerations for Children with Respiratory or Immunological Disorders

Treatment with oral corticosteroids and/or immune globulin for respiratory or immunological disorders requires special consideration when administering the chickenpox vaccine.

Oral Corticosteroids. Varicella vaccine should not be given to individuals on high doses of oral corticosteroids (2 mg/kg/day) for more than one month. According to general guidelines, children may be immunized after steroid use at this dosage has been discontinued for three months. However, most experts agree that vaccination after one month or more of discontinuation of steroid use is safe and acceptable. If at all possible, discontinuing systemic steroids for two to three weeks after immunization is suggested. Experts agree that children on inhaled steroids are not at increased risk of disease from the chickenpox vaccine.

Immune Globulin. As with other live viral vaccines, varicella vaccines should not be administered within at least five months after receipt of any form of immune globulin or other blood product.

Talk to your doctor or nurse about the new chickenpox vaccine. The vaccine is safe and effective against preventing this common childhood disease. You can receive the chickenpox vaccine at National Jewish or from your pediatrician. For more general information, please consult the American Academy of Pediatrics' brochure, (Chickenpox and the New Vaccine.)

Important Considerations when Your Dosage Changes

As the control of your disease improves, or if serious side effects develop, your health care provider may reduce your steroid dosage by tapering to prevent "breakthrough" symptoms and to allow the adrenal glands time to function again. Because the dose is highly individualized, follow your health care provider's recommendations.

As your body adjusts to a lower steroid dosage, you may experience some withdrawal side effects. These may include an increase in breathing difficulty due to worsening of your disease, fatigue, weakness, depression, and joint aches. If breathing difficulty occurs, or if any of the above symptoms are severe, notify your health care provider. The non-respiratory side effects usually disappear within a few weeks or months.

If your steroid dosage has recently been decreased or discontinued and you experience a serious illness, surgery or injury, you may temporarily require additional steroids. During this time, your adrenal glands may not be functioning at full capacity and cannot handle stress to the body. This is especially important if you have taken routine maintenance oral steroid therapy within the last year or completed a burst within the past two weeks. Inform all of your health care professionals that you have been on corticosteroid treatment. Some people choose to wear a medical alert bracelet or carry a card with specific information about their steroid use.

National Jewish and Research on Corticosteroids

National Jewish is the nation's leading research and treatment center for steroid dependent asthma. Since the 1960s, Center researchers have been helping patients manage severe asthma while developing innovative treatments to reduce patients' needs for these potent medications.

We currently have a number of programs to help people with steroid-dependent asthma:

- Testing new inhaled corticosteroids: Inhaled steroids have become a first-line treatment for asthma, because they carry a much lower risk of side effects than oral steroids. National Jewish researchers conduct studies on new inhaled steroids that may be safer and more effective than those already available.

- Studying mechanisms of steroid-resistant asthma: A small percent of asthma patients fail to respond to either oral or inhaled steroid therapy, despite high doses over prolonged treatment periods. National Jewish researchers study the basis of poor response to steroids. Their studies indicate that physiological changes at the molecular level contribute to this phenomenon in these individuals. The researchers speculate that steroid-resistant asthma may be due to more than one abnormality. These findings may have implications for the design of alternative treatment approaches for unmanageable asthma.

- Evaluating non-steroidal anti-inflammatory drugs: Some medications, alone or in combination with corticosteroids, may succeed in controlling airway inflammation in asthma while reducing the risk of steroid side effects. Center researchers perform clinical trials on non-steroidal anti-inflammatory drugs to determine whether they may be more effective than those already available (i.e., nedocromil). Testing with a 5-lipoxygenase inhibitor and newly engineered molecules, such as the interleukin-4 receptor antagonist, may hold promise for asthma sufferers in the future.

- Quality of life studies: We measure patients' quality of life—their medical conditions, emotional status, abilities to engage in activities of daily living—after treatment at National Jewish. This allows us to quantify the effectiveness of our care, so that we may provide patients even higher levels of well-being.

Note: This information is provided to you as an educational service of National Jewish. It is not meant to be a substitute for consulting with your own physician.

Chapter 43

Update on Theophylline

Theophylline has in the past been a mainstay in the treatment of moderate to severe asthma, but is less popular than it used to be. Recently, however, there has been a renewed enthusiasm for the use of theophylline in the treatment of asthma, because of newly identified anti-inflammatory and immunomodulatory effects. Several studies have demonstrated that theophylline inhibits histamine release and suppresses inflammatory cell activation. Recent studies have also found evidence of theophylline's effects in modulating T-cell counts in peripheral blood and biopsy specimens, reducing activated eosinophils in biopsy specimens, and attenuating allergen-induced histamine release from mast cells.

Theophylline is particularly effective in controlling the late-phase allergic reaction of atopic asthma. The late-phase reaction is thought to be the most important reaction involved in the development of airway hyperreactivity, and hyperreactive airways are prone to go into spasm at any insult, from cold air to strong perfume.

At therapeutic blood levels, theophylline reduces bronchoconstriction and associated airway hyperresponsiveness, inhibits both immediate and late bronchoconstriction following antigen challenge, and diminishes the influx of neutrophils. These anti-inflammatory and

From "Theophylline," by M. Eric Gershwin, M.D., in *Allergy and Asthma Magazine* (Professional Edition), Vol. 7, No. 1, [Online] April 1998. Available: http://www.healthline.com/articles/ap980101.htm. © 1998 by Healthline Publishing Inc., 830 Menlo Ave., Ste. 100, Menlo Park, CA 94025. Reprinted with permission.

mucociliary effects—together with the drug's ability to improve dia-phragmatic muscle functions—may also explain theophylline's ben-eficial effect in chronic obstructive pulmonary disease. It may be interesting to note that theophylline also relaxes spasms of the lower airways independent of the type of mediator that induces bronchocon-striction.

Maintaining therapeutic levels of theophylline while avoiding wide swings between toxic and subclinical dosage ranges has long been a chal-lenge. However, with the advent of controlled- and sustained-release theophylline preparations such as Theo-24, this challenge has become much simpler.

Sustained-release theophylline preparations require fewer daily doses. This not only enhances patient compliance, resulting in better asthma control, but also permits improved maintenance of therapeutic levels throughout the day and night.

Because asthma has such a strong inflammatory component, most clinicians treat asthma patients with aggressive anti-inflammatory medications in their initial regimens. However, as our understand-ing of asthma increases, it is important for clinicians to recognize that effective asthma regimens are often idiosyncratic, requiring drug regi-mens to be individualized to best meet the needs of the patient.

Reference

M. Weinberger and H. Hendeles, "Theophylline in Asthma," *New England Journal of Medicine,* vol. 334, no. 21 (May 23, 1996).

—by M. Eric Gershwin, M.D.

Dr. Gershwin is Chief of Allergy and Immunology and the Jack and Donald Chia Professor of Medicine at the University of California, Davis. He is board certified in internal medicine, allergy, and clinical immunology.

Chapter 44

Asthma Inhalation Therapy

Up to 5% of the U.S. population suffers from asthma, a respiratory condition characterized by airway inflammation, airway obstruction (at least partially reversible), and airway hyperresponsiveness to such stimuli as environmental allergens, viral respiratory-tract infections, irritants, drugs, food additives, exercise, and cold air. The major underlying pathology in asthma is airway inflammation. Inflammatory cells—eosinophils, CD4+ lymphocytes, macrophages, and mast cells—release a broad range of mediators, including interleukins, leukotrienes, histamine, granulocyte-colony-stimulating factor, and platelet-activating factor. These mediators are responsible for the bronchial hyperreactivity, bronchoconstriction, mucus secretion, and sloughing of endothelial cells. Because asthma is an inflammatory disease, early treatment with inhaled glucocorticoids is recommended for optimum long-term control. Beta-agonists, while effective for symptomatic control in the short term, do not control the inflammation; indeed, there is evidence that excessive use may exacerbate asthma and contribute to its worldwide increase in prevalence, morbidity, and mortality. (Barnes PJ. *Br Med J*. 1993; 307: 815-816. Kemp JP. *Arch Intern Med*. 1993; 153: 805-812.)

From "Asthma Inhalation Therapy," in *Medical Sciences Bulletin,* Vol. 19, No.3, 1996. © 1996 by Pharmaceutical Information Associates, Ltd., 2761 Trenton Rd., Levittown, PA 19056. All rights reserved. Reprinted with permission.

Glucocorticoid Therapy: Inhalation vs. Oral

Inhalation therapy with anti-inflammatory glucocorticoids is recommended for the initial treatment of asthma, with the addition of beta-agonists as needed. Glucocorticoids reduce the risk of fatal and near fatal asthma in both children and adults, and administration by inhalation (compared with oral administration) reduces the risk of systemic side effects. This is because the glucocorticoids available for inhalation therapy are highly active topically and only weakly active systemically, which minimizes effects on the pituitary-adrenal axis, the skin, and the eye. Side effects associated with inhalation therapy are primarily oropharyngeal candidiasis and dysphonia (due to atrophy of laryngeal muscles). Both side effects are less common when a spacer is used because less drug is deposited in the oropharynx and larynx. Oral glucocorticoids cause atrophy of the dermis—with thin skin, striae, and ecchymoses—but inhaled glucocorticoids do not cause similar changes in the respiratory tract.

Another advantage of inhaled over oral administration is that the direct deposition of steroid in the airways generally provides more predictable administration. The oral doses required for adequate control vary substantially, whereas inhaled glucocorticoids are usually effective within a narrower range. There are, however, a number of factors that influence the availability of inhaled glucocorticoids: extent of airway inflammation; degree of lung metabolism; amount of drug swallowed and metabolized in the GI tract; the patient's ability to coordinate the release and inspiration of the medication; type of glucocorticoid; and the delivery system. (When a spacer is used between the inhaler and the mouth, the inhaler is easier to manipulate and more drug reaches the lungs.)

The most widely used aerosol glucocorticoids are beclomethasone dipropionate (Vanceril/Schering) and budesonide (Rhinocort/Astra, similar to beclomethasone). These agents have a high affinity for intracellular glucocorticoid receptors but are rapidly metabolized to biologically inactive compounds. In one study comparing the efficacy of inhaled versus oral therapy for reducing respiratory symptoms and improving airway function, the ratio of the potency of inhaled budesonide versus oral prednisone was about 40 to 1. There is no evidence that efficacy diminishes with time. Asthma can usually be controlled with beclomethasone or budesonide 200 to 800 micrograms inhaled daily. Doses up to 1,000 micrograms daily have little effect on pituitary-adrenal secretion in adults; larger doses may cause some (variable) dose-dependent suppression of secretion. Doses of 2,000 micrograms/day in adults have been associated with thinning of the skin, slight glucose intolerance, psychiatric disturbances (rarely), and cataracts (with long-term therapy). Beclomethasone in doses of 1,000 to 2,000 micrograms/day (long-term) has been associated with decreases in bone density. Flunisolide (Aerobid/Forest) and triamcinolone (Azmacort/Rorer) are also available for inhalation therapy in the United States, but they haven't been studied as extensively. (Utiger RD. *N Engl J Med*. 1993; 329: 1731-1733.)

Inhaled Glucocorticoids in Young Children

Early treatment with inhaled glucocorticoids gives optimal long-term control of asthma. In children, there is some evidence that delaying the initiation of such therapy may result in irreversible changes in the airways. Moderate doses of glucocorticoids by inhalation have proved to be safe for children, even young children, and even when given over long periods of time. In their study of 15 children aged 2 to 7 years given budesonide 200 micrograms/day by inhalation, Volovitz, et al., found the drug to be remarkably safe and effective for up to 5 years. The severity of asthma decreased in the first month of therapy (58% reduction in the number of days with asthma symptoms and 75% reduction in use of bronchodilators), and improvement was maintained. At the end of the trial, asthma recurred in 13 of the 15 patients enrolled, and budenoside was required to control the symptoms.

Budesonide did not suppress pituitary-adrenal function; there was no documented effect on 24-hour serum cortisol concentration, serum cortisol responses to corticotropin, or urinary cortisol excretion. Growth patterns—height, weight, and bone age—were normal throughout the treatment period for all patients. Larger doses have been shown to delay growth and skeletal maturation, but then so can asthma. No cataracts were seen (although cataracts have been reported with glucocorticoid inhalation therapy). The investigators concluded that "prolonged administration of budesonide in a relatively low dose of 200 micrograms per day to young children with severe asthma is not only effective but also safe, as demonstrated by their normal linear growth and normal pituitary-adrenal function." (Utiger RD. *N Engl J Med*. 1993; 329: 1731-1733. Volovitz B et al. *N Engl J Med*. 1993; 329: 1703-1708.)

The Problem with Metered-Dose Inhalers

The standard device for asthma inhalation therapy is the metered-dose aerosol inhaler (MDI). One problem with these devices is the difficulty of determining when the inhaler is out of medication. Williams, et al., interviewed 51 asthmatic patients and examined their inhalers to see whether the patients were using their inhalers appropriately. They found that in this particular group of patients, the correct protocol was often ignored. Of the 81 inhalers assessed, 21 were at their "floating weight" (that is, the canisters had delivered the licensed number of doses) and 12 were at their "red weight" (canisters had enough expellant left for only 48 hours). Nineteen patients had no inhaler in reserve. During the interview, 37 of the 51 patients admitted to using an inhaler until it was almost or completely empty, and 36 occasionally or frequently ran out of inhalant (33 of whom became moderately or severely wheezy). Only three assessed their inhalers by flotation, and none asked to float their canister when given a nearly empty canister to use. Almost all the patients continued to use their inhalers after the canisters had delivered the licensed number of doses. Running out of medication unawares may provoke rebound bronchospasm and increase the risk of morbidity and even mortality, said the investigators. They concluded that "aerosol metered dose inhalers give insufficient information about the drug remaining in the inhaler and are therefore unsafe. A counter mechanism could rectify the problem." (Williams DJ et al. *Br Med J*. 1993; 307: 771-772.)

Bergner, et al., also believe that some exacerbations of asthma occur when patients continue to use MDIs beyond the specified number of sprays. The problem is that patients are unable to tell by sight, sound, or taste when the dose is no longer adequate, so they generally continue to use their inhalers until the canister is exhausted. "Our own unpublished trial indicated that the 'sink or float' test that some pharmaceutical companies recommend does not accurately reveal when the specified number of sprays has been actuated. When metered dose medications are taken at a regularly scheduled frequency, patients should calculate the finish date and mark their calendars. When an MDI is used 'as needed,' patients should keep a written tally, although this is cumbersome and unlikely to occur." (Bergner A et al. *JAMA*. 1993; 269: 1506.)

A second problem with canisters is the tendency for some inhalers to deliver less than promised. Bergner, et al., noted that many of their patients claim that some inhaler sprays decline in force, volume, or effectiveness before the specified number has been used, even though the device is shaken before use. (Bergner A et al. *JAMA*. 1993; 269: 2051.) Weiss noted that a decline in the force of spray may occur long before the end of the life of the canister as specified by the manufacturer. An asthmatic himself, Weiss has noted that his flunisolide

(AeroBid) inhaler loses spray strength after the 17th day of use, even though the product should last for 25 days. Weiss wrote to the manufacturer (Forest Pharmaceuticals), but his request for information was ignored. He wrote to the FDA, but waited 8 months before getting some (incomplete) information. He concluded that, "(1) the failure of MDIs to deliver the specified number of specified doses may be a cause of asthmatic exacerbations; (2) drug delivery by MDIs as a function of the number of inhalations used needs documentation and should be required by the FDA; and (3) it may be impossible to get desired information out of a pharmaceutical company and a long time to get a response of any sort from the FDA." (Weiss W. *JAMA*. 1993; 270: 2050.)

A Forest Pharmaceuticals spokesperson replied that failure to clean the inhaler system may have caused the "perceived" loss of efficacy. Cleaning involves removing the metal cartridge, rinsing the plastic inhaler and cap with briskly running warm water, drying thoroughly, and replacing cartridge and cap. Failure to clean the inhaler system properly may result in medication clogging the delivery system, which could lead to a decrease in the dose delivered. The FDA also commented that a number of factors may be involved in spray decrease, including priming (priming an inhaler before use is counted as one spray), temperature (the inhaler should be at room temperature), and agitation (the inhaler should be well shaken). (Bodenheimer S. *JAMA* 1993; 270: 2050. Nightingale SL. *JAMA*. 1993; 270: 2051.)

One reason for diminished dose administration is the design of the MDI itself. When only 15% or so of the original amount of suspension is left in the MDI, the meter chamber does not fill uniformly and the doses left are below acceptable levels. Manufacturers of some inhalers warn patients of this fact. However, "Patients generally do not count sprays and are not aware of how close they are to the end of the specified number of sprays," said Bergner. "Therefore, when their asthma exacerbates, they do not make the association between the exacerbation and the diminishing doses that may be delivered toward the end of the canister's 'life.'" Either they use more beta-agonist if the efficacy of the glucocorticoid is diminished, or vice versa, or they just assume their asthma got worse. Physicians don't usually ask how close patients are to the end of their inhalers but just assume that an asthma exacerbation is due to other causes (viral infection, pollen count, weather change, etc.). "It is our concern that the asthma patients most likely to be seriously affected by diminished doses are those with the most continuous, severe, and disabling asthma," said Bergner, and "the insidious reduction in doses delivered at the end of metered dose inhalers may be contributing, in part, to the increased mortality, hospitalizations, and morbidity of asthma in spite of the great advances made in our understanding and therapy of this common disorder." (Bergner A et al. *JAMA*. 1993; 270: 2051.)

Chapter 45

Your Metered-Dose Inhaler and Chlorofluorocarbons

Metered-dose inhalers (MDIs) are devices that people with asthma and chronic obstructive pulmonary disease (chronic bronchitis and emphysema) use to deliver medicine to their lungs. The medication is delivered by a propellant in the MDI whenever it is used. For most MDIs, the propellant is one or more gases called chlorofluorocarbons (CFCs).

Over the next few years, MDIs that contain CFCs are expected to be replaced by new inhaler devices that do not contain CFCs (non-CFC inhalers). This change has just begun and will continue for several years as more non-CFC options become available.

Patients and health care providers need to learn about the change to non-CFC inhalers. This [chapter] will help answer many of the questions that you may have about the change.

Why Will CFC MDIs Be Changing?

Although CFCs in medicines are safe for patients to inhale, CFCs are harmful to the environment. Scientists have found that when CFCs get into the upper regions of the earth's atmosphere (stratosphere), they reduce the amount of ozone in the ozone layer that surrounds the earth. The ozone layer acts as a shield to protect the earth

From "Your Metered-Dose Inhaler Will Be Changing...Here Are the Facts," [Online] Undated. Available: http://www.nhlbi.nih.gov/health/public/lung/ asthma/mdi.htm. Produced by the International Pharmaceutical Aerosol Consortium and the National Asthma Education and Prevention Program (NAEPP), National Heart, Lung, and Blood Institute (NHLBI). For complete contact information, please refer to Chapter 68, "Resources."

against the sun's harmful rays. With less ozone in the ozone layer, too many of these harmful rays reach the earth and can increase the risk of potentially serious health problems, such as skin cancer and cataracts, as well as other health and environmental problems. To lower the risk of health and environmental problems caused by ozone depletion and to help restore the ozone layer, most countries have agreed to stop using CFCs. The agreement was made in 1987 and is known as the Montreal Protocol.

CFCs are used in many types of products (such as air conditioners, refrigerators, etc.), not just MDIs. However, in response to the Montreal Protocol, the manufacture of CFCs for these purposes has already been stopped. Nonetheless, CFC MDIs have been given a special exemption because they are so important for treating asthma and chronic obstructive pulmonary disease. The manufacture of CFCs for use in MDIs will not be stopped until safe and effective replacements are available. But the goal is to one day replace CFC MDIs with alternatives that do not contain CFCs.

What Are the Benefits of Changing to Non-CFC Inhalers?

The change to non-CFC inhalers is one of many steps being taken worldwide to restore the ozone layer. A clear benefit of these efforts will be to help reduce the health and environmental risks caused by the sun's harmful rays.

The change is stimulating the development of many new types of non-CFC inhalers. Some of these will be new MDIs that have non-CFC propellants. Other inhalers are being developed that do not use propellants, such as dry powder inhalers and mini-nebulizers. This means that physicians may have several options to prescribe and patients may have additional choices in how their medicine is delivered. The safety and effectiveness of every new non-CFC inhaler will be reviewed by the U.S. Food and Drug Administration (FDA) before it is approved.

What Steps Have Been Taken to Change from CFC to Non-CFC Inhalers?

Many professional, public, and private groups are working to ensure that medicines are available to properly care for patients during the change from CFC to non-CFC inhalers. Although the conversion has been challenging, there has been a worldwide drive to develop non-CFC inhalers.

- The pharmaceutical industry has been working very hard to develop non-CFC MDIs. Companies around the world are testing inhalers containing new propellants instead of CFCs. These new propellants have been shown to be just as safe for patients as CFCs.

- Other non-CFC options not requiring propellants are being developed, including dry powder inhalers, mini-nebulizers, and other devices.

- The FDA and the U.S. Environmental Protection Agency (EPA) are working together to ensure that CFC MDIs remain available until safe and effective replacements are available.

- The National Asthma Education and Prevention Program (NAEPP), in collaboration with the International Pharmaceutical Aerosol Consortium, is developing educational materials regarding the change to non-CFC inhalers. Several NAEPP member organizations are also involved in patient education efforts, including the Allergy and Asthma Network/Mothers of Asthmatics, Inc.; the American Academy of Allergy, Asthma, and Immunology; the American Lung Association; the Asthma and Allergy Foundation of America; and representatives from the FDA and the EPA.

Which MDIs Will Be Available to Patients during the Change to Non-CFC Inhalers?

Concerns about patient health are important in the change from CFC to non-CFC inhalers. In order for patients and health care providers to have time to prepare for these changes, CFC MDIs will remain available until an adequate number of safe and effective non-CFC inhalers are available. However, we do not know how long this will take. All patients should have adequate choices of medicines during the change.

How Will the New Inhalers Differ from CFC MDIs?

There may be some differences in how CFC and non-CFC MDIs work, look, taste, or feel. Many new products will be produced and approved over time. It will be important for patients to talk with their doctor, nurse, pharmacist, respiratory therapist, or other health care provider when they get a new inhaler to make sure they know the correct way to use it. One non-CFC MDI for the medicine albuterol is available. Although patients may notice some minor differences in the feel or taste of the new product, the FDA has found it comparable in safety and effectiveness to the albuterol CFC MDIs. As with any change in therapy, patients should talk to their health care provider about non-CFC medication and other alternatives when they become available.

Will All Patients Have to Use Non-CFC Inhalers?

Yes. The goal is to phase out and ultimately eliminate the use of CFCs in MDIs. Although it will likely take a few years for this to happen, the process has already begun. It is important for patients and their health care providers to start making plans for the change now.

Where Can I Get More Information?

For information about asthma, other respiratory diseases, the Montreal Protocol, and the change to non-CFC inhalers, contact:

Allergy and Asthma Network/Mothers of Asthmatics, Inc.
Phone: 800-878-4403
Internet address: http://www.aanma.org

American Academy of Allergy, Asthma, and Immunology
Phone: 800-822-ASTHMA
Internet address: http://www.aaaai.org

American Association for Respiratory Care
Phone: 972-243-2272
Internet address: http://www.aarc.org

American College of Allergy, Asthma, and Immunology
Phone: 800-842-7777
Internet address: http://allergy.mcg.edu

American College of Chest Physicians
Phone: 847-498-1400
Internet address: http://www.chestnet.org

American Lung Association
Phone: 800-LUNG USA
Internet address: http://www.lungusa.org

American Pharmaceutical Association
Phone: 202-628-4410
Internet address: http://www.aphanet.org

American Society of Health-System Pharmacists
Phone: 301-657-3000
Internet address: http://www.ashp.org

American Thoracic Society
Phone: 212-315-8700
Internet address: http://www.thoracic.org

Asthma and Allergy Foundation of America
Phone: 800-7-ASTHMA
Internet address: http://www.aafa.org

European Federation of Asthma and Allergy Associations
Internet address: http://www.efanet.org

International Pharmaceutical Aerosol Consortium
Phone: 202-408-7189
Internet address: http://www.ipacmdi.com

National Association of School Nurses
Phone: 207-883-2117
Internet address: http://www.nasn.org

National Asthma Education and Prevention Program
Phone: 301-592-8573
Internet address: http://www.nhlbi.nih.gov/about/naepp

U.S. Environmental Protection Agency
Phone: 800-296-1996
Internet address: http://www.epa.gov/ozone

U.S. Food and Drug Administration
Phone: 301-827-4420
Internet address: http://www.fda.gov

Chapter 46

Adrenergic Bronchodilators

How you take a drug can affect how well it works and how safe it will be for you. Sometimes it can be almost as important as what you take. Timing, what you eat and when you eat, proper dose, and many other factors can mean the difference between feeling better, staying the same, or even feeling worse. This [chapter] is intended to help you make your treatment work as effectively as possible. It is important to note, however, that this is only a guideline. You should talk to your doctor about how and when to take any prescribed drugs.

This [chapter] is about adrenergic bronchodilators, most commonly used in metered-dose inhalers (small aerosol pumps). While doctors consider inhalers generally quite safe, these drugs can cause adverse effects if not used properly.

Conditions These Drugs Treat

Adrenergic bronchodilators alleviate the symptoms of asthma, chronic bronchitis, and emphysema by opening air passages in the lungs to allow easier breathing. While they are not a cure for asthma, adrenergic bronchodilators can temporarily relieve the classic symptoms of the disease: wheezing, coughing, shortness of breath, and

From "How to Take Your Medicines: Adrenergic Bronchodilators (Inhaled)," by Rebecca D. Williams, in *FDA Consumer* [Online] November 1991. Available: http://www.fda.gov. Produced by the U.S. Food and Drug Administration. For complete contact information, please refer to Chapter 68, "Resources."

tightness in the chest. They can also prevent bronchospasm when taken shortly before exercising.

How to Take

There are several devices that administer adrenergic bronchodilators. The metered-dose inhaler is the most common. A small aerosol pump, the inhaler sprays a controlled amount of medicated mist through a mouthpiece for the patient to inhale. The inhaler easily fits in a purse or bag to use anywhere.

Follow your doctor's directions for assembling and using the inhaler. For most brands, hold the inhaler bottle upside down and close your lips firmly over the mouthpiece. Press down firmly on the bottle as directed and inhale deeply. Then remove the mouthpiece and hold your breath a moment before exhaling slowly.

The prescribed dosage can vary, depending on the patient's symptoms and other factors. Always follow your doctor's instructions regarding the number and frequency of inhalations. Some patients are instructed to take two inhalations. Others are told to wait a minute or two and take another inhalation only if necessary.

Bronchodilators can also be taken using nebulizers or respirators to produce the spray, but these are almost always used only at a doctor's office or under strict medical supervision.

Most metered-dose inhalers require a doctor's prescription. Inhalers containing one type of bronchodilator, epinephrine, are available over the counter in brand names such as AsthmaHaler, Bronkaid, Primatene, and AsthmaNefrin. But do not use an over-the-counter inhaler unless your doctor recommends it and you have been diagnosed with asthma.

Missed Doses

For adults using inhalers, a typical dose of the medicine is two inhalations, four times a day. If you miss a dose, take it as soon as you remember, and consult your doctor about when to take the next dose. Be careful not to inhale more of the medicine than your doctor recommends. Large doses of bronchodilators might cause serious side effects.

Relief of Symptoms

Bronchodilators may provide relief in as quickly as a few seconds or as long as 30 minutes after using.

Side Effects and Risks

Side effects include nervousness, restlessness and trembling. Less common side effects include coughing, dizziness, indigestion, irritated mouth or throat, pounding heartbeat, headache, increased sweating, an increase in blood pressure, muscle cramps or twitching, nausea or vomiting, sleeplessness, paleness, and weakness.

Seek immediate medical attention if any side effects develop, including the following: bluish skin, severe dizziness or faintness, continuous flushing or redness of face or skin, increased wheezing or difficulty in breathing, skin rashes, hives or itching, and swelling of the face, lips, or eyelids.

Check with your doctor as soon as possible if you experience chest pain, irregular heartbeat, numbness in the hands or feet, or unusual breathing. If the inhaler medicine leaves an unpleasant taste in your mouth or changes your sense of smell or taste, contact your doctor immediately.

Precautions and Warnings

Check with your doctor at once if the bronchospasm continues after using an inhaler. Also, tell your doctor if you are pregnant or breast-feeding, and ask about any additional risks under those circumstances. Diabetics may find that their blood sugar levels rise after using this medicine. Diabetics who notice a change in their blood or urine sugar test results should tell their doctors.

Before Taking This Medicine

Before using an inhaler, tell your doctor if you have had adverse reactions to any drugs, especially other adrenergic bronchodilators. Also tell your doctor if you have any of the following medical problems:

- brain damage
- convulsions and seizures
- diabetes
- heart or blood vessel disease
- high blood pressure
- mental disease
- overactive thyroid
- Parkinson's disease

413

Inform your doctor of any prescription or over-the-counter drugs you are taking now or have taken in the last two weeks, especially any beta blockers, heart medicines, or mood-changing drugs.

Also, tell your doctor if you have ever used cocaine or other stimulants.

Some Commonly Used Metered-Dose Inhalers

- albuterol (Proventil, Ventolin)
- bitolterol (Tornalate)
- epinephrine (AsthmaHaler, Bronkaid Mist, Medihaler-Epi, Primatene Mist)
- isoetharine (Bronkometer)
- isoproterenol (Isuprel, Medihaler-Iso)
- metaproterenol (Alupent)
- pirbuterol (Maxair)
- terbutaline (Brethaire)

—by Rebecca D. Williams

Chapter 47

Stepwise Management of Symptoms

Stepwise Approach to Managing Asthma in Adults and in Children over 5 Years of Age

All patients need to have a short-acting inhaled beta$_2$-agonist to take as needed for symptoms. Patients with mild, moderate, or severe persistent asthma require daily long-term-control medication to control their asthma.

See Table 47.2. for the recommended pharmacologic therapy at each level of asthma severity and Chapter 40 for dosage information.

Gaining Control of Asthma

The physician's judgment of an individual patient's needs and circumstances will determine at what step to initiate therapy. There are two appropriate approaches to gaining control of asthma:

- Start treatment at the step appropriate to the severity of the patient's asthma at the time of evaluation. If control is not achieved, gradually step up therapy until control is achieved and maintained, or

Excerpted from "Pharmacologic Therapy: Managing Asthma Long Term," in *Practical Guide for the Diagnosis and Management of Asthma,* based on the *Expert Panel Report 2: Guidelines for the Diagnosis and Management of Asthma.* Produced by U.S. Department of Health and Human Services, National Heart, Lung, and Blood Institute (NHLBI), NIH Publication No. 97-4053, October 1997. For complete contact information, please refer to Chapter 68, "Resources."

- At the onset, give therapy at a higher level to achieve rapid control and then step down to the minimum therapy needed to maintain control. A higher level of therapy can be accomplished by either adding a course of oral steroids to inhaled steroids, cromolyn, or nedocromil, or using a higher dose of inhaled steroids.

- In the opinion of the Expert Panel, the preferred approach is to start with more intensive therapy in order to more rapidly suppress airway inflammation and thus gain prompt control.

If control is not achieved with initial therapy (e.g., within 1 month), the step selected, the therapy in the step, and possibly the diagnosis should be reevaluated.

Maintaining Control

Increases or decreases in medications may be needed as asthma severity and control vary over time. The Expert Panel's opinion is that followup visits every 1 to 6 months are essential for monitoring asthma. In addition, patients should be instructed to monitor their symptoms (and peak flow if used) and adjust therapy as described in the action plan (see Chapter 53).

Step Down Therapy

Gradually reduce or "step down" long-term-control medications after several weeks or months of controlling persistent asthma (i.e., the goals of asthma therapy are achieved). In general, the last medication added to the medical regimen should be the first medication reduced.

Inhaled steroids may be reduced about 25 percent every 2 to 3 months until the lowest dose required to maintain control is reached. For patients with persistent asthma, anti-inflammatory medications should be continued.

For patients who are taking oral steroids daily on a long-term basis, referral for consultation or care by an asthma specialist is recommended. Patients should be closely monitored for adverse side effects. Continuous attempts should be made to reduce daily use of oral steroids when asthma is controlled:

- Maintain patients on the lowest possible dose of oral steroids (single dose daily or on alternate days).

- Use high doses of inhaled steroids to eliminate or reduce the need for oral steroids.

Step Up Therapy

The presence of one or more indicators of poor asthma control (see Table 47.4.) may suggest a need to increase or "step up" therapy. Before increasing therapy, alternative reasons for poorly controlled asthma should be considered. Referral to a specialist for comanagement or consultation may be appropriate.

The addition of a 3- to 10-day course of oral steroids may be needed to reestablish control during a period of gradual deterioration or a

Table 47.1. Classification of Asthma Severity: Clinical Features before Treatment

	Days with symptoms	Nights with symptoms	PEF or FEV$_1$*	PEF variability
Step 4 Severe persistent	Continual	Frequent	≤60%	>30%
Step 3 Moderate persistent	Daily	≥5/month	>60%-<80%	>30%
Step 2 Mild persistent	3-6/week	3-4/month	≥80%	20-30%
Step 1 Mild intermittent	≤2/week	≤2/month	≥80%	<20%

*Percent predicted values for forced expiratory volume in 1 second (FEV$_1$) and percent of personal best for peak expiratory flow (PEF) (relevant for children 6 years old or older who can use these devices).

Patients should be assigned to the most severe step in which any feature occurs. Clinical features for individual patients may overlap across steps.

An individual's classification may change over time.

Patients at any level of severity of chronic asthma can have mild, moderate, or severe exacerbations of asthma. Some patients with intermittent asthma experience severe and life-threatening exacerbations separated by long periods of normal lung function and no symptoms.

Patients with two or more asthma exacerbations per week (i.e., progressively worsening symptoms that may last hours or days) tend to have moderate-to-severe persistent asthma.

moderate-to-severe exacerbation (see Chapter 57). If symptoms do not recur after the course of steroids (and peak flow remains normal), the patient should continue in the same step. However, if the steroid course controls symptoms for less than 1 to 2 weeks, or if courses of steroids are repeated frequently, the patient should move to the next higher step in therapy.

Special Considerations for Infants, Children, and Adolescents

Infants and Preschool Children

Treatment of acute or chronic wheezing or cough should follow the stepwise approach presented in Table 47.3. In general, physicians should do the following when infants and young children consistently require treatment for symptoms more than two times per week:

- Prescribe daily inhaled anti-inflammatory medication (inhaled steroids, cromolyn, or nedocromil) as long-term-control asthma therapy. A trial of cromolyn or nedocromil is often given to patients with mild persistent asthma.

- Monitor the response to therapy carefully (e.g., frequency of symptoms over 2 to 4 weeks).

- If benefits are sustained for at least 3 months, a step down in therapy should be attempted.

- If clear benefit is not observed, treatment should be stopped. Alternative therapies or diagnoses should be considered.

- Consider oral steroids if an exacerbation caused by a viral respiratory infection is moderate to severe. If the patient has a history of severe exacerbations, consider steroids at the onset of the viral infection.

Medication delivery devices should be selected according to the child's ability to use them. Be aware that the dose received can vary considerably among delivery devices:

- Children aged 2 or less—nebulizer therapy is preferred for administering cromolyn or high doses of short-acting inhaled beta$_2$-agonists. A metered-dose inhaler (MDI) with a spacer/holding chamber that has a face mask may be used to take inhaled steroids.

- Children 3 to 5 years of age—MDI plus spacer/holding chamber may be used by many children of this age. If the desired therapeutic effects are not achieved, a nebulizer or an MDI plus spacer/holding chamber with a face mask may be required.

Spacers/holding chambers are devices that hold the aerosol medication so the patient can inhale it easily. This reduces the problem of coordinating the actuation of the MDI with the inhalation. Spacers/holding chambers come in many different shapes. These devices are not simply tubes that put space between the patient's mouth and the MDI. Examples of spacers/holding chambers are illustrated in Chapter 48.

Parents or caregivers need to be instructed in the proper use of appropriately sized face masks, spacers with face masks, and holding chamber devices. Acceptable use of the delivery device should be demonstrated in the office before the patient leaves. The ability of children to use the devices may vary widely.

School-Age Children and Adolescents

The pharmacologic management of school-age children and adolescents follows the same basic principles as those for adults, but with special consideration of growth, school, and social development:

- Cromolyn or nedocromil is often tried first in children with mild or moderate persistent asthma. This is because these medications are often effective anti-inflammatory therapies and have no known long-term systemic effects.

- For children with severe persistent asthma, and for many with moderate persistent asthma, inhaled steroids are necessary for long-term-control therapy. Cromolyn and nedocromil do not provide adequate control for these patients. See stepwise approach to pharmacotherapy (Table 47.2.) for treatment recommendations.

Inhaled Steroids and Growth

The potential but small risk of adverse effects on linear growth from the use of inhaled steroids is well balanced by their efficacy. Poor asthma control itself can result in retarded linear growth. Most studies do not demonstrate a negative effect on growth with dosages of

419

Table 47.2. Stepwise Approach for Managing Asthma in Adults and Children over 5 Years Old: Treatment

Long-Term Control (preferred treatments are in bold print)

Step 4
Severe
persistent

Daily medications:
- **Anti-inflammatory: inhaled steroid (high dose)*** AND
- Long-acting bronchodilator: either **long-acting inhaled beta$_2$-agonist** (adult: 2 puffs q 12 hours; child: 1-2 puffs q 12 hours), sustained-release theophylline, or long-acting beta$_2$-agonist tablets AND
- Steroid tablets or syrup long term; make repeated attempts to reduce systemic steroid and maintain control with high-dose inhaled steroid.

Step 3
Moderate
persistent

Daily medication:
- Either **anti-inflammatory: inhaled steroid (medium dose)*** OR **inhaled steroid (low- to-medium dose)*** and add a long-acting bronchodilator, especially for nighttime symptoms: either **long-acting inhaled beta$_2$-agonist** (adult: 2 puffs q 12 hours; child: 1-2 puffs q 12 hours), sustained-release theophylline, or long-acting beta$_2$-agonist tablets.
- If needed **anti-inflammatory: inhaled steroids (medium- to-high dose)*** AND long-acting bronchodilator, especially for nighttime symptoms: either **long-acting inhaled beta$_2$-agonist,** sustained-release theophylline, or long-acting beta$_2$-agonist tablets.

Step 2
Mild
persistent

Daily medication:
- **Anti-inflammatory: either inhaled steroid (low dose)*** or **cromolyn** (adult: 2-4 puffs tid-qid; child: 1-2 puffs tid-qid) or **nedocromil** (adult: 2-4 puffs bid-qid; child: 1-2 puffs bid-qid) (children usually begin with a trial of cromolyn or nedocromil).
- Sustained-release theophylline to serum concentration of 5-15 mcg/mL is an alternative, but not preferred, therapy. Zafirlukast or zileuton may also be considered for those 12 years old, although their position in therapy is not fully established.

Step 1
Mild
intermittent

- No daily medication needed.

Quick-Relief

All patients
Short-acting bronchodilator: **inhaled beta$_2$-agonist** (2-4 puffs) as needed for symptoms. Intensity of treatment will depend on severity of exacerbation.

*See estimated comparative daily dosages for inhaled steroids in Chapter 40.

The stepwise approach presents general guidelines to assist clinical decision-making. Asthma is highly variable; clinicians should tailor medication plans to the needs of individual patients.

***Gain control** as quickly as possible. Either start with aggressive therapy (e.g., add a course of oral steroids or a higher dose of inhaled steroids to* *the therapy that corresponds to the patient's initial step of severity); or start at the step that corresponds to the patient's initial severity and step up treatment, if necessary.*

__Step down:__ Review treatment every 1 to 6 months. Gradually decrease treatment to the least medication necessary to maintain control.

__Step up:__ If control is not maintained, consider step up. Inadequate control is indicated by increased use of short-acting beta$_2$-agonists and in: step 1 when patient uses a short-acting beta$_2$-agonist more than two times a week; steps 2 and 3 when patient uses short-acting beta$_2$-agonist on a daily basis or more than three to four times in 1 day. But before stepping up: Review patient inhaler technique, compliance, and environmental control (avoidance of allergens or other precipitant factors).

A course of oral steroids may be needed at any time and at any step.

Patients with exercise-induced bronchospasm should take two to four puffs of an inhaled beta$_2$-agonist 5 to 60 minutes before exercise.

Referral to an asthma specialist for consultation or comanagement is recommended if there is difficulty maintaining control or if the patient requires step 4 care. Referral may be considered for step 3 care.

400 to 800 mcg a day of beclomethasone,[1-3] although a few short-term studies have.[4-5] Adverse effects on linear growth appear to be dose dependent. High doses of inhaled steroids have greater potential for growth suppression, but less potential than the alternative of oral steroids. Some caution (e.g., monitoring growth, stepping down therapy when possible) is suggested while this issue is studied further.

Action Plan for Schools

The clinician should prepare a written action plan for the student's school that explains when medications may be needed to treat episodes and to prevent exercise-induced bronchospasm. Recommendations to limit exposures to offending allergens or irritants and a written request for the child to carry quick-relief medications at school could be helpful. When possible, schedule daily medications so they do not need to be taken at school.

Table 47.3. Stepwise Approach for Managing Infants and Young Children (5 Years of Age and Younger) with Acute or Chronic Asthma Symptoms

Long-Term Control

Step 4 **Severe** **persistent**	**Daily anti-inflammatory medication** • High-dose inhaled steroid* with spacer and face mask • If needed, add oral steroids (2 mg/kg/day); reduce to lowest daily or alternate-day dose that stabilizes symptoms
Step 3 **Moderate** **persistent**	**Daily anti-inflammatory medication** • Either: medium-dose inhaled steroid* with spacer and face mask. Once control is established, consider: lower medium-dose inhaled steroid* with spacer and face mask and nedocromil (1-2 puffs bid-qid) • OR lower medium-dose inhaled steroid* with spacer and face mask and theophylline (10 mg/kg/day up to 16 mg/kg/day for children 1 year of age, to a serum concentration of 5-15 mcg/mL)**
Step 2 **Mild** **persistent**	**Daily anti-inflammatory medication** • Infants and young children usually begin with a trial of cromolyn (nebulizer is preferred—1 ampule tid-qid; or MDI—1-2 puffs tid-qid) or nedocromil (MDI only—1-2 puffs bid-qid) • OR low-dose inhaled steroid* with spacer and face mask
Step 1 **Mild** **intermittent**	No daily medication needed.

Quick-Relief

All patients	Bronchodilator as needed for symptoms: Short-acting inhaled beta$_2$-agonist by nebulizer (0.05 mg/kg in 2-3 cc of saline) or inhaler with face mask and spacer (2-4 puffs; for exacerbations, repeat q 20 minutes for up to 1 hour) or oral beta$_2$-agonist. **With viral respiratory infection,** use short-acting inhaled beta$_2$-agonist q 4 to 6 hours up to 24 hours (longer with physician consult) but, in general, if repeated more than once every 6 weeks, consider moving to next step up. Consider oral steroids if the exacerbation is moderate to severe or at the onset of the infection if the patient has a history of severe exacerbations.

* See estimated comparative dosages for inhaled steroids in Chapter 40.

** For children <1 year of age: usual max mg/kg/day = 0.2 (age in weeks) + 5.

The stepwise approach presents general guidelines to assist clinical decision-making. Asthma is highly variable; clinicians should tailor medication plans to the needs of individual patients.

__Gain control__ as quickly as possible. Either start with aggressive therapy (e.g., add a course of oral steroids or a higher dose of inhaled steroids to the therapy that corresponds to the patient's initial step of severity); or start

at the step that corresponds to the patient's initial severity and step up treatment, if necessary.

Step down: *Review treatment every 1 to 6 months. If control is sustained for at least 3 months, a gradual stepwise reduction in treatment may be possible.*

Step up: *If control is not achieved, consider step up. Inadequate control is indicated by increased use of short-acting beta$_2$-agonists and in: step 1 when patient uses a short-acting beta$_2$-agonist more than two times a week; steps 2 and 3 when patient uses short-acting beta$_2$-agonist on a daily basis OR more than three to four times a day. But before stepping up: review patient inhaler technique, compliance, and environmental control (avoidance of allergens or other precipitant factors).*

A course of oral steroids (prednisolone) may be needed at any time and step.

Referral to an asthma specialist for consultation or comanagement is recommended for patients requiring step 3 or 4 care. Referral may be considered for step 2 care.

Managing Asthma in Older Adults

Make adjustments or avoid asthma medications that can aggravate other conditions:

- Inhaled steroids. Give supplements of calcium (1,000 to 1,500 mg per day), vitamin D (400 units a day), and, where appropriate, estrogen replacement therapy, especially for women using high doses of inhaled steroids.

- Oral steroids may provoke confusion, agitation, and changes in glucose metabolism.

- Theophylline and epinephrine may exacerbate underlying heart conditions. Also, the risk of theophylline overdose may be higher because of reduced theophylline clearance in older patients.

Inform patients about potential adverse effects on their asthma from medications used for other conditions, for example:

- Aspirin and other oral nonsteroidal anti-inflammatory medications (arthritis, pain relief)

- Nonselective beta-blockers (high blood pressure)
- Beta-blockers in some eye drops (glaucoma)

Chronic bronchitis and emphysema may coexist with asthma. A 2- to 3-week trial with oral steroids can help determine the presence of reversibility of airway obstruction and indicate the extent of potential benefit from asthma therapy.

Managing Special Situations

Managing Exercise-Induced Bronchospasm

Exercise-induced bronchospasm generally begins during exercise and reaches its peak 5 to 10 minutes after stopping. The symptoms often spontaneously resolve in another 20 to 30 minutes.

A diagnosis of exercise-induced bronchospasm is suggested by a history of cough, shortness of breath, chest pain or tightness, wheezing, or endurance problems during and after vigorous activity. The

Table 47.4. Poor Asthma Control: Indicators and Reasons

Indicators of Poor Asthma Control—Consider Increasing Long-Term Medications*

- Awakened at night with symptoms
- An urgent care visit
- Patient has increased need for short-acting inhaled beta$_2$-agonists (excludes use for upper respiratory viral infections and exercise-induced bronchospasm) OR
  —At step 1: Used short-acting inhaled beta$_2$-agonists more than two times in a week
  —At steps 2-3: Used short-acting inhaled beta$_2$-agonists more than three to four times a day OR used this medication on a daily basis for a week or less
  —Patient used more than one canister of short-acting inhaled beta$_2$-agonist in one month

Assess Reasons for Poor Asthma Control before Increasing Medications—ICE

- Inhaler technique—Check patient's technique.
- Compliance—Ask when and how much medication the patient is taking.
- Environment—Ask patient if something in his or her environment has changed.

Also consider:
- Alternative diagnosis—Assess patient for presence of concomitant upper respiratory disease or alternative diagnosis.

* *This may mean a temporary increase in anti-inflammatory medication to regain control or a "step up" in long-term therapy. This will depend on the frequency of the above events, reasons for poor control, and the clinician's judgment.*

diagnosis can be confirmed by an objective measure of the problem (i.e., a 15 percent decrease in peak flow or FEV_1 between measurements taken before and after vigorous activity at 5-minute intervals for 20 to 30 minutes.)

For the vast majority of patients, exercise-induced bronchospasm should not limit either participation or success in vigorous activities. The following are the recommended control measures:

- Two to four puffs of short-acting beta$_2$-agonist 5 to 60 minutes before exercise, preferably as close to the start of exercise as possible. The effects of this pretreatment should last approximately 2 to 3 hours. A long-acting inhaled beta$_2$-agonist taken at least 30 minutes before exercise will last 10 to 12 hours.[6] Cromolyn or nedocromil can also be used before exercise with a duration of effect of 1 to 2 hours.[7-9]

- A 6- to 10-minute warmup period before exercise may benefit patients who can tolerate continuous exercise with minimal symptoms. The warmup may preclude a need for repeated medications.

- Increase in long-term-control medications, if appropriate. If symptoms occur with usual activities or exercise, a step up in long-term-control therapy may be warranted. Long-term control of asthma with anti-inflammatory medication (i.e., inhaled steroid, cromolyn, or nedocromil) can reduce the frequency and severity of exercise-induced bronchospasm.[10]

Teachers and coaches need to be notified that a child has exercise-induced bronchospasm. They should be told that the child is able to participate in activities but may need inhaled medication before activity. Athletes should disclose the medications they use and adhere to standards set by the U.S. Olympic Committee.[11] A complete, easy-to-use list of prohibited and approved medications can be obtained from the U.S. Olympic Committee's Drug Reference Hotline: (800) 233-0393.

Managing Seasonal Asthma Symptoms

- During the allergy season: Use the stepwise approach to the long-term management of asthma to control symptoms.

- Before the season: If symptoms during a season are predictable, start daily anti-inflammatory therapy (inhaled steroids, cromolyn, or nedocromil) just before the anticipated onset of symptoms and continue this throughout the season.

Managing Asthma in Patients Undergoing Surgery

- Evaluate the patient's asthma over the past 6 months.
- Improve lung function to predicted values before surgery, possibly with a short course of oral steroids.
- Give patients who have received oral steroids for longer than 2 weeks during the past 6 months 100 mg of hydrocortisone every 8 hours intravenously during the surgical period. Reduce the dose rapidly within 24 hours following surgery.

Managing Asthma in Pregnant Women

Management of asthma in pregnant women is essential and is achieved with basically the same treatment as for nonpregnant women. Poorly controlled asthma during pregnancy can result in reduced oxygen supply to the fetus, increased perinatal mortality, increased prematurity, and low birth weight.[12] There is little to suggest an increased risk to the fetus for most drugs used to treat asthma.

Drugs or drug classes with potential risk to the fetus include brompheniramine, epinephrine, and alpha-adrenergic compounds (other than pseudoephedrine),[13-15] decongestants (other than pseudoephedrine), antibiotics (tetracycline, sulfonamides, and ciprofloxacine), live virus vaccines, immunotherapy (initiation or increase in doses), and iodides.

References

1. Wolthers OD. Long-, intermediate- and short-term growth studies in asthmatic children treated with inhaled glucosteroids. *Eur Respir J* 1996;9:821-7.

2. Kamada AK, Szefler SJ, Martin RJ, et al., and the Asthma Clinical Research Network. Issues in the use of inhaled glucocorticoids. *Am J Respir Crit Care Med* 1996;153:1739-48.

3. Barnes PJ, Pedersen S. Efficacy and safety of inhaled steroids in asthma. *Am Rev Respir Dis* 1993;148:S1-S26.

4. Tinkelman DG, Reed CE, Nelson HS, Offord KP. Aerosol beclomethasone dipropionate compared with theophylline as

primary treatment of chronic, mild to moderately severe asthma in children. *Pediatrics* 1993;92:64-77.

5. Doull IJM, Freezer NJ, Holgate ST. Growth of pre-pubertal children with mild asthma treated with inhaled beclomethasone dipropionate. *Am J Respir Crit Care Med* 1995;51:1715-9.

6. Kemp JP, Dockhorn RJ, Busse WW, Bleecker ER, Van As A. Prolonged effect of inhaled salmeterol against exercise-induced bronchospasm. *Am J Respir Crit Care Med* 1994;150:1612-5.

7. Albazzaz MK, Neale MG, Patel KR. Dose-response study of nebulized nedocromil sodium in exercise induced asthma. *Thorax* 1989;44:816-9.

8. de Benedictis FM, Tuteri G, Pazzelli P, Bertotto A, Bruni L, Vaccaro R. Cromolyn versus nedocromil: duration of action in exercise-induced asthma in children. *J Allergy Clin Immunol* 1995;96:510-4.

9. Woolley M, Anderson SD, Quigley BM. Duration of terbutaline sulfate and cromolyn sodium alone and in combination on exercise-induced asthma. *Chest* 1990;97:39-45.

10. Vathenen AS, Knox AJ, Wisniewski A, Tattersfield AE. Effect of inhaled budesonide on bronchial reactivity to histamine, exercise, and eucapnic dry air hyperventilation in patients with asthma. *Thorax* 1991;46:811-6.

11. Nastasi KJ, Heinly TL, Blaiss MS. Exercise-induced asthma and the athlete. *J Asthma* 1995;32:249-57.

12. Nelson HS, Weber RW. Endocrine aspects of allergic diseases. In: Bierman CW, Pearlman DS, eds. *Allergic Diseases from Infancy to Adulthood.* Philadelphia: WB Saunders, 1988. ch. 15.

13. Schatz M, Zeiger RS, Harden KM, et al. The safety of inhaled beta-agonist bronchodilators during pregnancy. *J Allergy Clin Immunol* 1988;82:686-95.

14. *Federal Register.* 21 CFR Parts 201, 202. 1979;44(124):37434-37467.

15. Briggs GG, Freeman RK, Yaffe SJ. *Drugs in Pregnancy and Lactation: A Reference Guide to Fetal and Neonatal Risk,* 2nd ed. Baltimore, MD: Williams & Wilkins, 1986.

Chapter 48

How to Use Your Inhaler Effectively

Using an inhaler seems simple, but most patients do not use it the right way. When you use your inhaler the wrong way, less medicine gets to your lungs. (Your doctor may give you other types of inhalers.)

For the next 2 weeks, read these steps aloud as you do them or ask someone to read them to you. Ask your doctor or nurse to check how well you are using your inhaler.

Use your inhaler in one of the three ways pictured (Figures 48.1. or 48.2. are best, but Figure 48.3. can be used if you have trouble with Figures 48.1. and 48.2.).

Steps for Using Your Inhaler

Getting ready:

1. Take off the cap and shake the inhaler.

2. Breathe out all the way.

3. Hold your inhaler the way your doctor said (Figure 48.1., 48.2., or 48.3. below).

Excerpted from "How to Use Your Metered-Dose Inhaler the Right Way," in *Practical Guide for the Diagnosis and Management of Asthma,* based on the *Expert Panel Report 2: Guidelines for the Diagnosis and Management of Asthma.* Produced by U.S. Department of Health and Human Services, National Heart, Lung, and Blood Institute (NHLBI), NIH Publication No. 97-4053, October 1997. For complete contact information, please refer to Chapter 68, "Resources."

Breathe in slowly:

4. As you start breathing in slowly through your mouth, press down on the inhaler one time. (If you use a holding chamber, first press down on the inhaler. Within 5 seconds, begin to breathe in slowly.)

5. Keep breathing in slowly, as deeply as you can.

Hold your breath:

6. Hold your breath as you count to 10 slowly, if you can.

7. For inhaled quick-relief medicine (beta$_2$-agonists), wait about 1 minute between puffs. There is no need to wait between puffs for other medicines.

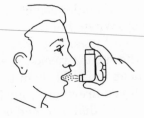

Figure 48.1. Hold inhaler 1 to 2 inches in front of your mouth (about the width of two fingers).

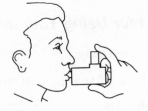

Figure 48.2. Use a spacer/ holding chamber. These come in many shapes and can be useful to any patient.

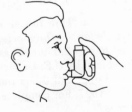

Figure 48.3. Put the inhaler in your mouth. Do not use for steroids.

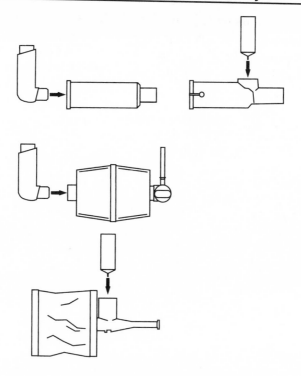

Figure 48.4. *Examples of spacer/holding chamber devices.*

Clean Your Inhaler as Needed

Look at the hole where the medicine sprays out from your inhaler. If you see "powder" in or around the hole, clean the inhaler. Remove the metal canister from the L-shaped plastic mouthpiece. Rinse only the mouthpiece and cap in warm water. Let them dry overnight. In the morning, put the canister back inside. Put the cap on.

Know When to Replace Your Inhaler

For medicines you take each day, [follow this example]. Say your new canister has 200 puffs (number of puffs is listed on canister) and you are told to take 8 puffs per day. [Divide 200 puffs by 8 puffs to find the number of days this canister will last. The answer is 25.] So this canister will last 25 days.

If you started using this inhaler on May 1, replace it on or before May 25. You can write the date on your canister.

For quick-relief medicine take as needed and count each puff.

Do not put your canister in water to see if it is empty. This does not work.

Chapter 49

Immunotherapy (Allergy Shots)

Immunotherapy (commonly called allergy shots) is a form of treatment to reduce your allergic reaction to allergens. Allergens are substances to which you are allergic. Research has shown that allergy shots can reduce symptoms of allergic rhinitis (hay fever) and allergic asthma. Remember, not all asthma is due to allergies. Allergy shots can be effective against grass, weed and tree pollens, house dust mites, cat and dog dander, and insect stings. Allergy shots are less effective against molds and are not a useful method for the treatment of food allergy.

Immunotherapy consists of a series of injections (shots) with a solution containing the allergens that cause your symptoms. Treatment usually begins with a weak solution given once or twice a week. The strength of the solution is gradually increased with each dose. Once the strongest dosage is reached, the injections are usually given once a month to control your symptoms. At this point, you have decreased your sensitivity to the allergens and have reached your maintenance level. Allergy shots should always be given at your health care provider's office.

When Is Immunotherapy Recommended?

If you are considering allergy shots, talk to your health care provider about a referral to a board certified allergist. A board certified allergist

From "Med Facts: Immunotherapy (Allergy Shots)," [Online] Undated. Available: http://www.njc.org/MFhtml/IMT_MF.html. © 1995 by the National Jewish Medical and Research Center, 1400 Jackson St., Denver, Colorado 80206. Reprinted with permission. For complete contact information, please refer to Chapter 68, "Resources."

will follow a number of steps to evaluate if allergy shots are appropriate for you.

First, the allergist will ask you questions about your environment and symptoms to determine if skin testing is necessary. Typically, prick skin testing is conducted to identify the specific allergens that are causing your symptoms. Skin testing should only be administered under the supervision of a board certified allergist.

Once an allergy has been identified, the next step is to decrease or eliminate exposure to the allergen. This is called environmental control. Evidence shows that allergy and asthma symptoms may improve over time, if the recommended environmental control changes are made. For example, removing furry or feathered pets or following control measures for house dust mites and cockroaches may decrease symptoms. Preventing your contact with grasses, weeds, and tree pollen may be more difficult but possible by keeping outside doors and windows closed and using air conditioning. If you would like more information on methods of environmental controls, call LUNG LINE® at 1-800-222-LUNG.

Next, your health care provider may recommend antihistamines and nasal medications as remedies. In general, allergy shots are recommended only for persons with a history of severe or prolonged allergic rhinitis and for persons with allergic asthma when the allergen cannot be avoided. Allergy shots should be prescribed only by a board certified allergist.

How Long Are Allergy Shots Given?

Six months to a year of immunotherapy may be required before you experience any improvement in symptoms. If your symptoms do not improve after this time, your allergist should review your overall treatment program. If the treatment is effective, the shots usually continue three to five years, until the individual is symptom-free or until symptoms can be controlled with mild medications for one year. In general, allergy shots should be stopped if they are not effective within two to three years.

Rush Immunotherapy

Rush immunotherapy is a variation of allergy shots which "rushes" the initial phase of the treatment. Steadily increasing doses of allergen extract are given every few hours instead of every few days or weeks. There is an increased risk of a reaction with this procedure.

Therefore, rush immunotherapy should only be done in a hospital under very close supervision.

Other Therapies

There are a number of alternative treatments which claim to "cure" allergies. These methods are not supported by scientific studies and are not approved by the American Academy of Allergy, Asthma and Immunology. Unapproved alternative treatments include:

- Desensitization to foods, chemicals, and environmental allergens with sublingual (under the tongue) drops
- High-dose vitamin and mineral therapy
- Urine injections
- Bacterial vaccines
- Exotic diets

It is easy to feel overwhelmed or confused by the many different methods of allergy testing and treatment. We encourage you to work with a board certified allergist to evaluate and determine what is appropriate for you.

Chapter 50

Asthma and the Leukotriene Receptor: New Options for Therapy

Asthma is a chronic inflammatory disease of the airways that is complicated by episodes of acute inflammation. Even patients with mild disease show airways inflammation, including infiltration of the mucosa and epithelium with activated T cells, mast cells, and eosinophils. T cells and mast cells release cytokines that promote eosinophil growth and maturation and the production of IgE antibodies, and these, in turn, increase microvascular permeability, disrupt the epithelium, and stimulate neural reflexes and mucus-secreting glands. The result is airways hyperreactivity, bronchoconstriction, and hypersecretion, manifested by wheezing, coughing, and dyspnea.

Traditionally, asthma has been treated with oral and inhaled bronchodilators. These agents help the symptoms of asthma, but do nothing for the underlying inflammation. Recognition during the last 10 years of the importance of inflammation in the etiology of asthma has led to the increased use of corticosteroids, but many patients continue to suffer from uncontrolled asthma. Now the FDA has approved the first of a new class of antiasthma drugs—the leukotriene inhibitors and antagonists—with the potential to interfere with the initial steps in the inflammatory cascade.

We first reported on leukotrienes in *MSB* back in 1979, when the so-called "slow reacting substance of anaphylaxis" was identified as

From "Focus on . . . New Receptor Antagonists," in *Medical Sciences Bulletin*, Vol. 19, No.3, 1996. © 1996 by Pharmaceutical Information Associates, Ltd., 2761 Trenton Rd., Levittown, PA 19056. All rights reserved. Reprinted with permission.

an arachidonic acid derivative and given the name "leukotriene C." Since that time, scientists have determined that the leukotrienes (of which there are A, B, C, D, and E subtypes) play a crucial role in asthma. They cause airways smooth muscle spasm, increased vascular permeability, edema, enhanced mucus production, reduced mucociliary transport, and leukocyte chemotaxis.

Like the related prostaglandins, leukotrienes are synthesized from arachidonic acid in the cell membrane. Arachidonic acid in mast cells, macrophages, monocytes, eosinophils, and basophils is released from membrane phospholipids by the activation of phospholipase A2. After its release, arachidonic acid undergoes metabolism via two major pathways: the cyclooxygenase pathway (which produces various prostaglandins and thromboxanes) and the 5-lipoxygenase pathway (which produces leukotrienes). The prostaglandins, thromboxanes, and leukotrienes are known collectively as eicosanoids.

There are a number of anti-leukotrienes under investigation that either block leukotriene receptors or prevent leukotriene synthesis by blocking the enzyme 5-lipoxygenase (just as aspirin and the nonsteroidal anti-inflammatory agents block the other enzyme—cyclooxygenase—involved in arachidonic acid metabolism). The leukotriene inhibitors are a varied lot: some block 5-lipoxygenase directly, some inhibit the protein that "presents" arachidonate to 5-lipoxygenase, and some displace arachidonate from its binding site on the protein. The leukotriene antagonists, by contrast, block the receptors themselves that mediate airways hyperreactivity, bronchoconstriction, and hypersecretion.

The market for the new leukotriene inhibitors and antagonists is in the billions of dollars. An estimated 13 million Americans have asthma, and many are not controlled with available bronchodilators and corticosteroids. Indeed, asthma mortality has risen 40% since 1982. Abbott, Merck, and SmithKline Beecham all have anti-leukotrienes in final clinical trial, and Zeneca's zafirlukast (Accolate) was approved in late September. Abbott's zileuton (Zyflo) was the first leukotriene to be reviewed by the FDA. It was rejected in October 1995 because of adverse effects on liver function tests, but Abbott refiled an application in June, and an FDA advisory committee has recommended the drug for approval with the suggestion that liver function be carefully monitored. SmithKline Beecham's pranlukast (Ultair) is a leukotriene receptor antagonist licensed from Ono Pharmaceutical and approved for marketing in Japan. Merck's montelukast (Singulair) is a long-acting agent that will be the subject of an NDA filing during the first part of 1997. A number of additional drugs are under investigation, including the leukotriene antagonists pobilukast, tomelukast, and verlukast, and several inhibitors of leukotriene synthesis. (Holgate ST et al. *J Allergy Clin Immunol.* 1996;98:1-13. Spector SL. *Annals of Allergy, Asthma, Immunol.* 1995;75:473- 474. Additional information from the manufacturers.)

Part Six

Asthma Management

Chapter 51

Role of the Allergist in Cost-Effective Treatment of Asthma

The prevalence, morbidity, and associated economic costs of asthma are increasing at an alarming rate. This has occurred despite ever-increasing knowledge about the pathophysiologic condition of asthma and despite the development of more specific and effective drugs. In this review, we will part from the traditional (and necessary) approach of which medicines to use and when to use them and consider instead the question of whether there are aspects of delivery of care in the current health care system that may be contributing to the suboptimal outcomes experienced by many asthmatics. Information was obtained from a Medline search of relevant articles from the last 10 years plus earlier references culled from those articles.

To answer this question, we will examine first evidence of dysfunction in the current system of care and then aspects of the current system that seem more likely to result in a better outcome than others.

We will frame the problem by reviewing some of the major literature about asthma management. We will concentrate on the available literature that deals with expert vs generalist care.

The Problem

It is estimated that asthma affects between 7 and 20 million Americans.[1-3] Although this may reflect in part increased recognition of the

From "Asthma: Better Outcome at Lower Cost? The Role of the Expert in the Care System," by Thaddeus Bartter and Melvin R. Pratter, in *Chest,* Vol. 110, No. 6, December 1996, pp. 1589-96. © 1996 by the American College of Chest Physicians, 3300 Dundee Rd., Northbrook, IL 60062-2348. Reprinted with permission.

disease, the evidence clearly demonstrates a true increase in the prevalence of patients with symptomatic asthma.[1]

Both the morbidity and the economic cost of asthma are huge. A published estimate put the total costs (direct and indirect) of asthma in the United States in 1990 at $6.2 billion per year.[4] The largest direct cost was that of hospitalization. The study cited 463,500 hospitalizations for asthma per year at an annual cost of $1 billion. The cost of medications was the second largest direct cost at $700 million. Emergency department (ED) visits, about 1.81 million visits per year, were more frequent than physician office visits, 1.5 million per year, and incurred significantly greater cost, estimated at $200.3 million per year. The largest indirect cost, $700 million, came from the costs associated with missed school days for children. Estimated loss of income from premature deaths accounted for $680 million.

Asthma mortality is on the rise. A number of reports from the United States[1,5-7] and around the world[8-10] have documented that death rates have been increasing for at least the last 15 years. Many factors may play a role in this increase, but the inescapable paradox is that our success in preventing death from this disease is declining at the same time that our knowledge and therapeutic options are increasing.

The Current Medical System

There is a great deal of evidence demonstrating that current approaches to the care of asthmatics are suboptimal. Diagnostic accuracy is often inadequate, there is not consistent use of objective assessment of severity of airflow obstruction, corticosteroids, particularly by inhalation, are underutilized, and both physicians and patients often fail to recognize when an asthmatic is at high risk for fatal asthma.

The diagnosis of asthma is often inaccurate. The primary reason appears to be that clinical diagnosis remains the most widespread technique despite repeated evidence that objective testing (i.e., presence or absence of reversible airflow obstruction or bronchial hyperresponsiveness) is critical for accurate diagnosis.[11-15] Dales, et al.,[11] studied 200 insulators with a detailed respiratory questionnaire and bronchoprovocation challenge. They demonstrated that the questionnaire was unable to identify those with objectively documented bronchial hyperresponsiveness and therefore to separate those whose symptoms may have been due to asthma from those whose symptoms were almost certainly not due to asthma. Pratter, et al.,[12] demonstrated that using history and physical examination, experienced pulmonologists were able to correctly diagnose the presence or absence of asthma in patients with a history of wheeze only 54% of the time. They also demonstrated that a history of asthma had been incorrect 38% of the time. Adelroth, et al.,[13] in a similar study of patients with suspected asthma but normal results of spirometry, showed that experienced pulmonologists, when restricted to clinical examination alone, were incorrect in predicting either the presence or absence of bronchial hyperresponsiveness on bronchoprovocation challenge 39% of the time.

Physicians appear at times to ignore even the clinical information. Bucknall, et al.,[15] did a prospective study of patients admitted to the hospital either as having acute asthma or wheezing in a nonsmoker. They followed up 86 patients who were admitted to general wards without a specialist internist and 64 admitted to general wards with a special interest in pulmonary medicine. Despite a lack of significant differences between the two groups on hospital admission, 42% of the patients on the general wards were discharged with a diagnosis of chronic obstructive airways disease rather than asthma vs. 16% from the expert care ward (p<0.005). Obviously, a lack of accurate diagnosis is one of a series of problems that can lead to suboptimal treatment of asthmatics.

Once asthma has been diagnosed, determining the degree of obstruction present is essential to management since obstruction is the physiology being treated; knowledge of degree of obstruction is the bridge between diagnosis and treatment. Ample information in the pulmonary literature demonstrates that neither the patient nor the physician can accurately assess the severity of airflow obstruction without objective studies. Rubinfeld and Pain[16] documented years ago that 15% of asthmatics with a markedly reduced FEV_1 (<50% of predicted) did not sense the airflow reduction and did not report dyspnea. Shim and Williams[17] compared physical examination with objective measurements of airflow obstruction and concluded that, "it is unreliable to rely on the physical examination in assessing asthma." McFadden, et al.,[18] reported that when patients treated for asthma in the ED became asymptomatic but could still be heard to wheeze, the average FEV_1 was only 49% of predicted. Even when results of the lung examination became normal, the average FEV_1 had risen to only 63% of predicted. Emerman and Cydulka[19] recently compared physician estimates of degree of airflow obstruction with measured FEV_1 in patients in the ED for asthma. The physicians tended to overestimate the FEV_1, such that actual measurement of FEV_1 led to changes in treatment in 20.4% of patients. The authors concluded that pulmonary function studies should be considered part of the routine approach to acute asthma.

There is a great deal of evidence demonstrating that even when diagnosed, asthma is not optimally treated. In a recent review of physician treatment of hospitalized patients, Spevetz, et al.,[20] demonstrated not only suboptimal treatment during hospitalization but also suboptimal preadmission and discharge medication regimens. Daley, et al.,[21] reviewed asthma care at three different hospitals and documented similar errors. Dales, et al.,[22] looked at patients who presented to the ED for asthma and found "evidence of chronically poor asthma control, ineffective strategies to manage exacerbations, and chronic exposure to known environmental triggers." The authors also found that control was poor despite the fact that 74% of the patients had a "usual physician whom they visited regularly and specifically for their asthma." The message is not new; similar findings were published in the 1980s.[1-3] Suboptimal management is a redundant theme in the literature on deaths from asthma, which will be reviewed in more detail below. Finally, three studies of asthmatics placed on mechanical ventilation[24-26] between 1979[24] and 1993[25] emphasize inadequate treatment as a major factor and show that undertreatment has been a persistent and a consistent theme.

Death from Asthma

Death from a potentially reversible condition is an irrevocable failure of the system and both serves to highlight its dysfunction and to point to potential areas where care can be improved. We would like to review the factors involved in death in some detail. Table 51.1. summarizes the most salient points of these studies.

The British Thoracic Society[27] conducted a confidential inquiry into 90 deaths that occurred in England. The authors noted that the patients usually had had asthma for years and that while slightly over half had been poorly compliant, 47% died despite having been compliant with medical advice. They found that the majority had poor baseline control of asthma and that inadequate follow-up after hospital discharge was a crucial factor in the ultimate fatal outcome.

Johnson, et al.,[28] examined 90 deaths from asthma. They judged that only 13 of the deaths were probably inevitable. They believed that 77% of the time patients did not recognize the severity of the fatal attack. There were also problems with patient compliance in 53% of cases. The medical system also received scorching scrutiny; the authors believed that some aspects of general practitioner care had been inadequate in 98% of cases. Many of the physicians failed to appreciate the severity of the fatal attack.

Carswell[29] retrospectively examined the deaths of 30 asthmatic children. In 13 cases in which the duration of the attack could be determined, 7 died more than 12 h after the onset of the attack, strongly suggesting that more effective treatment could have changed the outcome. Death from asthma was associated with a long history of

Table 51.1. Death from Asthma

Authors (yr.)	Subjects	Risk factors	Factors in death
Hills, et al. (1982)[27]	90 deaths	Severe chronic asthma, poor compliance (53%), inadequate baseline control	Infrequent follow-up (79%), lack of appreciation of severity of disease (63%), underuse of corticosteroids and beta-agonists
Johnson, et al. (1984)[28]	90 deaths	Poor compliance	Patient and physician inability to appreciate severity of attack, inadequate baseline treatment, delays in treatment during fatal attack, delays in ambulance transport
Carswell (1985)[29]	30 deaths (children)	Severe asthma (especially nocturnal), poor compliance, prior cyanotic attack	Inadequate treatment before and during fatal attack, parental lack of understanding of severity of disease
Rea, et al. (1986)[31]	44 deaths	ED visits within year, hospitalization(s) within year, prior respiratory arrest, prior life-threatening episode, noncompliance, below-average medical care, ≥3 Rxs for asthma medications within year	—
Rea, et al. (1987)[30]	271 deaths	Inadequate prefatal medical management	Misjudgment of severity of final attack, leading to delays in seeking assistance
Molfino, et al. (1992)[26]	12 fatality-prone asthmatics	Noncompliance, history of respiratory failure	Inadequate steroid therapy
Crane, et al. (1992)[32]	39 deaths	Hospital admission in the 12 mo. preceding death, use of psychotropic drugs, use of 3 or more categories of asthma drugs	—

asthma, prior corticosteroid use, nocturnal symptoms, a prior cyanotic attack, and a history of poor compliance. Lack of parental understanding of the severity of the disease and faulty medical treatment were judged to be important factors.

Rea, et al.,[30] did a study of 271 deaths from asthma in New Zealand over a 2-year period. They identified both long-term inadequacies in asthma care and inadequate care just before death. One disturbing finding was that 24% of the patients who died had no ongoing medical care. They judged that 70% of the deaths had been potentially preventable.

Rea, et al.,[31] did a case-controlled study of some of the patients in the study cited above; 44 patients with fatal asthma were matched with a group of patients hospitalized for asthma and a third group of asthmatics from the community. The authors were able to define multiple risk factors for fatal asthma; previous hospitalization for asthma within the last year (16-fold increased risk of death), 1 or more ED visits for asthma within the last year, 1 or more prior life-threatening attacks, 1 or more prior respiratory arrests, a history of psychosocial problems, noncompliance, below-average medical care, and a history of prescriptions for 3 or more categories of asthma drugs within the past year.

Molfino, et al.,[26] followed up 12 asthmatics for 18 months following respiratory failure involving mechanical ventilation. Seven of the 12 participated actively in a follow-up program; the remaining 5 declined but were followed up with chart review. Two of the five who declined regular follow-up died, while none of the seven who consistently complied with follow-up died and only one was intubated. Apart from the factor of compliance itself, the authors believed that underuse of corticosteroids contributed to death in the noncompliant patients.

Crane, et al.,[32] looked at 39 patients who died from asthma and at 226 asthmatics requiring hospital readmission after an index admission. The factor associated with the highest odds ratio for death, 8.8, was a history of 5 or more hospitalizations for asthma in the previous year. The odds ratio dropped to 3.0 if there had been only 1 or 2 hospital admissions in the preceding 12 months.

The studies on death document the consistent theme that patients at high risk can be identified prospectively. The question then is whether solutions exist.

Solutions

We have reviewed above many of the aspects of care associated with suboptimal outcomes. We will now review two areas which the literature suggests can lead to improved outcomes. The first is expert care.

The second is patient education. While there is overlap, what we mean by "expert care" is that the patient is largely cared for by a system dominated by asthma experts (who also educate patients). We consider "patient education" programs to be outreach programs apart from the interaction of a patient with a physician whose goal is to teach patients more about their disease and some "self-management" skills.

Expert-Based Systems vs. Generalists

In the current health care system, care of asthmatics is divided somewhat arbitrarily between experts and generalists. We would like to review the literature that looks at the effect of expertise on outcome. We use the word "expert" rather than "specialist" because we acknowledge that a physician with the interest can gain the knowledge and experience required to be an expert in a field regardless of "title." For pulmonologists and allergists, the knowledge and experience requisite to become an expert in the care of asthmatics are integral to specialty training, but neither the information nor the expertise is proprietary.

Hetzel, et al.,[33] compared differences in the rate of death and near death for a group of 1,169 asthmatics admitted either to an "expert care" or "routine care" group. Only one nonfatal respiratory arrest occurred in the expert care group despite the fact that it was comprised of the sickest patients. In contrast, there were nine respiratory arrests in the routine care group, three of which were fatal.

Bucknall, et al.,[15] prospectively studied 150 asthmatics admitted to a teaching hospital in England. Sixty-four were admitted to a pulmonary ward while 86 were admitted to general wards. There were no significant differences between the two groups on admission. Two weeks after hospital discharge, significantly fewer of the patients from the expert ward were still symptomatic. In the year after admission, 20% of the patients who had been admitted to the general ward had been readmitted, while only 2% of the group who had received expert care had been readmitted (p<0.005). The authors concluded that these dramatic differences were most related to differences in in-hospital treatment, differences in discharge medications, and differences in follow-up planning.

Mayo, et al.,[34] prospectively enrolled patients who had either been admitted for asthma at least 2 times within the preceding year or had 5 or more ED visits in the previous 2 years. They randomly assigned patients either to an expert-run asthma clinic or to a routine care

449

group who were followed up with standard care. The asthma clinic emphasized patient teaching, an open-door policy, the use of inhaled steroids, and some patient self-management. The expert care patients had significantly fewer subsequent hospital admissions than the routine care group. Nineteen patients were then crossed over from the routine group into the expert care group. These patients subsequently had an improvement in outcome similar to that of the patients initially assigned to the asthma clinic. A cost analysis demonstrated that the direct cost per patient in the expert care group averaged less than 50% of the cost of care of patients assigned to "routine care." Addition of indirect costs (days lost from work, etc.) would only have widened the gap further.

Zeiger, et al.,[35] did a prospective case-controlled study of asthmatics enrolled in a health maintenance organization. They prospectively accrued all asthmatics 6 to 59 years of age presenting for acute ED treatment. One group (n=149) had a facilitated referral to an asthma expert, while the control patients (n=160) received routine follow-up care with the patients' primary care physicians. The protocol for the expert care group included the routine use of pulmonary function testing, education about asthma including instruction on how best to use asthma medications, and the use of home peak flow monitoring. At the end of 6 months, patients in the expert treatment group were significantly less symptomatic and had a 50% reduction (p<0.05) in ED visits for asthma. There was a lower hospitalization rate for the treatment vs. the control group, but it did not reach statistical significance.

Mahr and Evans[36] followed up patients who had been seen in an asthma clinic over a 1-year period. They then did a follow-up 2 years later. The patients were divided into an expert care group that had continued follow-up in the asthma clinic and a nonexpert care group of patients who had left the asthma clinic and were treated exclusively by their primary care physicians. The groups were similar in most respects at time of entry into the study. Follow-up revealed that both ED visits and hospitalizations for the expert care group were less than half of those of the nonexpert care group (p<0.001 and p<0.005, respectively).

Freund, et al.,[37] evaluated patients being cared for by asthma experts (n=190), family practitioners (n=34), and pediatricians (n=103). Severity of disease was not similar; experts cared for patients with more severe disease. Despite the fact that they had more severe asthma, the patients cared for by experts reported less intrusion of asthma in their lives than did the patients cared for by nonexperts.

The expert care patients had fewer ED visits, fewer hospitalizations, and fewer days missed from work or from school. Outpatient cost was greater for expert than nonexpert care, but the authors measured only physician office visit costs and not the direct costs of ED visits and hospitalizations or the indirect costs.

Crompton, et al.,[38,39] have described an extended experience with a system that routed patients experiencing exacerbation of asthma directly to hospital-based specialty care with no medical gatekeeping. In their hospital, any patient who was admitted once with a life-threatening asthma attack was subsequently placed on a list that allowed him/her admission to the respiratory ward of the hospital at any time the patient requested, eliminating the need (standard in their medical system) to consult first with their general physicians. For ethical reasons, there was no control group. Once patients reached the respiratory ward, some went home after initial assessment and treatment while others were admitted. Despite the fact that they were treating a subgroup of high-risk patients, the authors were able to document asthma death rates for the expert care group which were lower than those for asthmatics in surrounding geographic areas.

Ignacio-Garcia and Gonzalez-Santos[40] did a prospective study of a program similar to that reported by Mayo, et al.,[34] All patients attending an asthma clinic who agreed to participate were randomly allocated to an expert care group (n=35) or a control group (n=35). Both groups received some expert care; all were seen and had medications adjusted by a specialist, but the control group patients received no formal education, were seen only at predetermined intervals, and were encouraged to follow up with their family physicians or go to the ED when symptoms became problematic. The expert care patients were taught about monitoring of peak flow, how to properly use different medications, what can trigger asthma attacks, how and when to institute changes in therapy, and when to seek medical advice based on peak flow. At study end, both groups showed significant decreases in asthma exacerbations and physician visits, while only the expert care group demonstrated decreases in days lost from work (p=0.004) and in ED visits (p<0.001).

The above represent all of the studies we could find that contrasted expert with generalist care, not a skewed subset. The studies strongly suggest that the level of expertise the physician has in treating patients with severe lung disease has a direct effect on outcome. Expert involvement also has a positive impact on the overall cost of care.

Teaching Programs: Bringing Education to the Patient

A complementary body of literature deals with the issues of educational programs and self-management by asthmatics. The core of the strategies is based on expert knowledge. The goal is to teach the patient how to monitor his/her disease, to recognize which changes are clinically significant, and to react to clinically significant changes either by making protocol-driven changes in medications or by taking the important information back to the physician. "Self-management" is actually a misleading term, as it should represent a fruitful collaboration between patient and physician.[3]

A number of patient education programs have been shown to have beneficial effects on patient outcome, including functional status, perceived quality of life, family adjustment to illness, and reductions in health care utilization.[3,41-49] Other programs have shown less clearcut benefits, particularly with respect to ED visits and hospitalizations, major expense points in asthma care.[47,49-51] How candidates are selected, who administers the program, exactly what is taught, and how the "educated" patient interacts with the health care system are probably crucial factors.

The literature on the effect of educating patients on the value and use of home monitoring of peak flow is divided.[40,48,49,51,52] Some studies show a definite benefit to peak flow monitoring,[40,48] while others show none.[49,51] This is particularly interesting given the recurrent documentation in the literature of the importance of a physiologic basis for clinical decisions. The outcome differences between studies highlight the importance of adequacy of patient performance in measuring peak flow and especially the importance of how the information is used. No matter how accurate the data, it is of little importance unless it affects care positively.

When asthmatics themselves have been asked what kind of education/self-management they are interested in, they give two main answers. First, they are interested in practical information about what to do when having asthma problems and how their medicines help them.[44,53] Second, they do not wish to be the prime decision-makers during exacerbations.[53] This is consonant with the interesting finding that self-management autonomy does not correlate with perceived quality of life for asthmatics.[53]

Although the preponderance of the evidence supports the value of patient education in conjunction with expert physician oversight, the first step in education is patient compliance with enrollment. In this regard, the literature suggests that a number of asthmatics, even following a hospitalization for asthma,[54] will either refuse outright to participate or will fail to follow through and attend a formal asthma program. This is a crucial and unsolved problem.

Discussion

A recent editorial in *Chest* entitled "Health-Care Reform and Pulmonary/Critical Care Medicine: A Revolution with or without Data" by McDonald and Martin[55] notes three nonphysician forces that are increasingly affecting patient care: "(1) capitation; (2) the systematic exclusion of certain physicians from certain care provider roles; and (3) the implementation of clinical guidelines within care plans." The authors argue that the role of the specialist in the system of care and any benefits that the specialist can provide need to be documented in a climate which is essentially hostile to the concept of specialty care because of concerns about its cost. We would argue that in the field of asthma, a great deal of research has already been done. We have cited extensive literature that begets certain conclusions.

Generalists have historically delivered the bulk of asthma care, and the changes in health care delivery systems may further limit expert participation in the care of asthma. This pattern has clinical and economic problems. The current system of asthma care, at least for those with more severe asthma, is clinically suboptimal and not cost-effective. This is evident in the huge number of ED visits, the high number of hospitalizations and, most clearly, the increasing death rates for asthma. Given our expanded knowledge of asthma, this situation clearly reflects a generic failure of the current system of care delivery and not of scientific understanding or available pharmacology.

This system failure has been consistent, redundant, and persistent. In 1978, Anthony Seaton,[56] referring to asthma, wrote the following:

> In almost no other field is the gap between diagnostic and therapeutic knowledge and its general application so great. It is hard to realize why this should be so as the principles of diagnosis—to demonstrate reversibility of airways obstruction—and of treatment—to reverse the obstruction by one or more of only three types of drug—are so simple.

That 18-year-old quote is sadly applicable today and could be inserted in context in several of the recent articles on management of asthma.[20,21,23] Similar consistent documentation of failure of the system is evident in the literature on death from asthma noted in Table 51.1.

Again quoting Seaton,[56] he said in 1978 that, "the major problem in asthma today is the education of the profession about the disease." Years of appreciation of this problem and of education appear not to have reached the majority of practitioners enough to optimize practice patterns. Suboptimal practice patterns are a prevalent theme in the literature on asthma 18 years later.

In contrast, there is a body of literature that clearly demonstrates that expert care of problematic asthma leads to better clinical outcome at lower cost. It follows that either we need to train primary care providers to be specialists in asthma care or we need to allow specialists to be the primary providers at least for patients with moderate or severe asthma. The former is probably unrealistic, while the latter is a viable solution.

Given the prevalence of asthma, it is unrealistic to expect that every asthmatic can be identified, tested, and followed up by an expert. We must therefore ask at what point(s) should the system identify asthmatics who most need expert care in order to have their treatment optimized? Can patients who are doing poorly or who are at risk be moved from one system of care to another? Review of previous asthmatic deaths can be used to teach us who is at risk for future death and thus make preemptive changes for asthmatics who share important characteristics with those who have died. But while prevention of death is an important goal, it is important to note that many patients with asthma of less than fatal severity suffer chronically and that for this vast majority of patients, the goal is to minimize morbidity and improve quality of life. Certain pragmatic "break points" allow us to identify system failure for many of these patients. ED visits and hospitalizations are the most obvious identification points; they represent quantum drops in respiratory function, risk factors for death, and quantum increases in cost to the health care system.[57] They are also the negative outcome points studied in most of the articles quoted above which demonstrate the value of expert care. Both the decline in function and the increases in cost are incentives for physicians and insurers alike to consider a different approach to care; when an asthmatic goes to the ED or is hospitalized, it would be reasonable to examine his/her care system and possibly to change it. Another reasonable break point, though harder to precisely pinpoint, is the persistence of symptoms that interfere with normal activities despite ongoing therapy.

In their editorial, McDonald and Martin[55] state that the evolution toward managed care is a move toward a model in which the system takes more responsibility for the patient and in many cases moves "control" of the patient away from an individual physician. This change brings both potential good and risk. Managed health care systems have the capacity to identify patients with problematic asthma and to move them into expert-based care. Ironically, they also have the capacity to lock patients into treatment patterns that have been persistently proven to be ineffective. The data demonstrate that restricting patient access to expert care may be self-defeating when asthma is the diagnosis.

It is not surprising that expertise can both improve outcome and reduce cost. This is true primarily because of the enormous cost of emergency and inpatient care, the needs for which are diminished when experts manage asthma. The consonance of outcomes means that there need be no conflict between patient care and economic interests.

Conclusion

We are in the midst of a revolution in health care, but we have not arrived without data about the care of asthma. The evidence suggests that the vehicle for a win-win solution is the expert-based system of asthma care. While not every asthmatic can be seen by a specialist, it is feasible to identify those who have made ED visits, who have required hospitalization for asthma, or who have persistent symptoms despite therapy, and to recognize that the system may be failing them. To make experts their primary physicians, at least as regards asthma, is technically possible, medically preferable, and economically smart.

References

1. Parker SR, Mellins RB, Sogn DD. Asthma education: a national strategy. *Am Rev Respir Dis* 1989; 140:848-53

2. Lenfant C, Hurd SS. National asthma education program. *Chest* 1990; 98:226-27

3. Clark NM. Asthma self-management education: research and implications for clinical practice. *Chest* 1989; 95:1110-13

4. Weiss KB, Gergen PJ, Hodgson TA. An economic evaluation of asthma in the United States. *N Engl J Med* 1992; 326:862-66

5. Robin ED. Risk-benefit analysis in chest medicine; death from bronchial asthma. *Chest* 1988; 93:614-18

6. Buist AS. Is asthma mortality increasing? *Chest* 1988; 93:449-50

7. Lang DM, Polansky M. Patterns of asthma mortality in Philadelphia from 1969 to 1991. *N Engl J Med* 1994; 331:1542-46

8. Whitlaw WA. Asthma deaths. *Chest* 1991; 99:1507-10

9. Buist SA. Asthma mortality: trends and determinants. *Am Rev Respir Dis* 1991; 143:1037-39

10. Jackson R, Sears MR, Beaglehole R, et al. International trends in asthma mortality: 1970-1985. *Chest* 1988; 94:914-19

11. Dales RE, Ernst P, Hanley JA, et al. Prediction of airway reactivity from responses to a standardized respiratory symptom questionnaire. *Am Rev Respir Dis* 1987; 135:817-21

12. Pratter M, Hingston DM, Irwin RS. Diagnosis of bronchial asthma by clinical evaluation: an unreliable method. *Chest* 1984; 1:42-6

13. Adelroth E, Hargreave FE, Ramsdale EH. Do physicians need objective measures to diagnose asthma. *Am Rev Respir Dis* 1986; 134:704-07

14. Pratter MR, Curley FJ, Dubois J, et al. Cause and evaluation of chronic dyspnea in a pulmonary disease clinic. *Arch Intern Med* 1989; 149:2277-82

15. Bucknall CE, Robertson C, Moran F, et al. Differences in hospital asthma management. *Lancet* 1988; 1:748-50

16. Rubinfeld AR, Pain MCF. Perception of asthma. *Lancet* 1976; 1:882-84

17. Shim CS, Williams H Jr. Relationship of wheezing to the severity of obstruction in asthma. *Arch Intern Med* 1983; 143:890-92

18. McFadden ER, Kiser R, DeGroot WJ. Acute bronchial asthma: relations between clinical and physiologic manifestations. *N Engl J Med* 1973; 288:221-25

19. Emerman CL, Cydulka RK. Effect of pulmonary function testing on the management of acute asthma. *Arch Intern Med* 1995; 155:2225-28

20. Spevetz A, Dubois J, Bartter T, et al. Inpatient management of status asthmaticus. *Chest* 1992; 102:192-96

21. Daley J, Kopelman RI, Comeau E, et al. Practice patterns in the treatment of acutely ill hospitalized asthmatic patients at three teaching hospitals. *Chest* 1991; 100:51-6

22. Dales RE, Kerr PE, Schweitzer I, et al. Asthma management preceding an emergency department visit. *Arch Intern Med* 1992; 152:2041-44

23. Osman J, Ormerod P, Stableforth D. Management of acute asthma: a survey of hospital practice and comparison between thoracic and general physicians in Birmingham and Manchester. *Br J Dis Chest* 1987; 81:232-41

24. Westerman DE, Benatar SR, Potgieter PD, et al. Identification of high-risk asthmatic patient: experience with 39 patients undergoing ventilation for status asthmaticus. *Am J Med* 1979; 66:565-72

25. Kallenbach JM, Frankel AH, Lapinsky SE, et al. Determinants of near fatality in acute severe asthma. *Am J Med* 1993; 95:265-72

26. Molfino NA, Nannini LJ, Rebuck AS, et al. The fatality-prone asthmatic patient: follow-up study, after near-fatal attacks. *Chest* 1992; 101:621-23

27. Hills EA, Somner AR, Adelstein AM, et al. Death from asthma in two regions of England. *BMJ* 1982; 285:1251-55

28. Johnson AJ, Nunn AJ, Somner AR, et al. Circumstances of death from asthma. *BMJ* 1984; 288:1870-72

29. Carswell F. Thirty deaths from asthma. *Arch Dis Child* 1985; 60:25-8

30. Rea HH, Sears MR, Beaglehole R, et al. Lessons from the national asthma mortality study: circumstances surrounding death. *N Z Med J* 1987; 100:10-3

31. Rea HH, Scragg R, Jackson R, et al. A case-control study of deaths from asthma. *Thorax* 1986; 41:833-39

32. Crane J, Pearce N, Burgess C, et al. Markers of risk of asthma death or readmission in the 12 months following a hospital admission for asthma. *Int J Epidemiol* 1992; 21:737-44

33. Hetzel MR, Clark TJH, Branthwaite MA. Asthma: analysis of sudden deaths and ventilatory arrests in hospital. *BMJ* 1977; 1:808-11

34. Mayo PH, Richman J, Harris WH. Results of a program to reduce admissions for adult asthma. *Ann Intern Med* 1990; 112:864-71

35. Zeiger RS, Heller S, Mellon MH, et al. Facilitated referral to asthma specialist reduces relapses in asthma emergency room visits. *J Allergy Clin Immunol* 1991; 87:1160-68

36. Mahr TA, Evans R III. Allergist influence on asthma care. *Ann Allergy* 1993; 71:115-20

37. Freund DA, Stein MS, Hurley R, et al. Specialty differences in the treatment of asthma. *J Allergy Clin Immunol* 1989; 84:401-06

38. Crompton GK, Grant IWB, Bloomfield P. Edinburgh emergency asthma admission service: report on 10 years' experience. *BMJ* 1979; 2:1199-1201

39. Crompton GK, Grant IWB, Chapman BJ, et al. Edinburgh emergency asthma admission service: report on 15 years' experience. *Eur J Respir Dis* 1987; 70:266-71

40. Ignacio-Garcia JM, Gonzalez-Santos P. Asthma self-management education program by home monitoring of peak expiratory flow. *Am J Respir Crit Care Med* 1995; 151:353-59

41. Clark CJ. The influence of education on morbidity and mortality in asthma. *Monaldi Arch Chest Dis* 1994; 49:169-72

42. Clark NM, Feldman CH, Evans D, et al. The impact of health education on frequency and cost of health care by low income children with asthma. *J Allergy Clin Immunol* 1986; 78:108-15

43. Ringsberg KC, Wiklund I, Wilhelmsen L. Education of adult patients at an 'asthma school:' effects on quality of life knowledge and need for nursing. *Eur Respir J* 1990; 3:33-7

44. Osman LM, Abdalla MI, Beattie JAG, et al. Reducing hospital admission through computer supported education for asthma patients, *BMJ* 1994; 308:568-71

45. Maiman LA, Green LW, Gibson G, et al. Education for self-treatment by adult asthmatics. *JAMA* 1979; 241:1919-22

46. Bailey WC, Richards JM Jr, Brooks M, et al. A randomized trial to improve self-management practices of adults with asthma. *Arch Intern Med* 1990; 150:1664-68

47. Wilson SR, Scamagas P, German DF, et al. A controlled trial of two forms of self-management education for adults with asthma. *Am J Med* 1993; 94:564-75

48. Beasley R, Cushley M, Holgate ST. A self-management plan in the treatment of adult asthma. *Thorax* 1989; 44:200-04

49. Garrett J, Fenwick JM, Taylor G, et al. Prospective controlled evaluation of the effect of a community based asthma education centre in a multiracial working class neighbourhood. *Thorax* 1994; 49:976-83

50. Hilton S, Sibbald B, Anderson HR, et al. Controlled evaluation of the effects of patient education on asthma morbidity in general practice. *Lancet* 1986; 1:26-9

51. Drummond N, Adballa M, Beattie JAG, et al. Effectiveness of routine self-monitoring of peak flow in patients with asthma. *BMJ* 1994; 308:564-67

52. Clark NM, Evans D, Mellins RB. Patient use of peak flow monitoring. *Am Rev Respir Dis* 1992; 145:722-25

53. Gibson PG, Talbot PI, Toneguzzi RC, et al. Self-management, autonomy, and quality of life in asthma. *Chest* 1995; 107:1003-08

54. Yoon R, McKenzie DK, Miles DA, et al. Characteristics of attenders and non-attenders at an asthma education programme. *Thorax* 1991; 46:886-90

55. McDonald RC, Martin WJ. Health-care reform and pulmonary/critical care medicine: a revolution with or without data. *Chest* 1995; 107:1190-92

56. Seaton A. Asthma—contrasts in care. *Thorax* 1978; 33:1-2

57. Vollmer WM, Osborne ML, Buist AS. Temporal trends in hospital-based episodes of asthma care in a health maintenance organization. *Am Rev Respir Dis* 1993; 147:347-53

Chapter 52

Role of the Pharmacist in Asthma Care

Preface

Whether they work in community pharmacies, hospitals, or clinics, pharmacists are in a pivotal position to contribute to the overall management of asthma. Every year, pharmacists fill more than 7 million prescriptions for asthma medications, which remain the principal treatment for the disease. Pharmacists have many other opportunities to assist in the management of asthma.

Pharmacists can educate patients by providing information on the types and purposes of asthma medications and by demonstrating how to use inhaled medications and peak flow meters. They can reinforce and clarify the instructions contained in a patient's individual asthma management plan. In addition, pharmacists can refer patients who use over-the-counter medications to physicians for medical care.

Pharmacists can be a valuable source of important information for other members of the health care team. They can monitor medication use and refill intervals and use this information to alert prescribers and help identify patients with poorly controlled asthma. Pharmacists also can share information about asthma medications and the National Asthma Education and Prevention Program guidelines on the

Excerpted from "The Role of the Pharmacist in Improving Asthma Care," [Online] July 1995. Available: http://www.nhlbi.nih.gov/health/prof/lung/asthma/asmapmcy.txt. Produced by the National Heart, Lung, and Blood Institute (NHLBI), NIH Publication No. 95-3280, Claude Lenfant, M.D., Director. For complete contact information, please refer to Chapter 68, "Resources."

diagnosis and management of asthma with members of the health care team.

Introduction

The National Asthma Education and Prevention Program Expert Panel Report, *Guidelines for the Diagnosis and Management of Asthma,* released in August 1991 concluded that asthma is under-diagnosed and undertreated in the United States.[1] Common reasons for underdiagnosis and undertreatment on the part of patients and clinicians include the following:

- Not recognizing that a person has asthma.
- Not expecting enough from therapy.
- Not understanding the benefits and risks of different therapies.
- Not appreciating the chronic nature of asthma and not using (or adhering to) preventive therapy.
- Not accurately assessing the severity of an episode.
- Not recognizing signs of deterioration.
- Not treating episodes adequately.
- Not identifying triggers associated with the patient's asthma and not taking action to minimize or prevent exposure to such triggers (e.g., cigarette smoke).

An important factor contributing to the undertreatment of asthma is not appreciating the necessity to treat the underlying inflammation in asthma. Patients may not understand that short-acting beta$_2$-agonists treat only bronchospasm and cannot reduce or prevent the underlying problem of inflammation. Patients with moderate or severe asthma should take anti-inflammatory medication on a daily basis to prevent symptoms. Further, for exacerbations that do not respond adequately to bronchodilator therapy, a short course of systemic corticosteroid therapy may be needed to reverse the inflammation and speed recovery.

Pharmacists' Role in Asthma Management

Federal regulations (Omnibus Budget and Reconciliation Act 1990) of pharmacists receiving Federal funds and new regulations in many states require pharmacists to perform certain education and monitoring tasks. These regulations offer new opportunities for pharmacists to counsel patients. Pharmacists may have contact with patients with asthma who refill their prescriptions without routine physician care or who medicate themselves with over-the-counter (OTC) asthma products. As members of the health care team, pharmacists are in an excellent position to recognize patients who are not under the care of a physician or whose asthma may be poorly controlled for a variety of reasons. Pharmacists who recognize any of the criteria listed [below] can contact the patient's physician and can advise patients without regular physician care to seek medical care.

Appropriate therapy and patient adherence will prevent most emergency department visits and hospitalizations for asthma. However, when ED visits or hospitalizations occur, they provide an opportunity for pharmacists to ask about the patient's treatment plan and to reinforce and clarify instructions that will help prevent the problem from recurring.

Action Plan for Pharmacists

There are numerous areas where pharmacists can contribute to improving health outcomes in patients with asthma.

Pharmacists can:

1. Educate patients about the role of each medication

Pharmacists can help patients understand that, with appropriate therapy, most patients can lead normal, productive, and physically active lives. Pharmacists can educate patients about the two broad categories of asthma medications:

Medications used to *prevent and/or decrease the frequency* of symptoms. Preventive medication should be taken on a regular basis even when the patient is free of symptoms. This type of long-term medication includes inhaled anti-inflammatory agents such as corticosteroids, cromolyn, and nedocromil, which are preferred therapy. It may include extended-release formulations of theophylline. Also included as long-term medication are extended-release oral and long-acting inhaled beta$_2$-agonists, which are added to inhaled corticosteroids when the recommended doses of inhaled corticosteroids are not sufficient to control chronic symptoms, especially nighttime symptoms. Preventive long-term medication also may include, for severe asthma, alternate day oral corticosteroid therapy. In addition, the use of a short- or long-acting inhaled beta$_2$-agonist or cromolyn before exercise to prevent exercise-induced bronchospasm falls into the "prevention" category.

Medications taken to *relieve* asthma symptoms. Medications in this category are designed to relieve symptoms and generally are prescribed to be taken only as needed (PRN). This therapy includes primarily short-acting inhaled beta$_2$-agonists (albuterol, bitolterol, pirbuterol, or terbutaline). In addition, a short course of oral corticosteroids for patients who are not fully responsive to inhaled bronchodilators may be used to treat acute exacerbations of asthma.

An effective asthma management plan should ensure that the patient is given written and verbal instructions that describe when and how a medication should be taken, how much to take, how to evaluate the response to therapy, when to seek medical care, and what to do when the desired effect is not achieved or side effects are encountered. Pharmacists can reinforce these instructions by reminding patients, for example, to contact their physician when acute symptoms are not relieved by using their short-acting beta$_2$-agonist inhaler as directed or when their peak expiratory flow rate (PEFR) drops below a predetermined value.

Any one of the following criteria may indicate the need for medication adjustment, improved medication administration technique, or patient education concerning asthma and its management:

- Adverse effects from medications.

- Waking up at night from symptoms of asthma more than twice a month.

- Increased use of inhaled, short-acting beta$_2$-agonists (e.g., more than three to four times in 1 day).

- Long-term overuse of inhaled, short-acting beta$_2$-agonists (e.g., refilling the prescription more often than one canister/month or more than one canister/2 months of a short-acting agent when it is used in addition to a long-acting agent).

- Overuse or misuse of inhaled long-acting beta$_2$-agonists.

- Nonadherence to anti-inflammatory medications (e.g., refilling the prescription less than half as often as would be required if the directions on the prescription were followed).

- Failure to achieve quick and sustained response (i.e., beginning within 10 to 20 minutes and lasting longer than 3 to 4 hours) to short-acting beta$_2$-agonists during an acute asthma episode (as measured by a decrease in symptoms or an increase in peak expiratory flow rate).

- Poor tolerance to physical activity (i.e., the patient experiences symptoms of exercise-induced asthma).

- Missing school or work because of asthma symptoms.

- An emergency department visit or hospitalization for asthma.

2. Instruct patients about the proper techniques for inhaling medications

Inhaled medications are preferred over oral therapies. However, a major limitation in their effectiveness is the patient's ability to use the device appropriately.[2] Studies suggest that members of the health care team (e.g., physicians, nurses, and pharmacists) may not adequately instruct patients on how to use a metered-dose inhaler (MDI).[3] Improper MDI technique can be one cause of a poor response to therapy. Pharmacists can play an important role on the health care team by teaching patients with asthma about proper medication technique [including] helpful tips for instruction on MDI techniques. Other devices, such as dry powder inhalers, breath-actuated inhalers, and nebulizers, are also available, and they require different techniques for administration. A placebo inhaler, which can be obtained from pharmaceutical manufacturers, and instructional videos may be useful in demonstrating proper technique.

Patients using inhalation therapies need careful instruction, including a step-by-step demonstration at the time of dispensing the medication, and observation of their technique. Because inhaler technique tends to decline without routine review,[4] pharmacists should reassess a patient's technique when prescriptions are refilled or renewed. Patients should be reminded that the most important steps in a proper MDI technique are gentle exhalation before breathing in, a slow inhalation, and holding the breath.[5]

Pharmacists also should assess whether using a valved spacer device with an MDI would be helpful. Spacers may be beneficial to any patient, but they are indicated especially for the patient who cannot master the optimal inhaler technique. Spacers are routinely indicated for most patients using a corticosteroid MDI because they improve particle deposition in the lungs and decrease local side effects such as thrush and hoarseness. In children too young to use an MDI attached to a spacer device, a compressed air-driven nebulizer can be used to administer medications.

465

3. Monitor medication use and refill intervals to help identify patients with poorly controlled asthma

During symptomatic periods, selective short-acting inhaled beta$_2$-agonists may be sufficient to relieve asthma symptoms. When asthma is stable, it is preferable to use these agents on an as-needed basis. Overuse and overreliance on short-acting inhaled beta$_2$-agonists can be signs that asthma is poorly controlled. During an exacerbation, patients may increase the dose and/or frequency of use, which may lead to a delay in seeking appropriate medical care.

Pharmacists may find indications of chronic overuse of short-acting inhaled beta$_2$-agonists by checking patients' medical history and the frequency of refills.[6] Overuse can be defined as using more than one canister per month of a short- or long-acting beta$_2$-agonist or more than one canister of a short-acting beta$_2$-agonist in 2 months when used in conjunction with a long-acting agent. Pharmacists should also monitor for overuse of a long-acting beta$_2$-agonist (e.g., salmeterol). In general, these agents should not be used more than twice a day and are not appropriate to relieve acute symptoms.

If overuse is noted, pharmacists should alert the physician, who can assess the need for reevaluation of the patient and consider whether the patient needs to initiate or intensify anti-inflammatory therapy. Before contacting the physician, pharmacists should have the patient demonstrate his or her MDI technique. Poor technique may be one of the causes of overuse of an MDI. The physician will find this information useful in making a decision on how to respond to the situation. Physicians also may want to evaluate recent trends in peak flow meter readings.

Physicians will consider several factors when deciding whether to initiate or increase anti-inflammatory therapy. In general, a short course of oral corticosteroids may be indicated if the excessive use of an MDI is (1) short term; (2) due to an acute, severe episode; or (3) the result of an isolated exacerbation caused by a common cold or other upper respiratory tract infections. The initiation or dose increase of an inhaled anti-inflammatory agent (corticosteroids, cromolyn, or nedocromil) as long-term therapy may be indicated if the patient relies on short-acting inhaled beta$_2$-agonists daily to relieve symptoms, has frequent fluctuations in the peak expiratory flow rate, or has other signs of poorly controlled asthma.

Patients on preventive therapy for asthma also should be monitored for signs of nonadherence to anti-inflammatory therapy. In some cases, patients do not adhere to anti-inflammatory therapy because they do not understand the purpose of or perceive any immediate benefit from this therapy. Some patients may be discouraged about following their prescribed regimen because they fear adverse reactions to the medications. Refilling the prescription at intervals longer than indicated by the directions for use on the prescription may indicate nonadherence. For example, if an inhaled anti-inflammatory agent contains 100 puffs and the directions are to take 2 puffs twice a day, a patient refilling the prescription once every 60 days is underusing the medication. In this example, the canister should be depleted in 25 days (100 puffs divided by 4 puffs per day = 25 days).

4. Encourage patients purchasing OTC asthma inhalers or tablets to seek medical care

Asthma is one of the very few potentially fatal diseases for which OTC products are available for self-treatment. Use of OTC inhalers may lead to a delay in seeking appropriate medical care. Pharmacists should refer anyone using an OTC product for respiratory symptoms to a physician for diagnosis, regular monitoring, and proper treatment. The physician can then determine the need for other therapies, such as an inhaled anti-inflammatory agent to prevent symptoms.

Over-the-counter inhalers contain epinephrine, which is a nonselective, weak, and extremely short-acting bronchodilator. Thus, if physicians determine that the PRN use of an inhaled bronchodilator is indicated, they can prescribe a selective short-acting inhaled beta$_2$-agonist that will provide greater efficacy and a longer duration of action. Oral OTC asthma medications contain ephedrine or a combination of ephedrine and theophylline. Generally, bronchodilators are less effective and cause more side effects when administered by the oral route,[7] and combinations of theophylline and ephedrine have the potential to cause synergistic toxicity.[8]

5. Help patients use peak flow meters appropriately

It is recommended that clinicians consider peak expiratory flow rate monitoring for patients over 5 years of age with moderate or severe asthma. Regular home monitoring may detect decreased lung function and signs of an impending asthma episode before it becomes more severe. The PEFR is the greatest flow velocity that can be obtained during a forced expiration starting with fully inflated lungs. It provides a simple, quantitative, and reproducible measure of airway obstruction with a relatively inexpensive device that is available without a prescription.

Measuring PEFR in a patient with asthma is analogous to measuring blood pressure with a sphygmomanometer or blood glucose to guide insulin dosage. The PEFR is used by the physician to assess the severity of asthma as a basis for adding medication, monitoring response to chronic therapy, and detecting deterioration in lung function before symptoms develop. The physician may consider more aggressive therapy if the patient's highest value is less than 80 percent of predicted value and/or daily variability is more than 20 percent.

Pharmacists should discuss the following items with patients: (1) the intended purpose of a peak flow meter and (2) how to use it and record the values. The patient's physician should develop an individualized plan for the use of the peak flow meter. The plan should include a threshold value and instructions on what the patient should do if the PEFR drops below this value (e.g., increase medication, call the physician, or seek emergency medical care).

6. Help patients discharged from the hospital after an asthma exacerbation understand their asthma management plan

Every patient being discharged from the hospital for the treatment of acute asthma should receive and understand an individualized asthma management plan. An asthma management plan should include specific written instructions for patients and families. Hospital pharmacists can discuss such a plan with a patient before discharge, reinforcing and clarifying instructions that have been designed to prevent subsequent hospitalizations or emergency department visits. Pharmacists also can review the patient's inhaler and peak flow meter technique and provide instruction, if needed.

Written guidelines should include the following points:

- Specific instructions about use of medications, including dose, frequency of administration, guidelines for changing dose or adding medications if appropriate, and adverse effects to report to the clinician.

- The importance of long-term preventive medications.

- How to monitor body signs or symptoms and/or PEFR to detect increasing airflow obstruction as early as possible; early signs of airflow obstruction vary according to the individual and should be identified for each patient.

- Criteria for initiating or modifying treatment: a drop in PEFR or early signs or symptoms.

- List of steps to take in managing an acute asthma episode (i.e., remove the precipitating trigger, give medication, avoid strenuous physical activity, and keep patient and family calm).

- Specific criteria for seeking emergency medical care, including a pattern of declining PEFR; failure of medications at home to control worsening symptoms; difficulty in breathing (wheeze may be absent), walking, or talking; intercostal retractions; blue fingernails or lips.

- Observable signs that long-term therapy is less than optimal, such as asthma symptoms that cause sleep interruption, consistently low or highly variable PEFR, and/or too frequent use of short-acting inhaled beta$_2$-agonist. Such signs should be promptly discussed with the clinician.

Summary

Our current understanding of the pathophysiology of asthma and the availability of potent, effective therapies mean that asthma can be well controlled. However, to achieve this goal, optimal therapy must be prescribed and the patient must be taught how and when to use it. Pharmacists, as part of the health care team, help improve the pharmacologic management of asthma by teaching patients about their medications, how to use them, and the importance of using them as prescribed. Alerting physicians to suspected problems, such as underusing anti-inflammatory therapy or overusing inhaled bronchodilators, will provide an opportunity for the physician to consider changes in a patient's management plan when appropriate. Acting in these educational and information-sharing roles, pharmacists contribute to improving the control of asthma and enabling patients to live full, active, and productive lives.

References

1. National Heart, Lung, and Blood Institute, National Asthma Education Program, Expert Panel Report. *Guidelines for the Diagnosis and Management of Asthma.* NIH Publication No. 91-3042, August 1991.

2. Self TH, Brooks JB, Lieberman P, Ryan MR. The value of demonstration and role of the pharmacist in teaching current use of pressurized bronchodilators. *Canadian Medical Association Journal* 1983; 128:129-31.

3. Kesten S, Zive K, Chapman KR. Pharmacist knowledge and ability to use inhaled medication delivery systems. *Chest* 1993; 104:1737-42.

4. De Blaquiere P, Christensen DB, Carter WB, Martin TR. Use and misuse of metered-dose inhalers by patients with chronic lung disease. *American Review of Respiratory Diseases* 1989; 140:910-6.

5. Hindle M, Newton DA, Chrystyn H. Investigations of an optimal inhaler technique with the use of urinary salbutamol excretion as a measure of relative bioavailability to the lung. *Thorax* 1993; 48(6):607-10.

6. Executive Committee, American Academy of Allergy and Immunology. Inhaled beta-adrenergic agonists in asthma. *Journal of Allergy and Clinical Immunology* 1993; 91:1234-7.

7. Larsson S, Svedmyr N. Bronchodilating effect and side effects of beta$_2$-adrenoceptor stimulants by different modes of administration (tablets, metered aerosol, and combinations thereof). *American Review of Respiratory Diseases* 1977; 116:861-9.

8. Weinberger M, Bronsky E. Interaction of ephedrine and theophylline. *Clinical Pharmacology and Therapeutics* 1975; 17:585-92.

Resources

The following publications are available from the National Asthma Education and Prevention Program (NHLBI Information Center, P.O. Box 30105, Bethesda, MD 20824-0105; Telephone: 301-592-8573):

- *Expert Panel Report: Guidelines for the Diagnosis and Management of Asthma (Executive Summary)* (1991)—A summary presentation of the latest asthma management guidelines from the National Asthma Education and Prevention Program.

- *Asthma Management Kit for Clinicians* (1992)—Containing "Teach Your Patients about Asthma: A Clinician's Guide," a poster, peak flow meter standards, "Your Asthma Can Be Controlled: Expect Nothing Less," and "Check Your Asthma 'I.Q.'"

- *Check Your Asthma "I.Q."* (1990)—An asthma quiz that can be used as a simple pretest or posttest tool to measure client knowledge about asthma. (2 pages)

- *Facts about Asthma* (1990)—An overview of asthma, the current theory on asthma medications, asthma triggers, and the need for chronic—not episodic—care of asthma. (8 pages) Available in English and Spanish.

- *Teach Your Patients about Asthma: A Clinician's Guide* (1992)— A three-part patient education guide that includes teaching notes and worksheets. This publication is designed to help clinicians teach adults and children with asthma and parents of children with asthma about the disease and its management. (98 pages)

- *Your Asthma Can Be Controlled: Expect Nothing Less* (1991)—A pamphlet for patients with asthma that explains how patients can become active partners with their doctors in asthma management. (20 pages)

Contributors

Leslie Hendeles, Pharm.D., Principal Writer, University of Florida, Gainesville, Florida; H. William Kelly, Pharm.D., University of New Mexico, Albuquerque, New Mexico; Teresa McRorie, Pharm.D., University of Washington, Seattle, Washington; Timothy Self, Pharm.D., University of Tennessee, Memphis, Tennessee; Dennis Williams, Pharm.D., University of North Carolina, Chapel Hill, North Carolina; Robert A. Barbee, M.D., F.C.C.P., University of Arizona, Tucson, Arizona; National Asthma Education and Prevention Program: Joan Blair, M.P.H., R.N., Patient and Professional Education Specialist, Office of Prevention, Education, and Control, National Heart, Lung, and Blood Institute; Robinson Fulwood, M.S.P.H., Coordinator, National Asthma Education and Prevention Program, National Heart, Lung, and Blood Institute; Virginia Silver Taggart, M.P.H., Health Program Specialist, Division of Lung Diseases, National Heart, Lung, and Blood Institute; Support Staff: R.O.W. Sciences, Inc., Ted Buxton, M.P.H.; Gale Harris

471

Chapter 53

Peak Flow Monitoring

What Is a Peak Flow Meter?

A peak flow meter is a small, easy-to-use instrument that enables you to measure lung function at home, at work, wherever you go. The peak flow meter measures how fast a person can blow out air after a maximum inhalation. This is called the peak expiratory flow rate, or PEFR.

Why Use a Peak Flow Meter?

People with asthma cannot always feel the early changes taking place in their airways because these changes often occur gradually. By the time symptoms of asthma develop, a person can be experiencing a 25 percent or greater decrease in lung function.

The peak flow meter can serve as an early warning sign and in some cases may show a decrease in lung function one to three days before other respiratory symptoms become evident. This is important because once you know your lung function is declining, you can take steps to prevent an episode. The peak flow numbers, along with early

From "Med Facts: Adult Peak Flow Monitoring," [Online] 1993. Available: http://www.njc.org/MFhtml/APF_MF.html. © 1993 by the National Jewish Medical and Research Center, 1400 Jackson St., Denver, Colorado 80206. Reprinted with permission. And excerpted from "Patient Handouts," in *Practical Guide for the Diagnosis and Management of Asthma*, based on the *Expert Panel Report 2: Guidelines for the Diagnosis and Management of Asthma*. Produced by U.S. Department of Health and Human Services, National Heart, Lung, and Blood Institute (NHLBI), NIH Publication No. 97-4053, October 1997. For complete contact information, please refer to Chapter 68, "Resources."

473

warning signs, can be used to make decisions about asthma treatment. Most asthma experts agree that people with asthma need an objective means of assessing the severity of their condition. Pulmonary function studies are costly and impractical for home use; the peak flow meter provides a good alternative. It is an inexpensive, practical way to measure lung function.

The peak flow meter measures how fast you can blow air out after taking a deep breath. This measurement, which is read as a number, may reflect the amount of obstruction in the airways. Monitoring the peak flow numbers can help you and your clinician assess your lung function and the state of your asthma. It is a valuable number to use in making decisions about the following:

1. Effectiveness of asthma medications.
2. Adding or stopping medication(s).
3. When to seek emergency care.
4. Environmental control measures.
5. Personal assessments.

Using Peak Flow Numbers to Make Treatment Decisions

Predicted peak flow values are determined by height, sex, and age. Manufacturers usually supply graphs with standard values. You can use these as initial guides until you and your clinician define your "personal best." Determine your "personal best" by recording the values for two weeks when your asthma is under good control. Use the highest number you can regularly blow (after a bronchodilator treatment if prescribed.) Asthma is controlled when you do not experience asthma symptoms (including nighttime symptoms) and you maintain a normal level of activity. Peak flow values typically are highest in the midday or early evening, so use these readings to determine your personal best.

Once you've determined your personal best, it may be helpful for you and your clinician to establish zones. Zones will cue you about how well you are breathing. The zone system can be compared to the colors of a traffic light:

- **Green Zone** (80%-100% of personal best) signals **ALL CLEAR.** This indicates good lung function. Follow the routine treatment plan for maintaining asthma control.
- **Yellow Zone** (50%-80% of personal best) signals **CAUTION.** You may need more aggressive medical management for

asthma. This may include a temporary increase in bronchodilator and inhaled steroid medicines, an oral steroid burst or other medicines as prescribed by your physician.

- **Red Zone** (50% or less of personal best) signals a **MEDICAL ALERT!** You need immediate treatment with an inhaled bronchodilator. Notify your physician or seek emergency care if peak flow numbers do not immediately return and stay in the yellow or green zones.

You can mark your peak flow meter with colored tape, dots, or lines to indicate the green, yellow, and red zones. Remember that the peak flow percentages we suggest are guidelines only. Establish your peak flow zones with your clinician.

It can be helpful to record peak flow values on a graph or [Asthma Action Plan as shown in Figure 53.1.]. The peak flow information should supplement record-keeping of your asthma symptoms, use of inhaled medications, activity level, and nighttime awakenings due to asthma. This allows you and your clinician to monitor trends that may indicate changes in lung function. Persons whose numbers frequently fluctuate or slowly drop may need a change in their daily medications.

When to Use a Peak Flow Meter

The frequency that you record peak flow numbers depends upon the severity of your asthma, the season, your pattern of symptoms, and other factors specific to you. Persons with moderate, severe, or unstable asthma may need to record peak flow values before and after bronchodilator treatment twice a day (morning and evening). Individuals with mild or stable asthma may only need to use their peak flow meters two to three times a week. However, peak flow readings should be taken daily when you:

- are exposed to asthma triggers (such as allergens, smoke, and other environmental irritants), or
- have a respiratory infection, or
- have changes in medical therapy.

How to Use the Peak Flow Meter

1. Place the indicator at the bottom or beginning of the numbered scale.
2. Stand up.

3. Take a deep breath in.

4. Place the meter in your mouth, close your lips around the mouthpiece. Do not put your tongue in the hole.

5. Blow out as hard and as fast as you can without bending over.

6. Write down the number that you get.

7. Repeat steps 1 through 6 two more times.

8. Keep a record of the highest of the three numbers.

It is important to know that peak flow numbers are effort dependent. This means you must put forth a good effort to have reliable, consistent results.

Remember to Reevaluate "Personal Best" every six months to one year and adjust zones as needed.

To clean your peak flow meter, follow the manufacturer's directions.

ASTHMA ACTION PLAN FOR_____ Doctor's Name _____ Date _____

Doctor's Phone Number_____ Hospital/Emergency Room Phone Number _____

GREEN ZONE: Doing Well
- No cough, wheeze, chest tightness, or shortness of breath during the day or night
- Can do usual activities

And, if a peak flow meter is used,
Peak flow: more than _____
(80% or more of my best peak flow)

My best peak flow is:_____

Take These Long-Term-Control Medicines Each Day (include an anti-inflammatory)

Medicine	How much to take	When to take it

Before exercise ❑_____ ❑ 2 or ❑ 4 puffs 5 to 60 minutes before exercise

YELLOW ZONE: Asthma Is Getting Worse
- Cough, wheeze, chest tightness, or shortness of breath, or
- Waking at night due to asthma, or
- Can do some, but not all, usual activities

-Or-

Peak flow: _____ to _____
(50% - 80% of my best peak flow)

FIRST Add: Quick-Relief Medicine – and keep taking your GREEN ZONE medicine

_____ ❑ 2 or ❑ 4 puffs, every 20 minutes for up to 1 hour
(short-acting beta₂-agonist) ❑ Nebulizer, once

SECOND If your symptoms (and peak flow, if used) return to GREEN ZONE after 1 hour of above treatment:
❑ Take the quick-relief medicine every 4 hours for 1 to 2 days.
❑ Double the dose of your inhaled steroid for _____ (7-10) days.

-Or-

If your symptoms (and peak flow, if used) do not return to GREEN ZONE after 1 hour of above treatment:
❑ Take: _____ ❑ 2 or ❑ 4 puffs or ❑ Nebulizer
(short-acting beta₂-agonist)
❑ Add: _____ _____ mg. per day For _____ (3-10) days
(oral steroid)
❑ Call the doctor ❑ before/ ❑ within _____ hours after taking the oral steroid.

RED ZONE: Medical Alert!
- Very short of breath, or
- Quick-relief medicines have not helped, or
- Cannot do usual activities, or
- Symptoms are same or get worse after 24 hours in Yellow Zone

-Or-

Peak flow: less than_____
(50% of my best peak flow)

Take this medicine:

❑ _____ ❑ 4 or ❑ 6 puffs or ❑ Nebulizer
(short-acting beta₂-agonist)
❑ _____ _____ mg.
(oral steroid)

Then call your doctor NOW. Go to the hospital or call for an ambulance if:
- You are still in the red zone after 15 minutes AND
- You have not reached your doctor.

DANGER SIGNS
- Trouble walking and talking due to shortness of breath
- Lips or fingernails are blue

- Take ❑ 4 or ❑ 6 puffs of your quick-relief medicine AND
- Go to the hospital or call for an ambulance (_____) NOW!

Figure 53.1. Asthma Action Plan

Chapter 54

Chronotherapy: Controlling Nocturnal Breathing Problems

How our bodies marshal defenses against disease depends on many factors, such as age, gender, and genetics. Recently, the role of our bodies' biological rhythms in fighting disease has come under study by some in the medical community.

Our bodies' rhythms, also known as our biological clocks, take their cue from the environment and the rhythms of the solar system that change night to day and lead one season into another. Our internal clocks are also dictated by our genetic makeup. These clocks influence how our bodies change throughout the day, affecting blood pressure, blood coagulation, blood flow, and other functions.

Some of the rhythms that affect our bodies include:

- ultradian, which are cycles shorter than a day (for example, the milliseconds it takes for a neuron to fire, or a 90-minute sleep cycle)

- circadian, which last about 24 hours (such as sleeping and waking patterns)

- infradian, referring to cycles longer than 24 hours (for example, monthly menstruation)

- seasonal, such as seasonal affective disorder (SAD), which causes depression in susceptible people during the short days of winter.

Excerpted from "A Time to Heal: Chronotherapy Tunes in to Body's Rhythms," by Isadora Stehlin, in *FDA Consumer* [Online] April 1997. Available: http://www.fda.gov. Produced by the U.S. Food and Drug Administration. For complete contact information, please refer to Chapter 68, "Resources."

"The biology of human beings is not constant throughout the day, the menstrual cycle, and the year," says Michael Smolensky, Ph.D., director of the Chronobiology Center at the University of Texas. "Instead, it varies predictably in time."

Coordinating biological rhythms (chronobiology) with medical treatment is called chronotherapy. It considers a person's biological rhythms in determining the timing—and sometimes the amount—of medication to optimize a drug's desired effects and minimize the undesired ones.

According to Smolensky, patients are more likely to follow schedules for taking their medications when those medications are formulated as chronotherapies because of better medical results and fewer adverse side effects. "With better compliance, the disease can be better contained, which means fewer doctor visits and potential trips to the hospital because of acute flare-ups," he says.

The area in which chronotherapy is most advanced—drug chronotherapy—for the most part does not involve new medicines but using old ones differently. Revising the dosing schedule, reformulating a drug so its release into the bloodstream is delayed, or using programmable pumps that deliver medicine at precise intervals are some of the simple changes that may reap enormous benefits. Drugs that are reformulated as chronotherapeutics are regulated by the Food and Drug Administration.

Here's a look at how chronotherapy is being used [for asthma].

Asthma

Normal lung function undergoes circadian changes and reaches a low point in the early morning hours. This dip is particularly pronounced in people with asthma.

Chronotherapy for asthma is aimed at getting maximal effect from bronchodilator medications during the early morning hours. One example is the bronchodilator Uniphyl, a long-acting theophylline preparation manufactured by Purdue Frederick Co. of Norwalk, Conn., and approved by FDA in 1989. Taken once a day in the evening, Uniphyl causes theophylline blood levels to reach their peak and improve lung function during the difficult early morning hours. There are other bronchodilators that act similarly to address the early morning dip in lung function, but the manufacturers have not sought or received FDA approval for chronotherapeutic labeling.

Writing in the April 15, 1996, issue of *Hospital Practice*, Richard Martin, M.D., who directs the division of pulmonary medicine at the

National Jewish Center for Immunology and Respiratory Medicine in Denver, stated his belief that "the key to managing [asthma] cases is chronotherapy. I have found that unless treatment improves night-time asthma, it is hard to improve its daytime manifestations." For people with severe asthma who wake up several times a night gasping for breath, a good night's sleep can be a dream come true.

Regulatory Implications

Chronotherapeutics present new challenges to regulators and scientists alike. For example, according to FDA's Sokol, chronotherapeutic clinical studies need to consider additional parameters not usually required of other clinical trials. Among additional factors that must be considered, he says, are:

- time of day a drug is administered
- time-related biological factors, such as seasonal disorders (for example, seasonal affective disorder)
- patients' normal routines (for example, eating times and sleep patterns).

Making chronotherapy the focus of more clinical trials would be welcome news to many in the medical community, according to a 1996 American Medical Association survey. The study found that about 75 percent of the doctors surveyed said they would like more treatment options to match a patient's circadian, or daily, rhythms.

But chronotherapy has a way to go, considering that only 5 percent of the doctors surveyed said they were "very familiar" with the subject.

"Chronotherapy is not well recognized in the medical community," Sokol says, "but awareness is increasing. The implications are broad in every area of medicine."

— by Isadora Stehlin

Isadora Stehlin is a member of FDA's public affairs staff.

Chapter 55

Managing Asthma in the Child Care Setting

Asthma is a chronic breathing disorder and is the most common chronic health problem among children. Children with asthma have attacks of coughing, wheezing, and shortness of breath, which may be very serious. These symptoms are caused by spasms of the air passages in the lungs. The air passages swell, become inflamed, and fill with mucus, making breathing difficult. Many asthma attacks occur when children get respiratory infections, including infections caused by common cold viruses. Attacks can also be caused by:

- exposure to cigarette smoke,

- stress,

- strenuous exercise,

- weather conditions, including cold, windy, or rainy days,

- allergies to animals, dust, pollen, or mold,

- indoor air pollutants, such as paint, cleaning materials, chemicals, or perfumes, or

- outdoor air pollutants, such as ozone.

From "What You Should Know about . . . Asthma in the Child Care Setting," in *The ABCs of Safe and Healthy Child Care,* [Online] Undated. Available: http://www.cdc.gov/ncidod/hip/abc/facts01.htm. Produced by the Hospital Infections Program, National Center for Infectious Diseases, Centers for Disease Control and Prevention (CDC). For complete contact information, please refer to Chapter 68, "Resources."

As with any child with a chronic condition, the child care provider and parents should discuss specific needs of the child and whether they can be sufficiently met by the provider. Some people believe that smaller-sized child care centers or family child care home environments may be more beneficial to a child with asthma because exposure to common respiratory viruses may be reduced. However, this has not been proven to be true.

Children with asthma may be prescribed medications to relax the small air passages and/or to prevent passages from becoming inflamed. These medications may need to be administered every day or only during attacks. Asthma medication is available in several forms, including liquid, powder, and pill, or it can be breathed in from an inhaler or compressor. The child care provider should be given clear instructions on how and when to administer all medications and the name and telephone number of the child's doctor.

The child care provider should be provided with and keep on file an asthma action plan for each child with asthma. An asthma action plan lists emergency information, activities or conditions likely to trigger an asthma attack, current medications being taken, medications to be administered by the child care provider, and steps to be followed if the child has an acute asthma attack. Additional support from the child's health care providers should be available to the child care provider as needed.

Most children with asthma can lead a normal life, but may often have to restrict their activity. Some preventive measures for reducing asthma attacks include:

- Avoiding allergic agents such as dust, plush carpets, feather pillows, and dog and cat dander. Installing low-pile carpets, vacuuming daily, and dusting frequently can help to reduce allergic agents. A child who is allergic to dogs or cats may need to be placed in a facility without pets.

- Stopping exercise if the child begins to breathe with difficulty or starts to wheeze.

- Avoiding strenuous exercise.

- Avoiding cold, damp weather. A child with asthma may need to be kept inside on cold, damp days or taken inside immediately if cold air triggers an attack.

If a child with asthma has trouble breathing:

1. Stop the child's activity and remove whatever is causing the allergic reaction, if you know what it is.

2. Calm the child; give medication prescribed, if any, for an attack.

3. Contact the parents.

4. If the child does not improve very quickly, and the parents are unavailable, call the child's doctor.

5. If the child is unable to breathe, call 911.

6. Record the asthma attack in the child's file. Describe the symptoms, how the child acted during the attack, what medicine was given, and what caused the attack, if known.

Chapter 56

Managing Asthma at School

How Asthma-Friendly Is Your School?

Children with asthma need proper support at school to keep their asthma under control and be fully active. Use the questions below to find out how well your school assists children with asthma:

1. Is your school free of tobacco smoke all of the time, including during school-sponsored events?

2. Does the school maintain good indoor air quality? Does it reduce or eliminate allergens and irritants that can make asthma worse? Allergens and irritants include pets with fur or feathers, mold, dust mites (for example, in carpets and upholstery), cockroaches, and strong odors or fumes from such products as pesticides, paint, perfumes, and cleaning chemicals.

3. Is there a school nurse in your school all day, every day? If not, is a nurse regularly available to the school to help write

Excerpted from "How Asthma-Friendly Is Your School?" [Online] Undated. Available: http://www.nhlbi.nih.gov/health/public/lung/asthma/friendly.htm. Produced by the National Asthma Education and Prevention Program (NAEPP), National Heart, Lung, and Blood Institute (NHLBI) Information Center; and from "Challenges for Parents of Asthmatics: Barriers to Cooperation at School; Part I," [Online] 1998. Available: http://www.allergyasthma.com/archives/asthma10.html. © 1998 by Louise H. Bethea, M.D., P.A., Board Certified Allergist/Immunologist, 17070 Red Oak Dr., Ste. 107, Houston, TX 77090. Reprinted with permission. For complete contact information, please refer to Chapter 68, "Resources."

plans and give guidance for students with asthma about medicines, physical education, and field trips?

4. Can children take medicines at school as recommended by
their doctor and parents? May children carry their own
asthma medicines?

5. Does your school have an emergency plan for taking care of a
child with a severe asthma episode (attack)? Is it made clear
what to do? Who to call? When to call?

6. Does someone teach school staff about asthma, asthma management plans, and asthma medicines? Does someone teach
all students about asthma and how to help a classmate who
has it?

7. Do students have good options for fully and safely participating in physical education class and recess? (For example, do
students have access to their medicine before exercise? Can
they choose modified or alternative activities when medically
necessary?)

If the answer to any question is no, students may be facing obstacles to asthma control. Asthma out of control can hinder a student's
attendance, participation, and progress in school. School staff, health
professionals, and parents can work together to remove obstacles and
to promote students' health and education.

Challenges for Parents of Asthmatics: Barriers to Cooperation at School

A lot has been written about the importance of parents coordinating health and educational plans for their asthmatic children with
teachers, school nurses, and their doctors. Statistics report that
asthma is the number one cause of school absenteeism, accounting
for at least 125 million school days lost each year. Parents say they
are frustrated by inflexible school policies in their attempts to help
their children perform up to their potential in a safe, encouraging,
and productive learning atmosphere.

Many parents complain that their asthmatic children are trapped
in a system which does not acknowledge their physical limitations and
special needs. Many school systems, it seems, have the desire to accommodate asthmatic children, but they don't have the tools to put
this responsibility into action.

When these barriers exist, it is necessary for parents, educators, and healthcare professionals to work at striking a balance between what parents of children with asthma can expect a school to provide and what educators can expect of parents. This means the establishment of an open and effective channel of communication becomes the first and most important task at hand.

The child's physician, parents, and the school staff all share one common goal—minimizing time the child must miss school due to illness. After a treatment plan has been reached, especially if it involves routine and episodic medications, it is critical that the school nurse and the child's teachers are briefed so they understand exactly what the child's limitations are and why the medication is necessary.

This may be more difficult to accomplish than it appears. According to a monthly newsletter distributed by Mothers Of Asthmatics, until a parent has an injured or chronically ill child, most parents are not aware of the limits of a school's health services and resources or the potential of encountering inflexible policies. Then, they are often frustrated in their negotiations for medication management or a modified physical education program these students require so they can maintain as normal a learning environment as possible as well as good peer relationships. Three years ago, 80 national child health and education leaders convened in Houston to examine the barriers that keep children with chronic illnesses from participating fully in school. This dialogue revealed that attendance varied widely within school districts and from state to state. In far too many instances, they discovered, students who had frequent absences could not obtain much needed back-up tutoring or the home schooling they needed to keep up with their classes. And, unfortunately, these students are often penalized for missing class or gym time.

Many schools do not allow students to adapt their activity level, such as attend classes, but not actively participate in gym class, using the tired argument that if a child is well enough to come to school, they are well enough to participate fully. This inflexibility sends kids home when they are capable of remaining in class.

Building Bridges

Parents, in their attempts to keep their children in school and manage their child's health, often overlook the school nurse as an important potential ally.

Many school nurses have attended special workshops geared to updating their knowledge about quality asthma care so that they can intervene more effectively when necessary. They deal with children with asthma nearly every day, so they have a lot of hands-on experience. Chances are, they will be familiar with medication schedules and special needs of asthmatic children and perhaps can offer some suggestions about coping strategies to the parents.

According to practicing school nurses, it is an unfortunate fact that many parents seem unaware of the need to share specific information about their child's medication plan with healthcare professionals at school, or they are too busy to follow up with routine communications. This can really shortchange the child who has enough challenges facing him or her already.

Legal Protection

Legally, under a federal law, Section 504 of the Rehabilitation Act, students with asthma and other chronic illnesses are entitled to health services and necessary modifications to their regular education program. Section 504 prohibits discrimination in education (and employment) on the basis of a "handicap"; which, by definition includes asthma. Policies and practices that create barriers for students with chronic illnesses violate Section 504, and may be disputed under law.

Promoting health, safety, and medical compliance in school are not new challenges to many school staffs. Administrators, teachers, school nurses, and health educators can be a parent's best allies in overcoming disparities in school health policies and resources.

If, after trying all other avenues of communication, a parent is unable to work out a mutually acceptable arrangement at school to accommodate the needs of an asthmatic child, section 504 can be an important tool for obtaining appropriate health services for individuals, as well as establishing system-wide standards to protect all students. Help is available through the local or state Section 504 Coordinator, or the Office for Civil Rights (OCR), Department of Education.

There is also a wealth of information available to parents and educators, along with support and advocacy groups [listed in Chapter 68, "Resources."]

Chapter 57

Controlling Asthma Exacerbations at Home, in the Emergency Department, and in the Hospital

Home Management: Prompt Treatment Is Key

Educating patients to recognize and treat exacerbations early is the best strategy. Education and preparation of patients to manage their exacerbations (e.g., episodes of progressively worsening shortness of breath, cough, wheezing, chest tightness, or some combination of these symptoms) are essential and should include:

- A written action plan and clear instructions on how to follow it. (See Table 57.2 below).

- Instructions on how to recognize signs of worsening asthma and signs that indicate the need to call the doctor or seek emergency care.

- Prompt use of short-acting beta$_2$-agonists (two puffs every 20 minutes for 1 hour) and, for moderate-to-severe exacerbations, the addition of oral steroids. Increased therapy should be maintained for several days to stabilize symptoms and peak flow.

- Monitoring the response to the medications.

Excerpted from "Managing Asthma Exacerbations at Home, in the Emergency Department, and in the Hospital," in *Practical Guide for the Diagnosis and Management of Asthma,* based on the *Expert Panel Report 2: Guidelines for the Diagnosis and Management of Asthma.* Produced by U.S. Department of Health and Human Services, National Heart, Lung, and Blood Institute (NHLBI), NIH Publication No. 97-4053, October 1997. For complete contact information, please refer to Chapter 68, "Resources."

- Followup with patients to assess overall asthma control, the need to increase long-term-control medications, and the need to remove or withdraw from allergens or irritants that precipitated the exacerbation.

Patients at high risk of asthma-related death (see Table 57.1. below) require special attention—intensive education, monitoring, and care. They should be counseled to seek medical care early during an exacerbation and instructed about when and how to call for an ambulance. Patients with moderate-to-severe persistent asthma or a history of severe exacerbations should have the medication (e.g., steroid tablets or liquid) and equipment (e.g., peak flow meter, compressor-driven nebulizer for young children) for assessing and treating exacerbations at home.

Prehospital Emergency Medicine/Ambulance Management

It is recommended that emergency workers administer short-acting inhaled beta$_2$-agonists and supplemental oxygen to patients who have signs or symptoms of asthma.[1] Subcutaneous epinephrine or terbutaline are NOT recommended but can be used if inhaled medication is not available.

Emergency Department and Hospital Management of Exacerbations

Treat without Delay

Assess patient's peak flow or FEV_1 and administer medication(s) upon patient's arrival without delay. After therapy is initiated, obtain a brief, focused history and physical examination pertinent to the exacerbation. Perform a more detailed history, physical, and lab studies only after therapy has started.

The goals for treating asthma exacerbations are rapid reversal of airflow obstruction, reduction in the likelihood of recurrence, and correction of significant hypoxemia. To achieve these goals, the management of asthma exacerbations in the emergency department and hospital includes:

- Oxygen for most patients to maintain SaO_2 ≥90 percent (> 95 percent in pregnant women, infants, and patients with coexistent heart disease). Monitor oxygen saturation until a significant clinical improvement has occurred.

- Short-acting inhaled beta$_2$-agonists every 20 to 30 minutes for three treatments for all patients. The onset of action is about 5 minutes.

Table 57.1. Risk Factors for Death from Asthma

History of Severe Exacerbations
- Past history of sudden severe exacerbations
- Prior intubation for asthma
- Prior admission for asthma to an intensive care unit

Asthma Hospitalizations and Emergency Visits
- ≥2 hospitalizations in the past year
- ≥3 emergency care visits in the past year
- Hospitalization or emergency visit in past month

Beta$_2$-Agonist and Oral Steroid Usage
- Use of >2 canisters per month of short-acting inhaled beta$_2$-agonist
- Current use of oral steroids or recent withdrawal from oral steroids

Complicating Health Problems
- Comorbidity (e.g., cardiovascular diseases or COPD)
- Serious psychiatric disease, including depression, or psychosocial problems
- Illicit drug use

Other Factors
- Poor perception of airflow obstruction or its severity
- Sensitivity to *Alternaria* (an outdoor mold)
- Low socioeconomic status and urban residence

Sources: Suissa S, Ernst P, Bolvin JF, et al. A cohort analysis of excess mortality in asthma and the use of inhaled beta$_2$-agonists. *Am J Respir Crit Care Med* 1994;149(3 Pt 1):604-10. Kallenbach JM, Frankel AH, Lapinsky SE, et al. Determinants of near fatality in acute severe asthma. *Am J Med* 1993;95:265-72. Rodrigo C, Rodrigo G. Assessment of the patient with acute asthma in the emergency department. A factor analytic study. *Chest* 1993;104:1325-8. Greenberger PA, Miller TP, Lifschultz B. Circumstances surrounding deaths from asthma in Cook County (Chicago) Illinois. *Allergy Proc* 1993;14:321-6. O'Hollaren MT, Yunginger JW, Offord KP, et al. Exposure to an aeroallergen as a possible precipitating factor in respiratory arrest in young patients with asthma. *N Engl J Med* 1991;324:359-63.

Table 57.2. Management of Asthma Exacerbations: Home Treatment (continued on next page)

Assess Symptoms/Peak Flow*

Mild-to-Moderate Exacerbation

PEF 50-80% predicted or personal best or

Signs and Symptoms:
- Cough, breathlessness, wheeze, or chest tightness (correlate imperfectly with severity of exacerbation), or
- Waking at night due to asthma, or
- Decreased ability to perform usual activities

Instructions to Patient
Inhaled short-acting beta$_2$-agonist:
- Up to three treatments of 2-4 puffs by MDI at 20-minute intervals, or
- Single nebulizer treatment
Assess symptoms and/or peak flow after 1 hour

Good Response (Mild Exacerbation)

PEF >80% predicted or personal best and/or

Signs and Symptoms:
- No wheezing, shortness of breath, cough, or chest tightness, and
- Response to beta$_2$-agonist sustained for 4 hours

Instructions to Patient
- May continue 2-4 puffs beta$_2$-agonist every 3-4 hours for 24-48 hours prn
- For patients on inhaled steroids, double dose for 7-10 days
- Contact clinician within 48 hours for instructions

Incomplete Response (Moderate Exacerbation)

PEF 50-80% predicted or personal best or

Signs and Symptoms:
- Persistent wheezing, shortness of breath, cough, or chest tightness

Instructions to Patient
- Take 2-4 puffs beta$_2$-agonist every 2-4 hours for 24-48 hours prn
- Add oral steroid**
- Contact clinician urgently (same day) for instructions

Poor Response (Severe Exacerbation)

PEF <50% predicted or personal best or

Signs and Symptoms:
- Marked wheezing, shortness of breath, cough, or chest tightness
- Cyanosis
- Trouble walking or talking due to asthma
- Accessory muscle use
- Suprasternal retractions
- Response to beta$_2$-agonist lasts <2 hours

Table 57.2. (continued) Management of Asthma Exacerbations: Home Treatment

Poor Response (Severe Exacerbation) (continued)
Instructions to Patient
IMMEDIATELY:
- Take up to 3 treatments of 4-6 puffs beta$_2$-agonist every 20 minutes prn
- Start oral steroid**
- Contact clinician
- Proceed to emergency department, or call ambulance or 9-1-1

* Patients at high risk for asthma-related death should receive immediate clinical attention after initial treatment. More intensive therapy may be required.

** Oral steroid dosages: Adult: 40-60 mg, single or 2 divided doses for 3-10 days. Child: 1-2 mg/kg/day, maximum 60 mg/day, for 3-10 days.

Subsequent therapy depends on response. Subcutaneous beta$_2$-agonists provide no proven advantage over inhaled medication.

NOTE: Anticholinergics added to albuterol may be considered. Adding high doses of ipratropium bromide (0.5 mg in adults, 0.25 mg in children) to albuterol in a nebulizer has been shown to cause additional bronchodilation in some but not all studies,[2-4] particularly in patients with severe airflow obstruction.

- Oral steroids should be given to most patients—those with moderate-to-severe exacerbations, patients who fail to respond promptly and completely to an inhaled beta$_2$-agonist, and patients admitted into the hospital. Oral steroids speed recovery and reduce the likelihood of recurrence. Onset of action is greater than 4 hours.[5-7] Often, a 3- to 10-day course of oral steroids at discharge is useful:

  1. For patients who take oral steroids long term, give supplemental doses, even if the exacerbation is mild.
  2. In infants and children, give oral steroids early in the course of an asthma exacerbation.
  3. Oral administration of prednisone is usually preferred to intravenous methylprednisolone because it is less invasive and the effects are equivalent.[8,9]

Repeat Assessment

The Expert Panel recommends repeat assessments of patients with severe exacerbations after the first dose and the third dose (about 60 to 90 minutes after initiating treatment) of short- acting inhaled beta$_2$-agonists. Evaluate the patient's subjective response, physical findings, and lung function. Consider arterial blood gas measurement for evaluating arterial carbon dioxide (PCO_2) in patients with suspected hypoventilation, severe distress, or with FEV_1 or peak flow ≤30 percent of predicted after treatment.

Effectiveness of MDI plus Spacer/Holding Chamber vs. Nebulizer

Equivalent bronchodilation can be achieved by a beta$_2$-agonist given by MDI with a spacer/holding chamber under the supervision of trained personnel or by nebulizer therapy.[10-12] Continuous administration with a nebulizer may be more effective in children and severely obstructed adults[13-16] and patients who have difficulty with an MDI plus spacer/holding chamber.

Special Considerations for Infants

Infants require special attention due to their greater risk for respiratory failure.

- Use oral steroids early in the episode.
- Monitor oxygen saturation by pulse oximetry. SaO_2 should be >95 percent at sea level.
- Assess infants for signs of serious distress, including use of accessory muscles, paradoxical breathing, cyanosis, a respiratory rate >60, or oxygen saturation <91 percent.
- Assess response to therapy. A lack of response to beta$_2$-agonist therapy noted by physical exam or oxygen saturation is an indication for hospitalization.

Therapies Not Recommended for Treating Exacerbations

Theophylline/aminophylline is NOT recommended therapy in the emergency department because it appears to provide no additional benefit to short-acting inhaled beta$_2$-agonists and may produce adverse effects.[17-21] In hospitalized patients, intravenous methylxanthines are not beneficial in children with severe asthma[22-24] and their addition remains controversial for adults.[25-26]

Chest physical therapy and mucolytics are not recommended. Anxiolytic and hypnotic drugs are contraindicated. Antibiotics are NOT recommended for asthma treatment but may be needed for comorbid conditions (e.g., patients with fever and purulent sputum or with evidence of bacterial pneumonia). Aggressive hydration is NOT recommended for older children and adults. Assess fluid status and make appropriate corrections for infants and young children to reduce their risk of dehydration.

Hospital Asthma Care

In general, the principles of care in the hospital are similar to those for care in the emergency department and involve treatment with aerosolized bronchodilators, systemic steroids, oxygen, and frequent assessments. Clinical assessment of respiratory distress and fatigue and objective measurement of airflow (peak flow or FEV_1) and oxygen saturation with pulse oximetry should be performed. Most patients respond well to therapy; however, a small minority will show signs of worsening ventilation.

Signs of impending respiratory failure include declining mental clarity, worsening fatigue, and a PCO_2 of ≥ 42 mm Hg. Respiratory failure tends to progress rapidly and is hard to reverse. The decision to intubate is based on clinical judgment; however, intubation is best done semi- electively, before the crisis of respiratory arrest. Therefore, the Expert Panel recommends that intubation should not be delayed once it is deemed necessary. Intubation should be performed by physicians with extensive experience in intubation and airway management. Consultation or comanagement by a physician expert in ventilator management is appropriate.

Patient Discharge from the Emergency Department or Hospital

Patients can be discharged from the emergency department and hospital when peak flow or FEV_1 is ≥ 70 percent of predicted or personal best and symptoms are minimal. Patients should be assessed for discharge on an individual basis if they have a peak flow or FEV_1 of ≥ 50 but <70 percent of predicted or personal best and mild symptoms. Take into consideration the risk factors for asthma-related death. Hospitalized patients should have their medications changed to an oral or inhaled regimen and then be observed for 24 hours before discharge.

Before discharge, provide patients with the following:

- Sufficient short-acting inhaled beta$_2$-agonist and oral steroids to complete the course of therapy or to continue therapy until the followup appointment. Patients given oral steroids should continue taking them for 3 to 10 days. Patients may be asked to start taking or to increase inhaled steroids in an attempt to improve the patient's long-term-control regimen.

- Written and verbal instructions on when to increase medications or return for care should asthma worsen. The plan provided in the emergency department can be quite simple. Before discharge from the hospital, patients should receive a more complete written action plan on when to take their medicines.

- Training on how to monitor peak flow should be provided in the hospital and considered for patients in the emergency department. Also, consider issuing peak flow meters. Patients in both settings should receive instruction on monitoring their symptoms.

- Training on necessary environmental control measures and inhaler technique, whenever possible.

- Referral for a followup medical appointment. Tell patients from the emergency department to go to a followup appointment within 3 to 5 days or set up an appointment for them. When possible, phone or fax a notice to the patient's physician that the patient came to the emergency department. For both emergency department and hospital patients, emphasize the need for continual, regular care in an outpatient setting. If patients do not have a physician, refer them or arrange a followup visit with a primary care physician, a clinic, or an asthma specialist.

References

1. Fergusson, RJ, Stewart CM, Wathen CG, Moffat R, Crompton GK. Effectiveness of nebulised salbutamol administered in ambulances to patients with acute severe asthma. *Thorax* 1995;50:81-2.

2. Schuh S, Johnson DW, Callahan S, Canny G, Levison H. Efficacy of frequent nebulized ipratropium bromide added to frequent

high-dose albuterol therapy in severe childhood asthma. *J Pediatr* 1995;126:639-45.

3. Kelly HW, Murphy S. Corticosteroids for acute, severe asthma. *DICP* 1991;25:72-9.

4. Karpel JP, Schacter EN, Fanta C, et al. A comparison of ipratropium and albuterol vs. albuterol alone for the treatment of acute asthma. *Chest* 1996;110:611-6.

5. Rowe BH, Keller JL, Oxman AD. Effectiveness of steroid therapy in acute exacerbations of asthma: a meta-analysis. *Am J Emerg Med* 1992;10:301-10.

6. Scarfone RJ, Fuchs SM, Nager AL, Shane SA. Controlled trial of oral prednisone in the emergency department treatment of children with acute asthma. *Pediatrics* 1993;2:513-8.

7. Connett GJ, Warde C, Wooler E, Lenney W. Prednisolone and salbutamol in the hospital treatment of acute asthma. *Arch Dis Child* 1994;70:170-3.

8. Harrison BD, Stokes TC, Hart GJ, Vaughan DA, Ali NJ, Robinson AA. Need for intravenous hydrocortisone in addition to oral prednisolone in patients admitted to hospital with severe asthma without ventilatory failure. *Lancet* 1986;1(8474):181-4.

9. Ratto D, Alfaro C, Sipsey J, Glovsky MM, Sharma OP. Are intravenous corticosteroids required in status asthmaticus? *JAMA* 1988;260:527-9.

10. Idris AH, McDermott MF, Raucci JC, Morrabel A, McGorray S, Hendeles L. Emergency department treatment of severe asthma. Metered-dose inhaler plus holding chamber is equivalent in effectiveness to nebulizer. *Chest* 1993;103:665-72.

11. Colacone A, Afilalo M, Wolkove N, Kreisman H. A comparison of albuterol administered by metered dose inhaler (and holding chamber) or wet nebulizer in acute asthma. *Chest* 1993;104:835-41.

12. Kerem E, Levison H, Schuh S, et al. Efficacy of albuterol administered by nebulizer versus spacer device in children with acute asthma. *J Pediatr* 1993;123:313-7.

13. Lin RY, Sauter D, Newman T, Sirleaf J, Walters J, Tavakol M. Continuous versus intermittent albuterol nebulization in the treatment of acute asthma. *Ann Emerg Med* 1993;22:1847-53.

14. Rudnitsky GS, Eberlein RS, Schoffstall JM, Mazur JE, Spivey WH. Comparison of intermittent and continuously nebulized albuterol for treatment of asthma in an urban emergency department. *Ann Emerg Med* 1993;22:1842-6.

15. Papo MC, Frank J, Thompson AE. A prospective, randomized study of continuous versus intermittent nebulized albuterol for severe status asthmaticus in children. *Crit Care Med* 1993;21:1479-86.

16. Kelly HW, Murphy S. Beta-adrenergic agonists for acute, severe asthma. *Ann Pharmacother* 1992;26:81-91.

17. Fanta CH, Rossing TH, McFadden ER Jr. Treatment of acute asthma: is combination therapy with sympathomimetics and methylxanthines indicated? *Am J Med* 1986;80:5-10.

18. Rossing TH, Fanta CH, Goldstein DH, Snapper JR, McFadden ER Jr. Emergency therapy of asthma: comparison of the acute effects of parenteral and inhaled sympathomimetics and infused aminophylline. *Am Rev Respir Dis* 1980;122:365-71.

19. Murphy DG, McDermott MF, Rydman RJ, Sloan EP, Zalenski RJ. Aminophylline in the treatment of acute asthma when beta$_2$-adrenergics and steroids are provided. *Arch Intern Med* 1993;153:1784-88.

20. Rodrigo C, Rodrigo G. Treatment of acute asthma. Lack of therapeutic benefit and increase of the toxicity from aminophylline given in addition to high doses of salbutamol delivered by metered-dose inhaler with a spacer. *Chest* 1994;106:1071-6.

21. Coleridge J, Cameron P, Epstein J, Teichtahl H. Intravenous aminophylline confers no benefit in acute asthma treated with intravenous steroids and inhaled bronchodilators. *Aust N Z J Med* 1993;23:348-54.

22. Strauss RE, Wertheim DL, Bonagura VR, Valacer DJ. Aminophylline therapy does not improve outcome and increases adverse effects in children hospitalized with acute asthmatic exacerbations. *Pediatrics* 1994;93:205-10.

23. Carter E, Cruz M, Chesrown S, Shieh G, Reilly K, Hendeles L. Efficacy of intravenously administered theophylline in children hospitalized with severe asthma. *J Pediatr* 1993;122:470-6.

24. DiGiulio GA, Kercsmar CM, Krug SE, Alpert SE, Marx CM. Hospital treatment of asthma: lack of benefit from theophylline given in addition to nebulized albuterol and intravenously administered corticosteroid. *J Pediatr* 1993;122:464-9.

25. Huang D, O'Brien RG, Harman E, et al. Does aminophylline benefit adults admitted to the hospital for an acute exacerbation of asthma? *Ann Intern Med* 1993;119:1155-60.

26. Self TH, Abou-Shala N, Burns R, et al. Inhaled albuterol and oral prednisone therapy in hospitalized adult asthmatics. Does aminophylline add any benefit? *Chest* 1990;98:1317-21.

Chapter 58

Asthma and Pregnancy

When you become pregnant you experience many physical and emotional changes. Joy and wonder are often mixed with concerns about your health and your unborn child, especially if you have asthma. It is reassuring to know that studies show having asthma does not increase your chances of birth defects or of having multiple births. Further studies show that control of asthma can be achieved during pregnancy with little or no risk to you or your baby.

Your Doctors

Most women with asthma do very well during pregnancy. Your doctor(s), in determining the best treatment for you, will weigh the benefits versus the risks to both you and your unborn baby. Your doctor will review your asthma history thoroughly, identify your asthma triggers and have you do a breathing test (spirometry).

Since uncontrolled asthma threatens your well-being and that of your baby, you and your doctors share a common goal throughout your pregnancy—to keep you healthy and breathing normally.

From "Med Facts: Asthma and Pregnancy," [Online] 1995. Available: http://www.njc.org/MFhtml/APR_MF.html. © 1995 by the National Jewish Medical and Research Center, 1400 Jackson St., Denver, CO 80206. Reprinted with permission. For complete contact information, please refer to Chapter 68, "Resources."

What You Need to Know

To help control your asthma, it's important to know what may trigger an asthma attack for you. These "triggers" can include any allergen or irritant such as: molds, pollens, animal danders, strong odors, aerosol sprays, and exercise.

A cold or the flu can trigger an asthma episode; therefore, we recommend frequent hand-washing to help prevent the spread of infections. In addition, avoid cigarette smoking or exposure to second-hand smoke as it is a major asthma trigger and is associated with significant risks for an unborn baby.

It is helpful to know the early warning signs of an asthma episode so it can be treated immediately. These warning signs may be experienced before your asthma symptoms begin and can vary with each person. Early warning signs may include: an itchy throat, cough, feeling of tiredness, sneezing, headache, or breathing changes.

Shortness of breath can be common in many pregnant women; therefore, it is important to know the difference between the expected shortness of breath in pregnancy and that in asthma. Using a Peak Flow Meter daily can help you monitor changes in your asthma.

Medications

Ideally, it would be best to avoid all medications during pregnancy. However, it is more important that your asthma be controlled to assure your baby's oxygen supply and decrease your health risk. Therefore, a "drugless" pregnancy is not always possible or desirable.

If your doctor prescribes medications for the management of your asthma, the main goal will be to use the least amount necessary to prevent or control your asthma. Review your medications and only take those prescribed by your doctor. Even some simple "over-the-counter" medications, available without a prescription, can be harmful to your baby. Ask your doctor about any medication you are considering taking.

Although medication studies are not done with pregnant women, there are a number of asthma medications used successfully during pregnancy. In general, inhaled medications are preferred because less medication reaches the baby. Also, we recommend medications that have been used for many years. As with any medicine used during pregnancy, your doctor and you need to weigh the benefits versus the risks.

The following list reviews medications that are commonly used during pregnancy.

Anti-Inflammatory Medications. Medications in this group help to prevent or lessen symptoms by reducing inflammation in the airways. They do not provide immediate relief of symptoms:

- Cromolyn Sodium (Intal™): This is a non-steroidal anti-inflammatory medication which is taken daily to prevent symptoms of chronic asthma. It is available in a metered-dose inhaler and nebulizer solution.

- Nedocromil Sodium (Tilade™): This medication, recently available in the United States, is similar to cromolyn. It is available in a metered-dose inhaler.

- Corticosteroids: These are the most effective anti-inflammatory medications for the treatment of asthma and can be prescribed as inhaled or oral medication.

A steroid inhaler which reduces inflammation in the airways is commonly prescribed to prevent symptoms of asthma. Although there are several different steroid inhalers available, one containing beclomethasone (Beclovent™, Vanceril™) is generally recommended.

An oral steroid or tablet preparation (prednisone or methylprednisolone) may be needed for more severe episodes. Intravenous steroids also may be given to control severe episodes.

Bronchodilator Medications. These medications temporarily relieve symptoms of asthma by relaxing the smooth muscle and opening the airways:

- Beta-Agonists: An inhaled beta-agonist has the advantage of working immediately with less medication for the baby. It also is an effective treatment to prevent asthma symptoms caused by exercise when taken 15 minutes before the activity. They are available as:

  1. Inhaled: Albuterol (Proventil™, Ventolin™); Pirbuterol (Maxair™); Terbutaline (Brethaire™); Metaproterenol (Alupent™, Metaprel™); Bitolterol (Tornalate™)

  2. Tablet: Albuterol (Proventil™, Proventil Repetab™, Ventolin™); Terbutaline (Brethine™, Bricanyl™); Metaproterenol (Alupent™, Metaprel™)

- Theophylline: This bronchodilator is available in timed-release preparations that are long-acting. This is useful for controlling nighttime symptoms. It is important to have a theophylline blood level checked periodically. Some available brands of theophyl-line include: Slo-bid™, Theo-dur™, Theolair™, and Uniphyl™.

- Anticholinergic: This inhaled bronchodilator is slower acting than inhaled beta-agonists. It is available as Atrovent™.

Treatment for Nasal/Sinus Conditions:

- Nasal Sprays: Steroid nasal spray—Beclomethasone (Beconase AQ™, Vancenase AQ™); Nasal Cromolyn spray—Nasalcrom™
- Antihistamines: Chlorpheniramine (Chlor-Trimeton™); Tripelennamine
- Decongestants: Pseudoephedrine (Sudafed™); Oxymetazoline nose drops
- Nasal Saline Wash: A salt water rinse to your nose may be helpful in clearing nasal congestion.

Other Asthma-Related Medication/Treatment:

- Antibiotic—Amoxicillin™
- Immunotherapy (Allergy Shots): Do not start immunotherapy during pregnancy. However, if you have been receiving allergy shots and have not shown any systemic reactions, you may continue.
- Influenza (Flu) Vaccine: We recommend that persons with moderate to severe asthma receive this yearly vaccine. Because this vaccine is based on a killed virus, it is not associated with risks during pregnancy.

Management of Severe Episodes

A small percentage of women with asthma may experience an asthma episode severe enough to require hospitalization. It is important for this treatment to relieve your respiratory distress and ensure that you and your baby receive adequate oxygen. Your treatment may include frequent nebulized treatments, oxygen, intravenous corticosteroids, and/or theophylline.

Management During Labor and Delivery

It is important for you to discuss the use of anesthesia with your doctor in advance of your delivery date. This is especially important in the case of a cesarean section. It is also necessary to plan the availability of asthma medication. You may choose to bring your own medication to the hospital, or perhaps the hospital will provide it.

If a cesarean section is required, you may need intravenous theophylline if you have been on theophylline. You may need intravenous corticosteroids if you are steroid-dependent or have been on steroid tablets during the past year.

An epidural block, a saddle block, or local anesthesia is preferred to general ("gas") anesthesia. If you receive anesthesia of this form, you may be able to use your inhaled medication as directed by your physician. Your baby may be monitored with a fetal monitor to make sure that he or she is not experiencing distress.

It is important to plan ahead and discuss these decisions and potential problems with your doctors. This will help decrease complications and fears which may arise once labor begins.

Breastfeeding

Research shows that breastfeeding for the first 6-12 months of life may help prevent or delay the development of certain allergies. The decision to breastfeed should be based on you and your baby's individual needs.

In general, when breastfeeding the use of most asthma medications does not affect your baby or interfere with your milk production. Of course, it is important to discuss your use of any medications with the doctor caring for your baby. The medications listed earlier for use during pregnancy are generally used while breastfeeding without problems. Remember, your blood stream absorbs less medication with inhaled medications; therefore, less medication passes into your breast milk. The following list of medications offers some additional information that can be discussed with your doctor:

- Steroid Tablets: Although this medication passes through breast milk in trace amounts (even at high dosages), it has not been associated with problems.

- Theophylline: This medication passes through breast milk in trace amounts but has occasionally been associated with jitteriness, feeding difficulties and vomiting in a nursing baby.

- Antihistamines: These medications pass through breast milk in small amounts and have not been associated with problems.

We hope this information is reassuring and helpful for you during this special time. Although you may have to pay more attention to your asthma care, it is definitely worthwhile for you and your baby! As always, review your questions and concerns with your physician.

Chapter 59

Asthma and Aging

Asthma should not limit your enjoyment of life, no matter what your age. When you work with your doctor, your asthma can be controlled so that you can do the things you enjoy.

What Is Asthma?

Asthma is a disease of the lung airways. With asthma, the airways are inflamed (swollen) and react easily to certain things, like viruses, smoke, or pollen. When the inflamed airways react, they get narrow and make it hard to breathe. Common asthma symptoms are wheezing, coughing, shortness of breath, and chest tightness. When these symptoms get worse, it's an asthma attack.

Asthma symptoms may come and go, but the asthma is always there. To keep it under control, you need to work with your doctor and keep taking care of it.

Asthma and Aging

Many older adults have asthma. Some people develop it late in life. For others, it may be a continuing problem from younger years. The cause is not known.

From "Living with Asthma: Special Concerns for Older Adults," [Online] 1998. Available: http://www.nhlbi.nih.gov/health/public/lung/asthma/ asth_ap.htm. Developed by the National Asthma Education and Prevention Program (NAEPP) of the National Heart, Lung, and Blood Institute (NHLBI). For complete contact information, please refer to Chapter 68, "Resources."

Asthma in older adults presents some special concerns. For example, the normal effects of aging can make asthma harder to diagnose and treat. So can other health problems that many older adults have (like emphysema or heart disease). Also, older adults are more likely than younger people to have side effects from asthma medicines. (For example, recent studies show that older adults who take high doses of inhaled steroid medicines over a long time may increase their chance of getting glaucoma.) When some asthma and nonasthma medicines are taken by the same person, the drugs can combine to produce harmful side effects. Doctors and patients must take special care to watch out for and address these concerns through a complete diagnosis and regular checkups.

Diagnosing Asthma

If you have episodes of coughing, wheezing, shortness of breath, or chest tightness, have a complete checkup to find out what the problem is. It could be asthma or another medical problem.

Several tests may be needed to tell what is causing your symptoms. These tests include spirometry (to measure how open your airways are), a chest x-ray, an electrocardiogram (to show whether you have heart disease), and a blood test. Accurate diagnosis is important because asthma is treated differently from other diseases with similar symptoms.

Controlling Your Asthma

You can help get your asthma under control and keep it under control if you do a few simple things.

1. Talk openly with your doctor.

Say what you want to be able to do that you can't do now because of your asthma. Also, tell your doctor your concerns about your asthma, your medicines, and your health.

If you take medicine that you must inhale, be sure that you are doing it right. It must be timed with taking your breath in. And such common problems as arthritis or loss of strength may make it more difficult. Your doctor should check that you are doing it right and help you solve any problems.

It's also important to talk to your doctor about all the medicines you take—for asthma and for other problems—to be sure they will not cause harmful side effects. Be sure to mention eye drops, aspirin, and other medicines you take without a prescription. Also, tell your doctor about any symptoms you have, even if you don't think they are related to asthma. Being open with your doctor about your medicines and symptoms can help prevent problems.

Finally, be honest about any problems you may have hearing, understanding, or remembering things your doctor tells you. Ask your doctor to speak up or repeat something until you're sure of what you need to do.

2. Ask your doctor for a written treatment plan. Then be sure to follow it.

A written treatment plan will tell you when to take each of your asthma medicines and how much to take. If you have trouble reading small print, ask for your treatment plan (and other handouts) in larger type.

3. Watch for early symptoms and respond quickly.

Most asthma attacks start slowly. You can learn to tell when one is coming if you keep track of the symptoms you have, how bad they are, and when you have them. Your doctor also may want you to use a "peak flow meter," which is a small plastic tool that you blow into that measures how well you are breathing. If you respond quickly to the first signs that your asthma is getting worse, you can prevent serious asthma attacks.

4. Stay away from things that make your asthma worse.

Tobacco smoke and viruses can make asthma worse. So can other things you breathe in, such as pollen. Talk to your doctor about what makes your asthma worse and what to do about those things. Ask about getting a flu shot and a vaccine to prevent pneumonia.

5. See your doctor at least every 6 months.

You may need to go more often, especially if your asthma is not under control. Regular visits will let your doctor check your progress and, if needed, change your treatment plan. Your doctor also can check other medical problems you may have.

Bring your treatment plan and all your medicines to every checkup. Show your doctor how you take your inhaled medicines to make sure you're doing it right.

If You Need Help

If you ever feel depressed or under stress because of your asthma or other reasons, ask for help. Talking to close friends, family members, support groups, or counselors can help you feel better and help you keep your asthma under control.

Resources

For more information on asthma, contact these organizations:

National Heart, Lung, and Blood Institute Information Center
(301-592-8573)
Internet: http://www.nhlbi.nih.gov

Allergy and Asthma Network/Mothers of Asthmatics, Inc.
(800-878-4403)
Internet: http://www.aanma.org

American Academy of Allergy, Asthma, and Immunology
(800-822-ASTHMA)
Internet: http://www.aaaai.org

American College of Allergy, Asthma, and Immunology
(800-842-7777)
Internet: http://allergy.mcg.edu

American Lung Association
(800-LUNG USA)
Internet: http://www.lungusa.org

Asthma and Allergy Foundation of America
(800-7-ASTHMA)
Internet: http://www.aafa.org

National Jewish Medical and Research Center
(800-222-LUNG)
Internet: http://www.njc.org

Part Seven

Other Aids to
Wellness and Prevention

Chapter 60

Home Air Cleaners: Preventative Therapy for Asthma

James and Donna Notorfrancesco and their two children are classic examples of how cleaner indoor air can pay off with healthier days and good nights' sleep. All four have allergies and the youngest, five-year old son Christopher, has allergy-induced asthma, too.

According to his mother, Christopher is allergic to pollen, grass, and leaves outside his home, and to many things inside—everything from dust to dust mites, 12 kinds of mold, and even Christmas trees. Christopher is also very temperature-sensitive. His problems are so severe that, "Our windows are never open and we run central air from Memorial Day to Labor Day," Donna said.

They sought medical advice.

In 17 years of medical practice, first as a pediatrician and then as an allergist, Dr. William Spiegel has become convinced that controlling indoor air pollution in a home is often a key prescription for many of his allergy and asthma patients. He's seen the results pay off many times in active, healthier patients who can reduce and sometimes eliminate medication.

"If the majority of allergens that a person is sensitive to are indoor allergens, then the chance that environmental control measures can be the major modality of therapy and be very effective is good," Dr. Spiegel said.

Excerpted from "Don't Force Your Lungs to Clean Your Home's Air," in *Air Conditioning, Heating and Refrigeration News,* Vol. 199, No. 6, October 7, 1996, pp. 22-23. © 1996 by Business News Publishing Co., 755 W. Big Beaver, Ste. 1000, Troy, MI 48084. Reprinted with permission.

"For people who are mostly allergic to indoor particulates—to dust, dust mites, pet dander, and mold spores—I very often will use only environmental measures, or initially use a majority of environmental measures and a little medication to see how they do. And many people do well with just that."

Getting a high-efficiency air cleaner is one simple control measure. Dr. Spiegel said he and the other physicians at Allergy and Asthma Specialists, P.C., always discuss this with appropriate patients at the firm's six offices in Philadelphia and its tri-county suburbs.

"I'm a big proponent of air cleaners. When the windows are shut in a house that does not have an air cleaner, the only air filter you really have is . . . your nose and lungs," Dr. Spiegel said. "I'd rather you not breathe those particles if they're going to make you suffer."

He said he almost always recommends a whole-house electronic air cleaner for homes that have forced-air heating and cooling. He recommends the use of a portable air cleaner with a high-efficiency particulate arrestance (HEPA) filter in homes without forced-air circulation.

In homes with a cat, he recommends both a whole-house air cleaner and a portable HEPA air cleaner because cat dander can be so troublesome.

In recent years, three different allergists in three cities, including Dr. Spiegel, gave the Notorfrancescos the same advice when they moved into new homes: Find a good heating and air conditioning dealer, get a high-efficiency whole-house air cleaner, and control the humidity inside to prevent mold and mildew.

They moved into their latest home, in Hockessin, Del., just before Thanksgiving, 1995. It did not have a whole-house air cleaner. Within days, the three oldest family members were stuffy and congested. But Christopher—despite being on four potent medications—was so sick that his parents spent 10 consecutive nights staying up watching over him.

At that point Donna Notorfrancesco, tired and worried, wanted an immediate house call—not from a doctor, but from Tom D'Andrea, president of Boothwyn Heating and Air Conditioning in nearby Newark.

"They needed a whole-house air cleaner and central humidifier," D'Andrea said. "They needed a service indicator to tell them when the air cleaner's cells need to be cleaned. They also needed an energy-efficient way to keep air circulating through the whole-house air cleaner even if the furnace or air conditioner was not running."

And because Christopher is so temperature-sensitive, the Notorfrancescos also needed an accurate thermostat, one that could automatically switch from heating to cooling.

514

Until recently, all those additions would have left the family with five separate controls on the wall—and a steep learning curve to memorize how to use them. D'Andrea solved that problem by installing a new automated, all-in-one temperature and indoor air quality control system, Honeywell's Perfect Climate Comfort Center.

The system, about the size of an ordinary thermostat, includes an advanced programmable thermostat, an accurate electronic humidity control for homes, an air filter-air cleaner service indicator, programmable ventilation system control, and programmable fan control.

The Notorfrancescos also ordered the Comfort Center's optional outdoor sensor. It lets them make sure the temperature outside is within Christopher's safety zone before they let him go outside to play. Within days of having the whole-house air cleaner and control system installed, the entire family was breathing easier and sleeping better. More importantly, Christopher's health improved to the point that his medication could be cut in half on all but his worst days.

"If you read articles on children with asthma and allergies, they all recommend having an air cleaner." Donna said. And, after her latest experience, "I don't think we would ever again not have this system in a house.

Dr. Spiegel has blunt advice for people who think their health or comfort may be affected by indoor air pollution. "Preventive therapy is a heck of a lot better than waiting till you're sick," he said. "My point is that indoor environmental control strategies should be instituted as soon as you know that there are allergies, if not before."

Chapter 61

Vitamin Supplements: Aid for Asthmatics against Air Pollution

Simply taking antioxidant vitamins could help asthmatics exposed to polluted air breathe easier.

Preliminary results of a double blind study indicate that adults with asthma who took daily supplements of both vitamins E and C showed improved pulmonary function, compared to when they took a placebo, after being exposed to two common air pollutants, ozone and sulfur dioxide.

Ozone is formed from precursors in automobile exhaust, while sulfur dioxide is emitted from pulp mills, coal burning, and other industrial processes.

"Our results show that a combination of antioxidant vitamins can benefit people with asthma who are sensitive to air pollutants," said lead author Dr. Carol Trenga, who conducted the study while completing doctoral research at the University of Washington School of Public Health and Community Medicine. Coauthor of the study is Dr. Jane Koenig, an international expert on the respiratory health effects of air pollution.

From "Vitamin Supplements May Help Asthmatics Cope with Air Pollution," [Online] May 20, 1997. Available: http://www-camra.ucdavis.edu/vitasthma.html. Produced by the Center for Complementary and Alternative Medicine Research in Asthma, Allergies and Immunology, University of California, Davis. Reprinted with permission. For complete contact information, please refer to Chapter 68, "Resources."

Trenga presented her preliminary findings on Tuesday, May 20, [1997] at the American Lung Association/American Thoracic Society International Conference.

The study monitored pulmonary function in 17 asthmatic volunteers, who took a daily course of vitamins E and C (400 I.U. and 500 mg., respectively) and a daily course of placebo for separate five-week periods. Near the end of each course, participants received separate, 45-minute exposures to purified air and ozone at the current National Ambient Air Quality Standard (0.12 p.p. million). To measure effects of ozone exposure, volunteers then were exposed to two 10-minute sulfur dioxide challenges.

Test results showed an overall decrease in sensitivity to ozone exposure when volunteers took vitamins as compared to placebo. Improvements in pulmonary function were especially dramatic in a subset of six volunteers. While on vitamin supplementation, this group had a 5 percent increase in peak expiratory flow during the sulfur dioxide challenges after ozone exposure compared to a 13 percent decrease in peak expiratory flow for the same period while on placebo. These volunteers were previously identified as more sensitive to sulfur dioxide.

Trenga explains vitamins E, which is fat soluble, and C, which is water soluble, complement one another, helping increase the potential to reduce oxidative damage in the lungs. When polluted air comes in contact with the lung lining fluid, vitamin C is part of the body's first line of defense, serving to reduce both ozone and free radicals formed by ozone exposure. Vitamin E helps reduce lipid radicals and can be regenerated by vitamin C.

People with asthma may not be the only ones who could benefit from antioxidant vitamin supplements. Increases in daily vitamin intake may also benefit others exposed to chronic oxidative stress— such as smokers or industrial workers, Trenga said.

She adds that future research should focus on linkages between nutritional factors and toxicity and disease. This would include investigating whether regular antioxidant vitamin intake could ultimately reduce the need for medication or frequency of use among people with asthma.

Chapter 62

Vitamin C's Role in Controlling Asthma

Some 800 years ago, the philosopher Maimonides said people with asthma should eat a diet rich in fruits and vegetables—the major food sources of vitamin C. And in the early 1800s, a scientist named F.D. Reisseissen noted that people with scurvy, a disease of vitamin C deficiency, suffered asthmatic symptoms that improved when vitamin C-containing items were added to their diets. Now researchers are finding scientific backing for the centuries-old advice.

Consider that asthma can develop when the lungs are weakened by contaminants in environmental pollutants such as dirty air, cigarette smoke, and the like. Called oxidants, these contaminants not only contribute to the development of asthma but also bring on the symptoms of asthma attacks once someone becomes asthmatic: wheezing, chest tightness, coughing, and gasping for air.

Vitamin C, on the other hand, is an antioxidant that keeps oxidants from doing damage. And it happens to be the most abundant antioxidant nutrient in the lungs' inner lining. Thus, scientists suspect, the more vitamin C we consume, the more we have on hand to squelch the contaminants that make their way to the lungs.

Research corroborates the theory. As vitamin C intake goes up, the risk for asthma and other respiratory diseases appears to go down. Furthermore, out of 11 studies conducted since 1973, seven showed

From "Vitamin C for Warding off Asthma?" in *Tufts University Diet & Nutrition Letter,* Vol. 13, No. 12, February 1996, p. 3. © 1996 by *Tufts University Diet and Nutrition Letter,* 50 Broadway, 15th Fl., New York, NY 10004. Reprinted with permission.

improved breathing in people with asthma who received vitamin C supplements. Other scientific work has shown 35 percent lower concentrations of vitamin C in the liquid part of asthmatics' blood than in the blood of nonsmokers and 50 percent less vitamin C in asthmatics' white blood cells.

To Supplement with C or Not

It's too early in the research game to say that people should take vitamin C supplements to ward off asthma or lessen its severity. However, Gary Hatch, Ph.D., a lung researcher at the Environmental Protection Agency, does believe that eating more vitamin C-rich foods may be in order and that, in fact, the Recommended Dietary Allowance for that nutrient—60 milligrams for adults—could be much too low.

Fortunately, it's easy to consume much more than 60 milligrams of vitamin C. One orange, a third of a cup of chopped sweet red pepper, six ounces of grapefruit juice, and one kiwifruit each have more than 60 milligrams. Other good sources include broccoli, strawberries, Brussels sprouts, tomato juice, and cauliflower.

Asthma Sufferers Top the 12 Million Mark

More than 12 Million Americans are believed to suffer from asthma, making it the seventh-ranking chronic condition in the nation and the leading serious chronic illness among children. It is also responsible for about 5,000 deaths a year. Unfortunately, between 1982 and 1992, the estimated total number of asthma cases increased by more than 57 percent, according to the American Lung Association.

While genetics plays a part in who develops asthma, children of smokers are twice as likely to suffer from the disease as children of nonsmokers. And, contrary to popular belief, they don't usually "outgrow" the condition. Only about one in four asthmatic children become asthma-free adults.

The basic symptom of an asthma attack—difficulty breathing when air flow into and out of the lungs is blocked—occurs for three reasons: cells in the air passages secrete excess mucus that is both thick and sticky; the air tubes themselves begin to swell; and the muscles that control and direct air flow tighten. All of these events narrow the passages through which air travels, causing the wheezing, coughing, shortness of breath, and tightness in the chest that accompany labored breathing.

The good news is that asthma sufferers can often prevent attacks by avoiding their "triggers." For some people the triggers are cold air or vigorous exercise without short rests to break up the activity. For others, dust, bad air-quality days, cigarette smoke, animal dander, or stress triggers asthma.

There are two types of drugs to control the condition. One, bronchodilators, helps stop attacks once they've begun by relaxing the muscles in the air tubes. The other, anti-inflammatories, helps prevent attacks from starting in the first place, both by reducing the swelling of the air tubes and by decreasing mucus.

For more information about asthma and how to control it, call the American Lung Association at 1-800-LUNG-USA (586-4872).

Chapter 63

Who Should Get the Flu Vaccine

Though flu is expected to make its usual rounds this winter, many Americans won't have to suffer its high fever, characteristic cough, and possibly serious complications. A safe, effective vaccine is available.

It was not always so.

In 1918-1919—during the worst flu epidemic of all time—doctors had meager resources to fight the disease. To relieve symptoms, they relied on aspirin and other simple remedies. An influenza vaccine and antibiotics to combat pneumonia and other flu complications were years away from development. It has been estimated that over 20 million people died and possibly half the world's population came down with the flu in this global epidemic, or pandemic.

Influenza epidemics spread quickly through large populations because flu viruses are highly contagious. During flu's acute phase, respiratory tract secretions are rich in infectious virus and the disease is transmitted easily by sneezing and coughing. The incubation period lasts one to three days. Then symptoms—such as chills and fever that develop within 24 hours, headache often accompanied by sensitivity to light, sore muscles, backache, weakness, and fatigue—appear suddenly. Respiratory tract symptoms may be mild at first with a dry, unproductive cough, scratchy sore throat, and runny nose. As the person's temperature rises—sometimes to as high as 104 degrees

Excerpted from "How to Avoid the Flu," by Evelyn Zamula, in *FDA Consumer,* [Online] November 1994. Available: http://www.fda.gov. Produced by the U.S. Food and Drug Administration (FDA). For complete contact information, please refer to Chapter 68, "Resources."

Fahrenheit—the muscle aches and headache get worse, and secondary bacterial infections, such as bronchitis and pneumonia, may move in. Ear infections are a common complication in children.

With no complications, acute symptoms usually subside after two or three days and the fever ends, although it may last as long as five days. Weakness and fatigue may persist for several weeks.

Vaccine Most Important Defense

Today, we have several ways to defend people from influenza. The most important tool is immunization by a killed virus vaccine. Flu vaccines are licensed by FDA, and the exact composition of the vaccine varies each year, depending on the flu strains scientists expect to be most common.

Influenza viruses have the ability to change themselves, or mutate, thereby becoming different viruses. Having the flu once does not confer lasting immunity, as is the case with some childhood viral diseases. The antibodies people produce in response to the one flu virus don't recognize and, therefore, don't provide immunity to a different flu virus. Because the immunity conferred by a flu shot lasts for only about a year—and because different flu strains may circulate each season—individuals who want to be protected from flu should be vaccinated annually.

It takes two to four weeks for antibodies to develop after the vaccine is given. Therefore, the ideal time to get the flu vaccine is mid-October to mid-November, before the start of the flu season, which lasts from about December to March in the Northern Hemisphere. (Travelers should be aware that flu season lasts all year in some tropical climates, and in the Southern Hemisphere occurs from April to September.)

Who Should Get the Vaccine?

Vaccination is available to anyone who wants it and whose doctor agrees it would be beneficial. The Public Health Service's Advisory Committee on Immunization Practices (ACIP) strongly recommends vaccination for:

- People age 65 or older. (Effective May 1993, Medicare Part B pays for flu shots.)

- People over 6 months who have underlying medical conditions that put them at increased risk for flu complications. These include:

1. Chronic cardiovascular disorders or lung disease, including asthma in children.

2. Chronic metabolic diseases requiring hospitalization during the preceding year or regular checkups. These diseases include diabetes, kidney disorders, blood disorders, and impaired immune systems due to HIV infection or chemotherapy.

3. Residents of nursing homes and other facilities that provide care for chronically ill persons of any age.

4. Children and teenagers (6 months to 18 years of age) who have to take aspirin regularly and therefore may be at risk of developing Reye's syndrome after influenza. (Children who have symptoms of flu or chickenpox should not be given products containing aspirin or other salicylates without consulting a doctor.)

To reduce the risk of transmitting flu to high-risk persons, such as the elderly, transplant patients, and people with AIDS (who may have low antibody response to the flu vaccine)—and also to protect themselves from infection—ACIP recommends vaccination for doctors, nurses, hospital employees, employees of nursing homes and chronic-care facilities, visiting nurses, and home care providers. Students, police, firefighters, and other essential workers and community service providers may also find vaccination useful.

In most cases, children at high risk for influenza complications may receive the flu vaccine when they receive other routine vaccinations, including DTP (diphtheria, tetanus, and pertussis) and pneumococcal vaccines. Pregnant women who have a high-risk condition should be immunized regardless of the stage of pregnancy; healthy pregnant women may also want to consult their health care providers about being vaccinated.

Side Effects

The flu vaccine cannot cause flu because it contains only inactivated viruses. Any respiratory disease that appears immediately after vaccination is coincidental. However, the vaccine may have some side effects, especially in children who have not been exposed to the flu virus in the past.

The most commonly reported side effect in children and adults is soreness at the vaccination site that lasts up to two days. Fever, malaise, sore muscles, and other symptoms may begin 6 to 12 hours after vaccination and may last as long as two days.

People should be aware that they may test HIV-positive with the ELISA test after a recent flu shot, says the national Centers for Disease Control and Prevention. CDC recommends retesting with the more accurate Western Blot test to rule out false positives.

The vaccine is not for everyone. People allergic to eggs—the vaccine is made from highly purified, egg-grown viruses that have been made noninfectious—or other vaccine components should consult a doctor before getting a flu shot because they may develop hives, allergic asthma, difficulty breathing, and other allergic symptoms. The vaccine should not be given to any person ill with a high fever until the fever and other symptoms have abated.

Drugs Help Some People

For these individuals, and persons expected to develop low levels of antibodies in response to the influenza vaccine because they have impaired immune systems, influenza-specific anti-viral drugs can be used for prevention during the flu season or after infection to relieve influenza symptoms.

The anti-viral agents Symmetrel (amantadine), approved by FDA in 1976, and Flumadine (rimantadine), a chemically similar drug approved by FDA in September 1993, are safe and effective in preventing signs and symptoms of infection caused by various strains of the influenza A virus in children over 1, healthy adults, and elderly patients. These drugs may also be used for family members or close contacts of influenza A patients and for elderly nursing home patients who have been vaccinated but may need added protection. When a vaccine is expected to be ineffective because an epidemic is caused by strains other than those covered by the vaccine, anti-viral drugs may be used to provide protection against infection.

Either drug may be used following vaccination during a flu epidemic to provide protection during the two- to four-week period before antibodies develop. If an adult has already come down with the flu, treatment with Symmetrel or Flumadine has been shown to reduce symptoms and shorten the illness if administered within 48 hours after symptoms appear. Children with the flu can be treated with Symmetrel

About 5 to 10 percent of people who take Symmetrel experience nausea, dizziness, and insomnia. There have been reports of more serious neurological adverse events, including seizures and aggravations

526

of psychiatric illnesses. Flumadine has similar side effects, but at a lower rate.

Though many flu victims use over-the-counter preparations, such as decongestants and fever reducers, to make them feel more comfortable, none of these products affects the course of the disease.

Prevention Worthwhile

Every year, about 20 percent of the U.S. population may become infected with flu, although each flu season is different. About 1 percent of those infected will require hospitalization because of complications, mostly bacterial pneumonia. Among those hospitalized, as many as 8 percent may die—about 20,000 people in an average year. But the 1957-1958 "Asian flu" caused 70,000 deaths, and the 1968-1969 "Hong Kong flu" carried off 34,000 persons. The toll is usually greatest among the elderly.

The economic costs run high, too. From 15 million to 111 million workdays are lost each year, depending on the severity of the epidemic. Added to that are the costs of over-the-counter and prescription medicines, physician visits, hospitalization, and lost productivity.

It's no contest between the cost of a flu shot and the physical and other costs exacted by a bad case of the flu. A yearly vaccination early in the flu season is the best way to avoid this miserable disease.

Formulating the Vaccine

FDA's Vaccines and Related Biologicals Advisory Committee meets in late January each year to decide which strains of influenza virus should be incorporated into the vaccine for the coming flu season, based on reports from national and international surveillance systems. A World Health Organization panel meets in Geneva in mid-February to make final recommendations for the next season's flu vaccine.

The vaccine choices for the United States take into consideration the predominant strain(s) circulating among the population in the current season (November, December, January) and any "new" strains that may have appeared both here and in other parts of the world. Another important part of the decision process is the examination of antibody levels in people vaccinated with the current year's vaccine to determine if they had a good immune response. Equally important is examining antibody levels in the same people to see if the vaccine offered any protection against recently identified "new" strains.

"You have to make this decision [about which strains to include in the vaccine] a year in advance before the flu season starts," says Helen Regnery, Ph.D., chief, strain surveillance section, influenza branch, national Centers for Disease Control and Prevention. "There is an inherent problem; FDA's advisory committee must decide for a future event, based on past and current knowledge of circulating strains, as well as the appearance of new strains of influenza."

Flu viruses are divided into three types—A, B, and C—though the C type is not common. Influenza A viruses cause the most severe and widespread outbreaks, while influenza B causes limited, milder illness.

Influenza A viruses are classified into subtypes on the basis of two surface antigens (substances that induce antibody formation) called hemagglutinin (H) and neuraminidase (N). Currently, the circulating subtypes of influenza A that have been identified as causing extensive human illness are influenza A (H3N2) and influenza A (H1N1). Influenza A (H3N2) viruses have been much more prevalent than influenza A (H1N1) during the last five years.

"Last year's flu season [1993-1994] was more severe than average," says Nancy Arden, chief, influenza epidemiology, CDC. "More than 99 percent of the influenza viruses isolated and characterized were type A(H3N2) and most were similar to the A/Beijing/32/92 strain. Although people of all ages are susceptible to type A(H3N2), compared with influenza type A (H1N1) and type B, the A(H3N2) viruses are associated with more illness, complications, and deaths among the elderly."

—by Evelyn Zamula

Evelyn Zamula is a free-lance writer in Potomac, Md.

Chapter 64

Estrogen Fluctuation and Asthma Severity

A new study suggests a strong relationship between phases of the menstrual cycle and asthma attacks requiring emergency treatment.[1] According to the data, a fall in estradiol levels may cause as much as a fourfold increase in the frequency of severe asthma attacks. The results also provide a reminder that a patient's gender may have profound effects on the presentation of disease and responses to treatment.

"I'm optimistic that manipulating estrogen levels during the last third of the menstrual cycle may really help women who have perimenstrual exacerbations of asthma," says principal investigator Emil M. Skobeloff, M.D. "But until we have strong clinical data to support this approach, I don't want to do anything that might increase women's risk of breast or endometrial cancer," he adds.

The investigators enrolled 182 women, 13-47 years (mean age, 28.5 years), who presented to an urban emergency department (ED) because of an asthma attack. All had regular menstrual cycles, and none were pregnant, had reached menopause, had undergone hysterectomy, or were taking oral contraceptives or other hormone replacement therapy. None had evidence of pulmonary embolism, congestive heart failure, or pneumonia.

From "Asthma in the ED: The Effect of Menstrual Phase," by Mary Desmond Pinkowish, in *Patient Care,* Vol. 30, No. 17, October 30, 1996, pp. 4-5. © 1996 by Medical Economics Publishing Co., Five Paragon Dr., Montvale, NJ 07645-1742. Reprinted with permission.

Based on the date of the last menstrual period (day 1 of the menstrual cycle), participants were assigned to one of four groups: preovulatory (days 5-11 of the cycle); periovulatory (days 12-18); postovulatory (days 19-25); or perimenstrual (days 26-4).

This division of the menstrual cycle corresponds to fluctuations in serum estradiol levels, which peak in the periovulatory phase, decrease, rise again in the postovulatory phase, and remain elevated for about seven days. Levels then drop quickly during the perimenstrual phase. Estradiol levels were not measured in the women in this study, however. To ensure that usual asthma treatment routines were followed, the ED physicians—all of whom were emergency medicine faculty members—did not know the purpose of the study.

Most of the patients (81%) were discharged after treatment in the ED. Overall, 20% of the participants were in the preovulatory phase of the menstrual cycle at presentation, 24% were in the periovulatory phase, 10% were in the postovulatory phase, and 46% were in the perimenstrual phase. This difference between the perimenstrual phase and the other phases was statistically significant.

Although an asthma attack requiring emergency treatment was more likely to occur during the perimenstrual phase than during other times of the cycle, the severity of attacks did not differ significantly according to menstrual cycle phase. The only difference was that corticosteroids were used least frequently among women who presented during the postovulatory phase.

Investigators believe that physicians should wait for further data before changing the way they treat women with asthma. "But some women clearly have terrible perimenstrual asthma," says Robert Silverman, M.D., a coinvestigator and Director of Research, Department of Emergency Medicine Long Island Jewish Medical Center, New Hyde Park, N.Y. He adds that some women may not have noticed a correlation between periodic worsening of asthma and menstrual phase, and it may be worthwhile for patients to use a peak flowmeter and keep an asthma and menstrual diary to see if a connection exists.

"These women may benefit from higher doses or more frequent use of inhaled corticosteroids during the few days before the onset of menstruation. Some may even be able to have medication holidays during the remainder of their cycles," says Dr. Silverman.

Although some studies have suggested an association between menstrual phases and worsening of asthma, these have been small and retrospective in design. Several years ago, Dr. Skobeloff, who is Clinical Assistant Professor of Emergency Medicine at Allegheny

University of the Health Sciences, Philadelphia, and Attending Emergency Physician, Crozer-Chester Medical Center, Upland, Pa., demonstrated that female asthma admissions outnumber male admissions by 3 to 1. His studies of estradiol dynamics in normal and asthmatic rabbits—in which the bronchospastic response was heightened when estradiol levels fluctuated—led to the current study.

The most intriguing aspect of these findings may be broader than the implications for asthma. The investigators state, "We are suggesting a novel concept not only in the consideration of asthma in adult women but also possibly in the evaluation of women's disease in general."

Reference

1. Skobeloff EM, Spivey WH, Silverman R, et al: The effect of the menstrual cycle on asthma presentations in the emergency department. *Arch Intern Med* 1996; 156:1637-1640.

Chapter 65

Breathing Method Reduces Asthma Attacks

Many people with asthma aren't able to detect a problem with their breathing until the asthma attack becomes severe. But a new training method developed by researchers at Ohio University could one day help asthma patients detect an attack as early as 30 minutes before its onset.

Self-management of asthma includes the ability to detect resistance to air flow that is caused by constricted air passages. But research suggests that many people with asthma are unable to detect this breathing difficulty in time to stop the attack.

Researchers at Ohio University have developed a training method that helps asthma patients improve their perception of air flow resistance. In a study of 45 asthma patients who took part in the training, researchers found that participants had fewer asthma attacks because they detected the problems earlier and took medication before the onset of an attack.

"Breathing is so natural to us, we do it without thinking, and that's true for asthma patients as well," said Harry Kotses, professor of psychology at Ohio University and coauthor of the study. "If people with asthma can learn to be sensitive to changes in resistance to air flow,

From "New Training Method Helps Reduce Asthma Attacks," [Online] September 3, 1997. Available: http://www-camra.ucdavis.edu/trainasthma.html. Produced by the Center for Complementary and Alternative Medicine Research in Asthma, Allergies and Immunology, University of California, Davis. Reprinted with permission. For complete contact information, please refer to Chapter 68, "Resources."

they might be able to detect the early stages of an asthma attack and stop it before serious breathing difficulty occurs."

Asthma, the most common chronic childhood illness, affects nearly 15 million Americans, 5 million of whom are under the age of 19. According to the Centers for Disease Control and Prevention, asthma accounted for an estimated 198,000 hospitalizations and 342 deaths in 1993.

During an asthma attack, air flow into and out of the lungs is restricted by inflammation and swelling of the bronchial tubes and by bronchial narrowing caused by smooth muscle contraction.

An attack can be triggered by exercise, infection, respiratory irritants, stress, or an allergy to things such as pollen, dust mites, or animal dander. The illness usually is controlled by steroids that reduce inflammation of tissues in the airway, by bronchial dilators that relax constricted muscles, or both.

Because an asthma attack is costly to the patient in terms of health risk and hospital cost, physicians emphasize prevention through self-management. An attack can happen any time, Kotses said, and it's important that asthma patients learn to judge the illness' warning signs and take preventative measures early.

For the study, researchers interviewed 20 men and 25 women ages 18 to 24, all Ohio University undergraduate students. Each had been diagnosed with asthma by a physician and used prescribed medication for the illness.

Before undergoing training, study participants were interviewed about the frequency and severity of their asthma attacks. Sixteen had at least four asthma attacks a month, 20 had two or three attacks a month and nine had fewer attacks.

During the study, asthma patients were asked to breath through nylon mesh screens. Each screen had a different weave—some allowed for greater resistance to air flow and some for less resistance. Participants judged the level of difficulty they experienced while breathing through each of the screens.

At the beginning of the study, some participants said that widely woven screens caused more air flow resistance than those more tightly woven, which added support to theories that asthma patients are unable to determine air flow resistance accurately. But by the end of the study, most participants were able to identify correctly those screens that presented the most problems.

"It is possible that change in air flow obstruction associated with asthma occurs so gradually that it goes unnoticed until it is severe," Kotses said. "But the wide range we observed in ability to predict asthma suggests this is not the case. Some of our subjects reported ability to forecast occurrence of asthma by 30 minutes or more. A primary benefit of perception training may be that it increases the length of the warning period a patient has prior to the onset of an attack."

Although self-management of asthma has been part of asthma control for many years, the idea of adding perception training is new, Kotses said. Many of the study participants reported that breathing through the different mesh screens was very similar to an actual asthma attack, which suggests this method may be useful in a perception training program.

"The fact that our subjects were able to detect the onset of an attack earlier than before is very promising, but now we want to study the method using a larger group of asthma patients and examining them over a longer period of time," Kotses said.

The study, published in a recent issue of the *Journal of Psychosomatic Medicine,* was coauthored by Thomas Creer, a former professor of psychology who retired in 1996, and Cynthia Stout, a former psychology graduate student, both from Ohio University.

Chapter 66

Exercise for Asthma Patients

In Brief: The standard exercise recommendation—20 to 30 minutes at 60% to 85% of maximum heart rate four or five times a week—should be part of asthma management. Not only will patients benefit in a general way, but improved fitness is likely to reduce airway reactivity and medication use. The capacity to exercise, however, requires good general control of asthma, including use of inhaled corticosteroids and avoidance of triggers. In addition, patients must be taught to prevent exercise-induced bronchoconstriction by using inhaled medications and strategies like avoiding cold-weather exercise.

Not so many years ago, to prescribe exercise for people with asthma would have been regarded as imprudent, if not irresponsible. Strenuous physical activity can trigger bronchospasm, cause an attack, and put the asthma patient at risk, the reasoning went. Patients were routinely counseled to play it safe and avoid exertion.

But the thinking about asthma and its management has changed dramatically in recent years. It is now universally recognized that chronic asthma, which affects 14 million to 15 million Americans[1], is fundamentally a disease of airway inflammation, and that with appropriate focus on that component, symptoms can be effectively controlled in nearly all cases.

From "Exercise for Asthma Patients: Little Risk, Big Rewards," by Vincent Disabella, D.O., with Carl Sherman, in *The Physician and Sportsmedicine,* Vol. 26, No.6 [Online] June 1998. Available: http://www.physsportsmed.com/issues/1998/06jun/disabell.htm. © 1998 by The McGraw-Hill Companies, c/o *The Physician and Sportsmedicine,* 4530 W. 77th St., Minneapolis, MN 55435. All rights reserved. Reprinted with permission.

How Exercise Helps

With the management modalities currently available, virtually all asthma sufferers not only can but should exercise. They stand to reap the same benefits as others from regular physical activity through a reduced risk of cardiovascular disease, diabetes, and other health problems. In addition, some studies have found that exercise can improve the course of the disease itself. Reductions in airway responsiveness have been shown in patients who followed aerobic exercise programs[2]. Some research[3] also suggests that asthma sufferers who exercise regularly have fewer exacerbations, use less medication, and miss less time from school and work.

When they are physically fit and free from significant airway obstruction, people who have asthma respond to exercise very much like others, and their maximal heart rate, ventilation, blood pressure, and work capacity fall within the normal range[4]. Sedentary asthma sufferers, on the other hand, produce more lactate and are more subject to acidosis than unfit individuals without asthma who undertake similar physical exertion[5].

It is unfortunate, then, that asthma sufferers tend to be inactive and deconditioned[6]. The reasons for this most likely have more to do with fear, misinformation, and inadequate management than with intrinsic limitations imposed by the disease. That things could be otherwise is suggested by the substantial numbers of active children and adults, recreational athletes, and even elite athletes whose exertions are not deterred by their disease. In the 1984 Olympics, for example, 26 of 597 athletes had a documented history of chronic asthma[7].

There is abundant evidence that when asthma is untreated, tolerance for even mild activity is curtailed, but with effective management even patients who have fairly severe asthma are able to exercise and, in many cases, participate in competitive sports[8]. One essential means to this end is a protocol that keeps asthma generally under control, with an emphasis on anti-inflammatories, other medications when needed, and environmental interventions as described below. The other is treatment targeted specifically to patients who experience exercise-induced asthma (EIA).

Exercise as Trigger

Exercise is one of the well-known triggers of bronchoconstriction. Almost all individuals who have chronic asthma will have symptoms when they exercise at a sufficient intensity[9], and many people with no other asthma symptoms experience EIA.

Symptoms may be obviously pulmonary—chest tightness, shortness of breath, coughing—but for many patients they take the form of stomachache, chest pain, or nausea[10]. EIA symptoms typically appear after 8 to 10 minutes of vigorous exercise and may worsen after activity is terminated. Episodes usually remit completely within 30 to 60 minutes and do not increase airway reactivity or induce long-term deterioration in lung function. Whether EIA induces a late-phase reaction 4 or more hours after the initial episode in some patients is a matter of controversy[11].

One interesting feature of EIA is the occurrence in about half of individuals of a "refractory" period: If exercise is repeated within 1 hour of the first bout, bronchial narrowing recurs but is less severe than the previous episode. Within this period it may be possible to exercise longer and more strenuously without difficulty[12].

Although the exact mechanism of EIA is obscure, most investigators believe that changes in temperature and moisture levels within the airway are responsible. Airway temperature falls as respiration increases during exertion, then rises rapidly when exercise ends—a process that appears to eventuate in bronchial narrowing. Rapid breathing may increase evaporation of water from the surface of the bronchial mucosa, leading to mast-cell degranulation and smooth-muscle contraction[13].

These observations have useful clinical implications: Because EIA is usually less of a problem when patients exercise in warm, moist air [rather] than in cold, dry air, patients may be counseled to exercise indoors in cold weather, or to adopt strategies like covering the mouth and nose with a scarf to reduce airway temperature fluctuations when exercising outdoors. It may be helpful to induce a refractory period by timing strenuous exercise to begin after a warm-up and an interval of rest.

But even with intelligent precautions, most asthma patients need pharmacotherapy to prevent EIA. Pretreatment with inhaled beta-adrenergic agonists, generally considered the drugs of choice for this purpose, will reduce or eliminate symptoms in about 90% of patients[14], but other agents may need to be added or substituted in resistant cases. Studies have shown that the use of long-acting beta-2-agonists such as salmeterol xinafoate have protective effects against EIA, especially when used with concomitant inhaled glucocorticoid therapy. The use of salmeterol only once daily to prevent tolerance has been shown to be effective in minimizing the symptoms of EIA[15]. The use of long-acting beta-2-agonists has also been shown to improve the symptoms of nocturnal asthma[16].

While improved fitness does not abolish EIA, it has a positive impact on it. Whatever the mechanism, increased ventilation appears to be the EIA trigger; fit individuals use oxygen more efficiently and need to move less air at a given level of exercise intensity.

Untreated EIA is a potent barrier to exercise, but with proper management it need not be a limiting factor. A study[17] of 31 children who had asthma found no correlation between cardiovascular fitness and EIA: Even many in whom EIA (when assessed without preexercise medication) was severe were capable of achieving normal fitness. The same study attested to the efficacy of good general asthma management: The 12 children who regularly received inhaled corticosteroids had significantly less severe symptoms than the other children, which "confirms the importance of inhaled steroids in the prevention of exercise-induced asthma," the authors concluded.

Managing Chronic Asthma

Inhaled medications. Both for the general control of asthma and to enhance the capacity for exercise, daily anti-inflammatory therapy has emerged as the keystone. As recommended in the revised guidelines for asthma diagnosis and management issued last year by the National Heart, Lung, and Blood Institute (NHLBI)[1], I almost always prescribe an inhaled corticosteroid as first-line therapy for my patients of any age who have persistent asthma.

One of the new additions to the asthma armamentarium, the leukotriene modifiers zafirlukast and zileuton, may replace inhaled corticosteroids in selected cases. These drugs show great promise for treating patients who have known allergic triggers of their asthma exacerbations. Epidemiologic studies suggest that inhalation of environmental allergens is the most important cause of asthma. Leukotrienes also play a very important role in aspirin-induced asthma[18].

Cromolyn sodium or nedocromil sodium is an alternative for patients who have persistent problems with corticosteroids (i.e., oral candidiasis), or these drugs may be added to the regimen. The addition of these drugs should be entertained in patients who suffer from allergies or for whom inhaled glucocorticoid or beta-2-agonist therapy is failing.

Beta-agonists are no longer considered first-line drugs for chronic treatment, although a long-acting agent of this class (salmeterol) may be added for moderate to severe asthma that does not respond adequately to other drugs. A study by Pauwels, et al.,[19] shows that the use of long-acting beta-2-agonists increased lung function, decreased symptoms, and decreased the need for beta-2-agonist rescue therapy in patients on inhaled glucocorticoid therapy. Short-acting beta-agonists (albuterol and terbutaline sulfate) are still recommended as "rescue treatment" for rapid relief of acute symptoms.

Patient education is essential in asthma management, particularly when inhaled corticosteroids are used. Patients should be carefully instructed in inhaler technique, including the use of a spacer to optimize deposition and to prevent oral candidiasis. To this end, patients should also be taught to rinse their mouths with water or an antimicrobial mouthwash after each application of inhaled steroids.

Oral medications. I reserve oral corticosteroids for severe asthma exacerbations and withdraw them as soon as acceptable control has been reestablished. In the absence of other conditions contributing to airway obstruction (such as emphysema or lupus erythematosus), asthma patients should not need long-term systemic corticosteroids.

Allergy control. Allergy is a factor in most cases of asthma, so all patients should be tested to identify triggers. The following actions should be taken, as needed, to minimize exacerbating conditions:

- When sensitivity has been documented, take steps to reduce exposure to dust mites: Have carpets cleaned professionally and often, encase mattresses and pillows in plastic, and wash sheets and blankets weekly in very hot water;

- Keep indoor humidity below 50% to reduce exposure to mold as well as dust mites;

- Use poison bait, traps, and careful housekeeping to minimize cockroaches, often a problematic antigen;

- Ideally, because animal dander is a frequent trigger, remove pets from the house, or at least keep them out of the room where the patient sleeps; and

- Avoid, to the extent possible, exposure to nonspecific irritants such as tobacco smoke, wood smoke, air pollution, and cleaning agents.

When the allergic component of asthma is prominent, I often prescribe a second-generation nonsedating antihistamine or inhaled ipratropium bromide for use on a regular basis. Immunotherapy (allergy shots) may be indicated for patients whose allergies are due to known triggers and cannot be controlled by avoidance, antihistamines, and inhaled steroids.

Testing. The importance of testing in asthma control is emphasized in the NHLBI guidelines[1]; office spirometry is recommended when the disease is first diagnosed, when peak expiratory flow has stabilized, and every 1 to 2 years thereafter. Patients who have moderate to severe asthma should be taught to monitor their own peak flow daily and take preventive measures when a decline heralds an imminent attack.

The Exercise Prescription

Preexercise assessment. In addition to testing for asthma control, testing is also important before beginning an exercise program. A patient's asthma should be well controlled as indicated by both peak flow monitoring and a 1-second forced expiratory volume (FEV1) at or above 80% of expected levels. For middle-aged and older patients who have been inactive, stress testing to assess cardiovascular fitness is also indicated.

Exercise goals. The exercise goal for people who have asthma, as for most people, should be 20 to 30 minutes of activity that raises heart rate to 60% to 85% of maximum, four or five times a week. To the extent possible, I try not to discourage patients from any exercise they find congenial. Still, they should know that they are less likely to encounter difficulties if they make sensible modifications of their exercise practices, such as running indoors when the weather is cold or air pollution is high.

Cautions. Patients should be counseled to skip their exercise sessions on days when they are wheezing, when allergies are particularly troubling, or when peak flow testing suggests a decline in lung function. The importance of using a hand-held peak flow meter to assess airway hypersensitivity and determine the potential for a difficult day should be made clear to patients who have moderate to severe asthma.

I also emphasize the importance of inducing a refractory period. This can be accomplished by various methods, including 20 to 30 minutes of low-intensity exercise, seven 30-second periods of sprinting separated by short intervals, or a 15-minute warm-up at 60% of VO2 max. These maneuvers should be performed a half-hour before more strenuous exercise[20]. After warming up, patients should pretreat themselves with two puffs of a short-acting beta-agonist inhaler to protect against an attack for 2 to 6 hours.

After exercise, a cool-down period of several minutes of stretching or less strenuous activity will allow a gradual rewarming of the airways and make postexercise symptoms less likely.

Patients should be taught to deal with EIA symptoms if they appear despite preventive measures. While some well-trained athletes can "break through" their symptoms (continue to exercise until symptoms remit), this carries unacceptable risks for most patients. They should stop and take two more puffs of the beta-agonist inhaler and seek medical attention if this does not relieve symptoms.

The few patients who continue to be troubled by EIA despite preventive measures might be advised to try activities that have less asthmogenic potential, such as swimming, which exposes the exerciser to warm, moist air that tempers the effect on the airways. Sports that involve short bursts of strenuous activity, such as tennis or half-court basketball, provide less aerobic benefit than more continuous activities like running or biking, but may be more fitting for patients with persistent EIA.

Encourage and Educate

Even when asthma is well-controlled, some patients may need active encouragement and education to overcome their fears. It should be emphasized that far from being contraindicated by their disease, exercise is a valuable adjunct to its management.

References

1. Highlights of the Expert Panel Report 2: Guidelines for the Diagnosis and Management of Asthma, National Institutes of Health publication No. 97-4051A. Bethesda, MD, National Institutes of Health, National Heart, Lung, and Blood Institute, May 1997

2. Cochrane LM, Clark CJ: Benefits and problems of a physical training programme for asthmatic patients. *Thorax* 1990;45(5): 345-351

3. Szentagothai K, Gyene I, Szocska M, et al: Physical exercise program for children with bronchial asthma. *Pediatr Pulmonol* 1987;3(3):166-172

4. Bundgaard A: Exercise and the asthmatic. *Sports Med* 1985;2(4):254-266

5. McFadden ER Jr: Exercise performance in the asthmatic. *Am Rev Respir Dis* 1984;129(2 pt 2):S84-S87

6. Gong H Jr: Breathing easy: exercise despite asthma. *Phys Sportsmed* 1992;20(3):159-167

7. Voy RO: The US Olympic Committee experience with exercised-induced bronchospasm, 1984. *Med Sci Sports Exerc* 1986;18(3):328-330

8. Cypcar D, Lemanske RF Jr: Asthma and exercise. *Clin Chest Med* 1994;15(2):351-368

9. McFadden ER Jr: Exercise-induced asthma: assessment of current etiologic concepts. *Chest* 1987;91(6 suppl):151S-157S

10. Spector SL: Update on exercise-induced asthma. *Ann Allergy* 1993;71(6):571-577

11. McFadden ER Jr, Gilbert IA: Exercise-induced asthma. *N Engl J Med* 1994;330(19):1362-1367

12. Anderson SD: Exercise-induced asthma, in Middleton E, Reed CE, Ellis EF, et al (eds): *Allergy: Principles and Practice*, ed 4. St Louis, Mosby, 1993, pp 1343-1367

13. Anderson SD: Is there a unifying hypothesis for exercise-induced asthma? *J Allergy Clin Immunol* 1984;73(5 pt 2):660-665

14. Lemanske RF Jr, Henke KG: Exercise-induced asthma, in Gisolfi C, Lamb DR (eds): *Youth, Exercise and Sport: Perspectives in Exercise Science and Sports Medicine*. Indianapolis, Benchmark Press, 1989, vol 2, pp 465-511

15. Simons FE, Gerstner TV, Cheang MS: Tolerance to the bronchoprotective effect of salmeterol in adolescents with exercise-induced asthma using concurrent inhaled glucocorticoid treatment. *Pediatrics* 1997;99(5):655-659

16. D'Urzo AD: Long-acting beta-2-agonists: role in primary care asthma treatment. *Can Fam Physician* 1997;43(Oct):1773-1777

17. Thio BJ, Nagelkerke AF, Ketel AG, et al: Exercise-induced asthma and cardiovascular fitness in asthmatic children. *Thorax* 1996;51(2):207-209

18. O'Byrne PM, Israel E, Drazen JM: Antileukotrienes in the treatment of asthma. *Ann Intern Med* 1997;127(6):472-480

19. Pauwels RA, Lofdahl CG, Postma DS, et al: Effect of inhaled formoterol and budesonide on exacerbations of asthma: Formoterol and Corticosteroids Establishing Therapy (FACET) International Study Group. *N Engl J Med* 1997;337(20):1405-1411

20. Wilkerson LA: Exercise-induced asthma. *J Am Osteopath Assoc* 1998;98(4):211-215

—by Vincent Disabella, D.O., with Carl Sherman

Dr. Disabella is the assistant director of primary care sports medicine and the primary care sports medicine fellowship program for Crozer-Keystone Health System in Springfield, Pennsylvania. Mr. Sherman is a freelance writer in New York City. Address correspondence to Vincent Disabella, D.O., 196 W. Sproul Rd., Ste. 110, Springfield, PA 19064; e-mail: vdisabel@crozer.org.

Part Eight

Additional Help
and Information

Chapter 67

Glossary

A

acute: Having a short and relatively severe course. In opposition to chronic Type I Hypersensitivity or Anaphylactic Shock.

adrenal gland: The adrenal gland sits directly on top of the kidneys and consists of 2 separate organs, the cortex and the medulla. The medulla (inner portion) produces and secretes the catecholamine hormones, epinephrine (adrenaline) and norepinephrine (noradrenaline). The cortex (outer portion) produces the corticosteroids, glucocorticoids (such as cortisol), and mineralocorticoids (aldosterone).

airway: Air enters through the mouth and nose and passes down the pharynx (throat) and through the larynx (voice box). Air then continues

Excerpted from "HON Allergy Glossary," [Online] July 2, 1998. Available: http://www.hon.ch/Library/Theme/Allergy/Glossary/a.html. © 1998 by Health On the Net Foundation, c/o Medical Information Division, University Hospital of Geneva, 1211 Geneva 14, Switzerland. Reprinted with permission. From "Glossary," in *Global Strategy for Asthma Management and Prevention,* NHLBI/WHO Workshop Report. Produced by National Institutes of Health (NIH), National Heart, Lung, and Blood Institute (NHLBI), Global Initiative for Asthma. NIH Publication No. 95-3659, January 1995. From "Environmental Genome Project Glossary and Acronyms," [Online] November 1999. Available: http://www.niehs.nih.gov/envgenom/glossary.htm. Produced by the National Institute of Environmental Health Sciences (NIEHS), P.O. Box 12233, Research Triangle Park, NC 27709. For complete contact information, please refer to Chapter 68, "Resources."

down through the trachea (windpipe) which branches into two bronchi (singular: Bronchus) to each of the two lungs. The inflammation of the bronchus is called bronchitis.

allele: An alternate form of a gene.

allergen: An antigen (substance that elicits an antibody response) that is responsible for producing allergic reactions by inducing IgE formation. IgE antibodies, bound to basophils in circulation and mast cells in tissue, cause these cells to release chemicals when they come into contact with an allergen. These chemicals can cause injury to surrounding tissue—the visible signs of an allergy. An allergen can be almost anything which acts as an antigen to stimulate such an immune response. Common allergens: food (the most common are milk, fruit, fish, eggs, and nuts); pollen (especially ragweed, which causes hay fever); mold (from plants and food, which are most likely to cause asthma); house dust (which contains mites as well as dander from house pets); venom (from insects such as bees, wasps, and mosquitoes, or scorpions); and plant oils (especially poison ivy, oak, or sumac). Additionally, feathers, wool, dyes, cosmetics, and perfumes may also act as allergens.

allergic rhinitis: Characterized by an inflammation of the nasal mucous membranes due to an allergic response. The most common of all atopic diseases in the United States, affecting up to 10% of the adult population. While no one dies directly as a result of allergic rhinitis, the economic impact is substantial. Clinically, information is gained from a nasal examination which may reveal pale, boggy turbinate as well as clear to greenish rhinorrhea. When colored nasal secretions are stained and examined, they typically reveal large numbers of eosinophils as the main inflammatory cell. In many instances (particularly in children) complications such as chronic otitis media, rhino sinusitis, and conjunctivitis can be traced to chronic obstruction from allergic rhinitis. Concerning the treatment of allergic rhinitis, corticosteroid nasal sprays are very effective agents, especially for symptoms of congestion, sneezing, and runny nose.

allergy: Allergies are hypersensitivity reactions of the immune system to specific substances called allergens (such as pollen, stings, drugs, or food) that, in most people, result in no symptoms. The most severe form of allergy is Anaphylactic shock, which is a medical emergency. Allergy has different names depending upon where in the body it occurs.

allergy tests: Abdominal x-rays after lactose-barium meal; Allergy Skin Test; Breath Hydrogen Level (BHL) Test; Breath Methane Test; Fecal pH and reducing substances; Intestinal biopsy for lactase activity; Intestinal perfusion studies; Lactose tolerance test; Pulmonary Function Test (PFT); Radioallergosorbent Test (RAST); Skin Endpoint Titration (SET); Stool Acidity Test; and Urinary tests.

amino acid: Small organic molecule containing both a carboxyl group and an amino group bonded to the same carbon atom. For example: histamine; serotonin; epinephrine; norepinephrine.

anaphylaxis: The severest form of allergy which is a medical emergency. An often severe and sometimes fatal systemic reaction in a susceptible individual upon exposure to a specific antigen (such as wasp venom or penicillin) following previous sensitization. Characterized especially by respiratory symptoms, fainting, itching, urticaria, swelling of the throat or other mucous membranes, and a sudden decline in blood pressure.

angioedema: A vascular reaction involving the deep dermis or subcutaneous or submucal tissues, the histological features of which include vasodilation, superficial (papillary) dermal edema, increased permeability of the capillaries, a sparse perivascular infiltrate of lymphocytes and rare neutrophils and eosinophils. Characterized by the development of giant wheals.

antibiotic: Drug (such as penicillin, tetracycline, or cephalosporin) that is able to kill or inhibit the growth of certain micro-organisms (bacteria). Used to combat disease and infection. Some of the most common antibiotics are ampicillin, amoxicilin, and penicillin.

antibiotic allergy: An antibiotic may cause an allergic reaction, as is often the case with penicillin.

anticholinergic: Drugs of this class, such as ipratropium bromide and atropine, block acetlycholine from causing smooth muscle contractions and from producing excess mucus in the bronchi. These drugs further widen the airways of people who are already taking $beta_2$-adrenergic receptor agonists.

551

antigen: A substance that elicits an antibody response.

antihistamine: Drugs which block the action of histamine, thus preventing or alleviating the major symptoms of an allergic response. Antihistamines are typically combined with a decongestant to help relieve nasal congestion. Examples include Alkylamines (Chlorpheniramine, Brompheniramine); Ethanolamines (Diphenhydramine, Dimenhydranate, Clemastine); Piperazines (Hydroxyzine, Meclozine, Compazine); Piperadines (Azatadine, Triprolidine); Ethylenediamines (PBZ); Phenothiazines (Thorazine, Temaril); Tricyclic antidepressants (Imipramine, Doxopin, Amitryptoline); and others (Terfenadine, Astemizole, Loratadine, Acrivastine).

anti-inflammatories: Drugs used to reduce inflammation—the redness, heat, swelling, and increased blood flow found in infections and in many chronic noninfective diseases such as [asthma], rheumatoid arthritis, and gout.

asthma: Asthma can be defined clinically as a condition of intermittent, reversible airway constriction, due to a hyperreactivity to certain substances producing inflammation. In an asthma attack the smooth muscles of the lungs go into spasm with the surrounding tissue inflamed and secreting mucus into the airways. Thus, the diameter of the airways is reduced causing the characteristic wheezing as the person affected breathes harder to get air into the lungs. Attacks can vary in intensity and frequency.

asthma management: A comprehensive approach to achieving and maintaining control of asthma. It includes patient education to develop a partnership in management, assessing and monitoring severity, avoiding or controlling asthma triggers, establishing plans for medication and management of exacerbations, and regular follow-up care.

asymptomatic: Infection without symptoms. Someone who is asymptomatic has antibodies (for example, to HIV) but does not have any visible signs or symptoms (example, of HIV infection).

atopy: A type of inherited allergic response involving elevated immunoglobulin E. Sometimes called a reagin response, it means that you have hay fever, bronchial asthma, or skin problems like urticaria or eczema. It can also be acquired, sometimes following hepatitis or extended contact with solvents or alcohol.

B

bacteria: Microscopic organism (free-living single cells), sometimes parasitic, that take various forms and often cause disease (infection). Contain no nucleus and are therefore classed as prokaryotes. Bacteria come in one of three shapes: coccal (spherical); bacillary (rod-shaped), or spirochetal (spiral/helical). The shape of a bacteria is determined by the shape of the rigid cell wall. Bacteria are also generally classified into either gram-positive (blue) or gram-negative (pink) depending on their color following a laboratory procedure called a Gram Stain. Gram-negative bacteria are characterized by having two outer membranes, which makes them more resistant to conventional treatment. This class of bacteria also easily mutate and transfer these genetic changes to other strains, making them more resistant to antibiotic treatment. Examples of infections caused by this class of bacteria include the plague, rabbit fever, cholera, typhoid fever, and salmonella. Gram-positive bacteria are rarer and treatable with penicillin. Gram-positive bacteria can cause damage by either releasing toxic chemicals (e.g., clostridium botulinum) or by penetrating deep into tissue (e.g., streptococci). Infections caused by this class of bacteria include anthrax and listeriosis.

basophil: A type of leukocyte (white blood cell), also called a granular leukocyte, filled with granules of toxic chemicals, that can digest micro-organisms. Basophils are responsible for the symptoms of allergy. Despite similarities, basophils appear to be a distinct cell type from mast cells. Basophils are derived from bone marrow progenitors (psc) and contain granules that bind basic dyes. They are capable of synthesizing many of the same mediators as mast cells. Both express the same high affinity for Fce receptors (FceRI) and can be triggered by antigen binding to IgE. Basophils, like other inflammatory granulocytes, enter tissues only when they are recruited into inflammatory sites. Basophils, like neutrophils, express a number of adhesion molecules important for homing, such as LFA-1 (CD11aCD18), Mac-1 (CD11bCD18), and CD44. When basophils are triggered, they release two kinds of mediators: 1. Preformed granule-associated mediators such as histamine, serotonin, bradykinin, heparin, and cytokines. 2. Newly-generated mediators, prostaglandins, and leukotrienes, made from arachidonic acid in surrounding tissues.

B-cell (B lymphocyte): White blood cells which develop from B stem cells into plasma cells which produce immunoglobulins (antibodies).

An antibody-producing B-cell has reached the end of its differentiation pathway.

beta-adrenergic receptor agonists: These are the drugs used most commonly to relieve a sudden asthma attack or to prevent an attack during exercise. This type of bronchodilator stimulates beta-adrenergic receptors to widen the airways. Beta-adrenergic receptor agonists act on all beta-adrenergic receptors (e.g., adrenaline) which can cause side effects such as headache, muscle tremors, and restlessness. However there also exist drugs of this class that act only on beta$_2$-adrenergic receptors in the lungs, thus causing fewer side effects.

bronchiole: The branching airways connecting the bronchi with the alveolar ducts.

bronchitis: Bronchitis is an inflammation of the bronchus usually caused by an infection. This often includes the trachea and the bronchioles. Bronchiolitis is an inflammation of the bronchioles. Generally a mild condition that eventually heals totally, however, bronchitis can also be chronic. In this condition there is diffused inflammation of the air passages in the lungs, leading to decreased uptake of oxygen by the lungs and increased mucus production. Two main types of bronchitis exist: Infectious Bronchitis, caused by viruses and bacteria (e.g., Mycoplasma pneumoniae and Chlamydia). Most frequent in winter. Smokers and those with chronic sinusitis, bronchiectasis, and allergies, and children with enlarged tonsils and adenoids may experience recurrent infections; and Irritative Bronchitis, caused by dust, pollen, strong acid fumes, ammonia, chlorine, hydrogen sulfide, sulphur dioxide, ozone, tobacco smoke. Treatment includes aspirin for adults, acetaminophen for children, and antibiotics for those whose bronchitis is due to a bacterial infection.

bronchodilator: Anything that opens or expands the bronchi (that part of the body that conveys air to and from the lungs). Bronchodilating drugs are usually prescribed if a cough occurs with airway narrowing and can reduce coughing, wheezing, and shortness of breath. Bronchodilators can be taken orally, injected, or inhaled, and begin to act almost immediately but with the effect only lasting 4-6 hours. The most common bronchodilators are beta-adrenergic receptor agonists. These are the drugs used most commonly to relieve a sudden asthma attack or to prevent an attack during exercise. This type of bronchodilator stimulates beta-adrenergic receptors to widen the airways.

Beta-adrenergic receptor agonists act on all beta-adrenergic receptors (e.g., adrenaline) which can cause side effects such as headache, muscle tremors, and restlessness. However there also exist drugs of this class that act only on beta$_2$-adrenergic receptors in the lungs, thus causing fewer side effects. Anticholinergic drugs: Drugs of this class, such as ipratropium bromide and atropine, block acetylcholine from causing smooth muscle contractions and from producing excess mucus in the bronchi. These drugs further widen the airways of people who are already taking beta$_2$-adrenergic receptor agonists. Theophylline: Drug used in asthma treatment and prevention.

bronchus: The bronchi branch many times until becoming much smaller airways called "bronchioles." At the end of each bronchiole are tiny air-filled cavities called alveoli. Each alveolus is surrounded by many blood capillaries which allow oxygen to move into the bloodstream and carbon dioxide out. This exchange of substances is the primary function of the respiratory system.

C

cat allergy: One of the most common pet allergies. A tiny protein particle, the Fel d 1 allergen, found in the cat's skin flakes and saliva, causes this allergy.

causal factors: Risk factors that sensitize the airways and cause the onset of asthma. The most important of these factors are allergens and chemical sensitizers.

chronic: Long-lasting and severe, opposite of Acute. Examples include Chronic Atopic Dermatitis; Chronic Bronchitis; Chronic Cough; Chronic Rhinitis; and Chronic Ulcerative Colitis.

contributing factors: Risk factors that either augment the likelihood of asthma developing upon exposure to them, or may even increase susceptibility to asthma. These factors include smoking, viral infections, small size at birth, and environmental pollutants.

corticosteroid: Corticosteroids are a group of anti-inflammatory drugs similar to the natural corticosteroid hormones produced by the cortex of the adrenal glands. Among the disorders that often improve with corticosteroid treatment are asthma, allergic rhinitis, eczema, and rheumatoid arthritis. How these anti-inflammatory agents inhibit late phase allergic reactions occurs via a variety of mechanisms, including decreasing the density of mast cells along mucosal surfaces, decreasing chemotaxis and activation of eosinophils, decreasing cytokine production by lymphocytes, monocytes, mast cells, and eosinophils, inhibiting the metabolism of arachidonic acid, and other mechanisms. But for the side effects, corticosteroids would be the only drug needed for treating most allergic reactions. Much effort is underway to develop safer corticosteroids including topical application and modifying the molecules to preserve the anti-inflammatory properties while minimizing the undesirable side effects.

cytokine: Cytokines are soluble glycoproteins released by cells of the immune system, which act nonenzymatically through specific receptors to regulate immune responses. Cytokines resemble hormones in that they act at low concentrations bound with high affinity to a specific receptor. Common cytokines in allergology include Interleukins, Lymphokine, Interferon, Colony Stimulating Factor, Platelet-Activating Factor, and Tumor Necrosis Factor.

D

decongestant: The three most common oral decongestants are pseudoephedrine, phenylpropanolamine, and phenylephrine. These work by shrinking blood vessels in the nose, thus reducing congestion. Unfortunately, their effect is not confined to the nose as decongestants can worsen hypertension (high blood pressure), Raynaud's phenomenon, and can act as a stimulant. Due to this last side effect, decongestants are frequently combined with sedating antihistamines. However, the stimulant and sedative effects do not always cancel each other out, resulting in an upset in one's daily cycle.

desensitization therapy: A method where the body is repeatedly exposed to small amounts of an allergy causing substance, an allergen, in order to reduce the allergic reaction. For instance, if a person with diabetes has a bad reaction to taking a full dose of beef insulin, the doctor gives the person a very small amount of the insulin at first. Over a period of time, larger doses are given until the person is taking the full dose. This is one way to help the body get used to the full dose and to avoid an allergic reaction.

diagnostic techniques: The process of identifying a disease by its characteristic signs, symptoms, and laboratory findings. With cancer, the earlier the diagnosis is made, the better the chance of a cure.

DNA: A polymer composed primarily of units of deoxyribonucleic acids; DNA serves as the primary storage form of genetic information.

drug allergy: Certain drugs can cause a severe allergic reaction, known as an anaphylactic reaction. First exposure to a drug does not cause this reaction but subsequent exposure may. However an anaphylactoid reaction can occur following the first injection of certain drugs (e.g., polymyxin, pentamidine, opioids and contrast media used for x-rays). Although many organ systems can be involved in an allergic drug reaction, the skin is most commonly affected. Dermatologic reactions include urticaria, angioedema, dermatitis (allergic contact dermatitis, photodermatitis, exfoliative dermatitis), fixed drug eruption, and erythema multiforme (characterized by a rash and patches of red skin all over the body). Common antibiotics that can cause allergic reactions: Penicillin, Cephalosporin, Sulfonamide, and others, including Aztreonam, Isoniazid, and nitrofurantoin.

dust: Dust is a common allergen. House dust contains mites (which are the primary cause of dust-related allergies), microscopic particles of animal dander, pollen, mold, fibers from clothing and other fabrics, and detergents.

dust mites: The primary cause of dust allergy, dust mites are microscopic organisms found in homes. It is actually the excrement of these mites to which people are allergic, thus dust mites can cause allergic reactions even when dead.

E

edema: An accumulation of fluid between cells, causing swelling of the involved area. Edema is most often seen in the lower legs, the feet, and around the eyes. Examples include Laryngoedema and Angioedema.

environmental control: Removal of risk factors from the environment.

environmental response gene: A gene that has a specific reaction to environmental exposures, for example a drug metabolizing gene.

eosinophil: One of the five different types of white blood cell (WBC) belonging to the subgroup of WBCs called Polymorphonuclear Leukocytes. Characterized by large red (i.e., eosinophilic) cytoplasmic granules. Eosinophil function is incompletely understood. They are prominent at sites of allergic reactions and with parasitic larvae infections (helminths). Eosinophil secretory products inactivate many of the chemical mediators of inflammation and destroy cancer cells. This phenomenon is most obvious with mast cell-derived mediators. Mast cells produce a chemotactic factor for eosinophils. Produced in the bone marrow, eosinophils then migrate to tissues throughout the body. When a foreign substance enters the body, lymphocytes and neutrophils release certain substances to attract eosinophils which release toxic substances to kill the invader.

eosinophilia: An abnormally high number of eosinophils in the blood. Not a disease in itself but usually a response to a disease. An elevated number of eosinophils usually indicates a response to abnormal cells, parasites, or allergens.

epinephrine: A hormone released by the adrenal gland, which is the drug of choice for the treatment of anaphylaxis. Indeed those who are allergic to insect stings and certain foods should always carry a self-injecting syringe of epinephrine. Epinephrine increases the speed and force of heart beats, and therefore the work that can be done by the heart. It dilates the airways to improve breathing and narrows blood vessels in the skin and intestine so that an increased flow of blood reaches the muscles and allows them to cope with the demands of exercise. Usually treatment with this hormone stops an anaphylactic reaction. Epinephrine has been produced synthetically as a drug since 1900.

epitope: An alternative term for an antigenic determinant. These are particular chemical groups on a molecule that are antigenic, i.e., that elicit a specific immune response.

etiology: The scientific study or theory of the causes of a certain disease.

exacerbation: Any worsening of asthma. Onset can be acute and sudden, or gradual over several days. A correlation between symptoms and peak flow is not necessarily found. "Exacerbation" replaces the words "attack" and "episode."

extrinsic asthma: Asthma triggered by external agents such as pollen or chemicals. Most cases of extrinsic asthma have an allergic origin and are caused by an IgE mediated response to an inhaled allergen. This is the type of asthma commonly diagnosed in early life. Many patients with extrinsic asthma may respond to immunotherapy.

F

food allergy: A food allergy is any adverse reaction to a food or food component involving the body's immune system. A true allergic reaction to a food involves two primary components: contact with food allergens (part of the food that stimulates the immune system); Immunoglobulin E (IgE: an antibody in the immune system that reacts with allergens) and mast cells (tissue cells) as well as basophils (blood cells), which release histamine or other substances causing allergic symptoms when IgE antibodies attach onto these cells. Although most Americans consume a wide variety of food additives daily, only a small number have been associated with reactions. These reactions do not involve the immune system and therefore are examples of food intolerance rather than food allergy. While most allergic reactions to food are relatively mild, a small percentage of food-allergic individuals have severe reactions that can be life-threatening. Symptoms of a food allergy are highly individualistic and usually begin within minutes to a few hours after having eaten the offending food. The most common food allergens involved in food allergy are shellfish, milk, fish, soy, wheat, peanuts, egg, and tree nuts such as walnuts.

food intolerance: Food intolerance is an adverse reaction to food which does not involve the body's immune system. It can be caused by a metabolic reaction to an enzyme deficiency such as the inability to digest milk properly (lactose maldigestion), by food poisoning such as ingesting contaminated or spoiled fish, or a food idiosyncrasy such as sulfite-induced asthma.

G

gastrointestinal (GI): Relating to the stomach and intestines.

gene: Located in the nucleus of the cell, genes contain hereditary information that is transferred from cell to cell.

genetic: Refers to the inherited pattern located in genes for certain characteristics, while congenital refers to conditions existing prior to or at birth, but which are not inherited.

genetic predisposition: A latent susceptibility to disease at the genetic level, which may be activated under certain conditions.

genome: The complete chromosomal genetic complement.

glucocorticoid: Glucocorticoids are anti-inflammatory, immunosuppressive, and catabolic to skin tissue. Long-term use has inhibitory effects on DNA synthesis and cell division, which is considered to be causal to the side effects. Many people suffer the symptoms of Cushing's syndrome because they take glucocorticoid hormones such as prednisone for asthma, rheumatoid arthritis, lupus, or other inflammatory diseases.

glycoprotein: A protein coated with sugars, for example, cytokines.

H

hapten: A compound, usually of low molecular weight, that is not itself immunogenic [producing an immune response] but, when bound to a carrier protein or cell, becomes immunogenic and induces antibodies, which can bind the hapten either alone or in the presence of a carrier.

helper T-cell: A subset of T-cells that carry the T4 marker and are essential for turning on antibody production, activating cytotoxic T-cells, and initiating other immune responses. The number of T4 cells in a blood sample is used to measure the health of the immune system in people with HIV. T-helper lymphocytes contain two subsets, TH1 and TH2 cells.

heredity: A term used to describe conditions that are passed genetically from parents to children.

histamine: A hormone/chemical transmitter (biogenic monoamine, similar to Serotonin, Epinephrine, Norepinephrine) involved in local immune responses, regulating stomach acid production and in allergic reactions as a mediator of Immediate Hypersensitivity. When released from mast cells, histamine causes vasodilation and an increase in permeability of blood vessel walls. These effects, in turn cause the familiar symptoms of allergy including a runny nose and watering eyes. When released in the lungs, histamine causes the airways to swell shut in an attempt to close the door on offending allergens and keep them out. Unfortunately, the ultimate result of this response is the wheezing and difficulty in breathing seen in people with asthma— an occasionally deadly allergic complication which kills an estimated 4,000 Americans yearly.

hormone: Hormones are substances released into the bloodstream by glands or organs, which affect activity in cells at another site. Most are proteins composed of amino-acid chains of various lengths. Others are steroids. Hormones (similar to the cytokines and other mediators) act at low concentrations with very large responses in the body and bind with high affinity to specific receptors. These receptors are on the surface or inside the cell and the result of such binding causes an alteration in the cell's functioning. Hormones control growth and development, reproduction, and sexual characteristics as well as exercising a large influence over the body's use of energy. Examples include the Catecholamines (such as Epinephrine and Norepinephrine) and the Corticosteroids released by the adrenal glands.

hymenoptera: Hymenoptera are the most common insects which cause allergy (anaphylaxis). Scientists estimate that there are more than 300,000 species of Hymenoptera in the world, though only 120,000 have been identified and named so far. Examples include bees, honey-bees, yellow jackets, yellow hornets, wasps, and white-faced hornets.

hypersensitivity: State of reactivity to an antigen that is far greater than the antigenic challenge presented. Hypersensitivity is another term used for an allergic reaction and denotes a deleterious outcome rather than a protective one.

I

immune system: The immune system is a collection of cells (such as B-Cells, T-Cells, etc.), chemical messengers (e.g., cytokine), and proteins (such as immunoglobulin) that work together to protect the body from potentially harmful, infectious micro-organisms (microscopic life-forms), such as bacteria, viruses, and fungi. The immune system plays a role in the control of cancer and other diseases, but is also the culprit in the phenomena of allergies, hypersensitivity, and the rejection of transplanted organs, tissues, and medical implants.

immunoglobulin E (IgE): One of five classes of immunoglobulins made by humans (the others being IgA, IgD, IgG, and IgM). Its main function seems to be to protect the host against invading parasites. While parasitic disease may not be a major clinical issue in most industrialized nations, it is a major public health problem in developing nations. The antigen-specific IgE interacts with mast cells and eosinophils to protect the host against the invading parasite. However, the same antibody-cell combination is also responsible for typical allergy or immediate hypersensitivity reactions such as hay fever, asthma, hives, and anaphylaxis. There are two major types of receptor for the Fc portion (back) of the IgE or IgG4 molecule on cells. One, a high affinity receptor, is found primarily on mast cells and basophils. The other is a low affinity receptor found on CD23 cells. IgE attaches to these and acts as an antigen receptor. This class of immunoglobulins is distributed throughout the body, although cells synthesizing IgE are found predominantly in association with mucosal tissues. Reagin is the allergist's term for IgE antibodies.

immunotherapy: When an allergen can not be avoided, allergen immunotherapy is often the only viable solution. Here, tiny amounts of the allergen are injected under the skin in gradually increased doses until a maintenance level is reached. This stimulates the body to block or neutralize certain antibodies (cf. IgE) that are produced in response to the allergen and are thus responsible for the allergic symptoms experienced. This form of treatment varies in efficacy among different types of allergy and between individuals. Dust, pollen, mite, dander, and insect venom allergic reactions usually respond best. Researchers are trying to determine exactly which mechanisms are active in a specific patient so allergen immunotherapy can be better tailored to the individual. Also, work is ongoing to better chemically define the treating allergens, make allergen immunotherapy safer, and safely increase the interval between injections.

incidence: The number of new cases of a disease in a specified population over a defined period of time.

inflammation: When damage to tissue occurs, the body's immunologic response to the damage is usually inflammation. The damage may be due to trauma, lack of blood supply, hemorrhage, or infection.

This generalized response by the body includes the release of many components of the immune system (e.g., IL1 and TNF), attraction of cells to the site of the damage, swelling of tissue due to the release of fluid and other processes. Examples of conditions where inflammation is present include [Asthma,] Bronchiolitis, Bronchitis, Colitis, Dermatitis, Conjunctivitis, Rhinitis, and Rhinoconjunctivitis. Symptoms and signs of inflammation are reduced by anti-inflammatory medications such as non-steroidal anti-inflammatory drugs and Corticosteroids.

insect sting allergy: Allergic reactions to insect stings can be so severe that death may occur within the few minutes following a sting. Even if not fatal, sting allergy symptoms can be frightening, including dizziness, itchy welts or massive swelling of the body, inability to breathe, swallow or speak, fainting from low blood pressure, and shock.

interaction: Altered reaction of the body to one drug when another is taken as well.

interferon (IFN): A group of cytokine proteins with antiviral properties, capable of enhancing and modifying the immune response. Interferon is released to coat uninfected cells so that they don't become infected. Some interferons induce antiviral activity, others enhance the immune response. There are three main classes of interferon: alpha, beta, and gamma. IFN alpha is produced by virus-infected monocytes and lymphocytes. IFN beta is produced by virus-infected fibroflasts (and some other cell types). IFN gamma is produced by stimulated T and NK cells. IFN gamma increases MHC II expression, activates macrophages, neutrophils and NK cells as well as activating vascular endothelium, promoting T and B cell differentiation and increasing IL1 and IL2 synthesis. It also increases IgG2a and decreases IgE, G1, G2b, and G3 (opposite of IL4). All IFNs induce cell growth, activate CTL and NK cells as well as increasing MHC I expression. IFN alpha and beta bind to the same receptor while IFN gamma binds to another.

interleukin (IL): Glycoproteins secreted by a variety of leukocytes [white blood cells] which have effects on other leukocytes (Interleukin = between leukocytes). The ultimate purpose of the host defense system is to eliminate invading micro-organisms. Once an invading organism is recognized as foreign, elimination is accomplished through phagocytosis and antibody formation (in the case of bacteria) and cytotoxic attack (for viral, fungal, or other intracellular pathogens). How the immune system recognizes a foreign antigen has been the focus of intense investigation over the years. Immunologists have also been interested in how the immune system forms a long-term "memory" from antigen exposure so that future contact will stimulate an immediate defense against that particular antigen. In recent years they have determined that an important component of immunologic memory is interleukin-2, one of the cytokines produced by the lymphocyte series of white blood cells. The principal types of interleukins are IL1, IL2, and IL4.

intrinsic asthma: Asthma triggered by boggy membranes, congested tissues, and other native causes such as adrenalin stress or exertion. Intrinsic asthma generally develops later in life and virtually nothing is known of its causes. It carries a worse prognosis than extrinsic asthma and tends to be less responsive to treatment. Intrinsic bronchial hyperactivity can be triggered by infection, exercise, or drugs such as aspirin.

L

latex: Latex is the milky sap from the rubber tree Hevea brasiliensis. A polymer of cis 1-4 isoprene.

latex allergy: Patients who are allergic to latex may also be allergic to certain fruits (such as bananas, avocados, chestnuts, and kiwi) due to cross reacting elements in these fruits. IgE-mediated latex allergy clinical manifestations include Contact Urticaria or Generalized Urticaria, Conjunctivitis, Rhinitis, Bronchospasm, and Anaphylaxis.

leukocyte: Leukocytes or white blood cells (WBC) are cells in the blood that are involved in defending the body against infective organisms and foreign substances. Like all blood cells, they are produced in the bone marrow. There are 5 main types of white blood cell, subdivided between 2 main groups: Polymorphonuclear Leukocytes (granulocytes): (Neutrophils, Eosinophils, Basophils) and Mononuclear Leukocytes: (Monocytes and Lymphocytes). White blood cells are the principal components of the immune system and function by destroying "foreign" substances such as bacteria and viruses. When an infection is present, the production of WBCs increases. If the number of leukocytes is abnormally low (a condition known as leukopenia), infection is more likely to occur and it is more difficult for the body to get rid of the infection.

leukotriene: A mediator of Immediate Hypersensitivity. Leukotrienes are derived from the action of enzyme 5-lipoxygenase on arachidonic acid and are the chemicals which cause asthma symptoms. Leukotriene modifiers such as Zileuton (a 5-lipoxygenase inhibitor), Zafirlukast, and Montelukast prevent the synthesis or action of leukotrienes and thus, are often used to treat asthma.

lymphocyte: A white blood cell of the mononuclear leukocyte subgroup (like macrophage/monocytes). Lymphocytes identify foreign substances and germs (bacteria or viruses) in the body and produce antibodies and cells that specifically target them. It takes from several days to weeks for lymphocytes to recognize and attack a new foreign substance. The main lymphocyte sub-types are: B-Cells (special B-cells produce specific antibodies, proteins that help destroy foreign substances); T-Cells (T-cells attack virus-infected cells, foreign tissue, and cancer; they also produce a number of substances that regulate the immune response); NK Cells (among other functions, natural killer cells destroy cancer cells and virus-infected cells through phagocytosis and by producing substances that can kill such cells); Null cells (an early population of lymphocytes bearing neither T-cell nor B-cell differentiation antigens). Lymphocytes are small cells with virtually no cytoplasm, found in the blood, in all tissue, and in lymphoid organs, such as lymph nodes, the tonsils, thymus gland, spleen, and Peyer's patches.

M

macrophage: A large white blood cell, derived from monocytes (a subclass of Mononuclear Leukocytes). Properties include phagocytosis and antigen presentation to T-cells. Macrophages contain granules or packets of chemicals and enzymes (such as IL1) which serve the purpose of ingesting and destroying microbes, antigens, and other foreign substances. Macrophages are not found in the bloodstream but at locations where body organs interface with the environment or the bloodstream, for example, in the lungs, spleen, bone marrow, and liver. Similar cells in the blood are the monocytes.

mast cell: Mast cells (which are Leukocytes) contain metachromatic granules which store a variety of inflammatory mediators. These include histamine and serotonin; proteolytic enzymes that can destroy tissue or cleave complement components; heparin or chondroitin sulfate, which are anticoagulants; chemotactic factors, such as eosinophil chemotactic factor of anaphylaxis (an important regulator of eosinophil function), and neutrophil chemotactic factor. Normally, mast cells are not found in circulation.

mediator: An object or substance by which something is mediated, such as a structure of the nervous system that transmits impulses eliciting a specific response; a chemical substance (transmitter substance) that induces activity in an excitable tissue, such as nerve or muscle (e.g., hormones); or a substance released from cells as the result of an antigen-antibody interaction or by the action of antigen with a sensitized lymphocyte (e.g., cytokine). Concerning mediators of Immediate Hypersensitivity, the most important include Histamine, Leukotriene (e.g., SRS-A), ECF-A, PAF, and Serotonin. There also exist three classes of lipid mediators which are synthesized by activated mast cells through reactions initiated by the actions of phospholipase A2. These are Prostaglandins, Leukotrienes, and Platelet-activating factors (PAF).

mold: Molds are naturally occurring clusters of microscopic fungi which reproduce by releasing airborne spores. Certain individuals will develop asthma and nasal symptoms if they breathe in these spores and thus have a mold allergy.

mold allergy: Many people are allergic to mold. Mold spores are carried in the air and may be present all year long. Mold is most prevalent indoors, in damp locations, and in swamp coolers, bathrooms, washrooms, fabrics, rugs, stuffed animals, books, wallpaper, and other "organic" materials. Outdoors, mold lives in the soil, on compost, and on damp vegetation.

monoclonal antibodies: Laboratory-produced antibodies, which can be programmed to react against a specific antigen in order to suppress the immune response.

N

neutrophil: Neutrophils are Leukocytes (white blood cells) of the Polymorphonuclear Leukocyte subgroup. Neutrophils form a primary defense against bacterial infection. Like all the cells of the immune system, neutrophils are produced in the bone marrow and circulate in the bloodstream. However, neutrophils move out of blood vessels into infected tissue in order to attack the foreign substance (allergen, bacteria, etc.). Normally a serious bacterial infection causes the body to produce an increased number of neutrophils, resulting in a higher than normal WBC count. Neutrophils perform their function partially through phagocytosis, a process by which they "eat" other cells and foreign substances. The pus in a boil (abscess) is made up mostly of neutrophils.

P

peanut allergy: Peanut hypersensitivity is one of the most common food allergies and one of the most common causes of death by food anaphylaxis. Allergic reactions can vary from mild urticaria to severe, even fatal, anaphylaxis, but more generally are acute and dramatic.

PEF (peak expiratory flow) home monitoring: Measurement of PEF on a regular basis at home with a portable peak flow meter. PEF home monitoring is especially useful to patients over 5 years of age with moderate persistent to severe persistent asthma.

peptide: A molecule formed by joining two or more amino acids, for example, ECF-A.

pet allergy: Many people are allergic to animals. Most people are not allergic to the animal's fur or feathers. The allergy is more usually an immune reaction to a protein (an allergen) found in the saliva, dander (dead skin flakes), or the urine of an animal. The allergen gets carried in the air or in dust on very small, invisible particles. It then lands on the lining of the eyes (conjunctiva) and nose. It may also be inhaled directly into the lungs, causing allergic symptoms. Allergen contact with an allergic person's skin may also cause itching and hives.

placebo: An inactive compound having no physiological effect; an inert substance identical in appearance to the treatment drug used in clinical studies. A form of safe but non-active treatment frequently used as a basis for comparison with pharmaceuticals in research studies.

placebo effect: An apparently beneficial result of therapy that occurs because of the patient's expectation that the therapy will help.

pollen: Microscopic grains produced by plants in order to reproduce. Each plant has a pollinating period.

pollen allergy: A hypersensitive reaction to pollen. Such reactions include Extrinsic Asthma, Rhinitis, and Bronchitis.

polypeptide: Many peptides joined together, for example, insulin.

prevalence: The number of all new and old cases of a disease in a defined population at a particular point in time.

preventive treatment: Treatment intended to preserve health and prevent the occurrence or recurrence of a disease. Taking a drug to prevent yourself from getting an illness.

prognosis: Prediction of the future course of the disease.

prophylaxis: Measures taken (treatment, drugs) to prevent the onset of a particular disease ("primary" prophylaxis) or recurrent symptoms in an existing infection that have be brought under control ("secondary" prophylaxis, maintenance therapy).

protein: A molecule composed of many amino acids and with a complex structure, for example, immunoglobulin, casein.

R

receptor: A protein molecule (most commonly on the surface of a cell) which reacts to a substance which stimulates it. This leads to further biochemical changes within the cell itself. Cell-surface receptors are proteins in, on, or traversing the cell membrane that recognize and bind to specific molecules in the surrounding fluid. The binding may serve to transport molecules into the cell's interior or to signal the cell to respond in some way. Examples of such receptors include the alpha and beta receptors on blood vessels; the beta-1 receptor of the heart; the histamine receptor on mast cells; and cytokine specific receptors.

respiratory system: The respiratory system is the system by which oxygen, essential for life, is taken into the body and the waste product, carbon dioxide, is expelled from the body. The respiratory system consists of the mouth and nose, airways, and lungs.

rhinitis: Rhinitis is an inflammation of the nasal mucosa (the mucous membrane that lines the nose and the sinus), often due to an allergic reaction to pollen, dust, or other airborne substances (allergens). Although the pathophysiology of many types of rhinitis is unknown, an accurate diagnosis is necessary, since not all types of rhinitis will respond to the same treatment measures. Classification of chronic rhinitis: Atopic Rhinitis, Seasonal Allergic Rhinitis (also known as hay fever), Perennial Rhinitis (year-round) with Allergic Triggers, Perennial Rhinitis with Non-Allergic Triggers, Idiopathic Non-Allergic Rhinitis, Infectious Rhinitis, Rhinitis Medicamentosa, Mechanical Obstruction, Hormonal, and Allergic (seasonal and perennial) Rhinitis.

risk factor: An agent that when present increases the probability of disorder expression. There are two types of risk factors: Risk factors involved in the development of the condition of asthma can be inherited, such as atopy. Alternatively, a risk factor can be due to environmental exposure. See "causal factors," "contributing factors," and "triggers."

S

sinus: Sinus means 'cavity.' Many structures of the human body are thus called sinuses. However, the term generally refers to the paranasal sinus. The Paranasal Sinuses are air cavities within the facial bones. They are lined by mucous membranes similar to those in other parts of the airways. The Paranasal sinuses consist of the following: Ethmoid Sinus, Frontal Sinus, Maxillary Sinus, and Sphenoid Sinus. An inflammation of the sinuses is called Sinusitis.

sinusitis: Inflammation of the sinuses, with causes ranging from dust to hay fever. Obstinate cases can be caused by chronic sinus infections or the continued exposure to allergens from food, pets, or environmental irritants. The most commonly affected sinus is the maxillary sinus.

steroid: Hormone o r drug. A large family of structurally similar chemicals. Various steroids have sex determining, anti-inflammatory, and growth-regulatory roles. Examples include Corticosteroid, Glucocorticoid.

systemic: Throughout the body. Sometimes applies to medications that are taken orally or parenterally that saturate the entire body.

T

T-cell or T-lymphocyte: A lymphocyte (white blood cell) that develops in the bone marrow, matures in the thymus, and expresses what appears to be antibody molecules on their surfaces but, unlike B-cells, these molecules cannot be secreted. This is called a T-Cell Receptor (CD3 and CD4 or CD8). It works as part of the immune system in the body and produces cytokine to help B-lymphocytes produce immunoglobulin.

TH1/TH2 cells: Subsets of T-helper lymphocytes, involved in cell-mediated immune responses. TH1 cells secrete IL-1 and gamma interferon, which enhance cell-mediated responses and inhibit both TH2 subset cell activity and the humoral immune responses. TH1 is inflammatory, produces IL2, IFN gamma, TNF beta, provides help to B-cells in IgG2a production, activates macrophages and CTL, and stimulates delayed type hypersensitivities. TH2 cells, the other subset of T-helper cells, are also involved in cell-mediated immune responses. TH2 cell activity and secretions are thought to inhibit cell-mediated responses and to enhance the humoral response. TH2 cells produce IL4, IL5, IL6, IL10, and IL13, which provide help to B-cells and induce class switch to IgE and IgG1, as well as supporting eosinophils and mast cells.

theophylline: A drug used in asthma treatment and prevention. Theophylline is a bronchodilatory drug and comes in various forms such as short-acting tablets and syrups, as well as longer-acting sustained release capsules and tablets. It can also be given intravenously if a serious asthma attack is taking place. The dose of Theophylline must be closely monitored as too little has little effect, while too much can cause side effects such as abnormal heart rhythms, nausea, insomnia, and seizures.

T killer cell: An effector lymphocyte with Fc receptors which allow it to bind to and kill antibody-coated target cells by antibody-dependent cell-mediated cytotoxicity (ADCC). T killer cells are a subset of CD8+ lymphocytes and are not to be confused with natural killer cells.

trigger: A risk factor that causes exacerbation of asthma; a stimulus that causes an increase in asthma symptoms and/or airflow limitation.

U

urticaria (hives): Urticaria is a skin symptom that accompanies many allergic disorders. It is a relatively common disorder caused by localized mast-cell degranulation, with resultant dermal venular hyperpermeability culminating in pruritic wheals. Mostly results from an antigen-induced (pollens, foods, drugs, insect venom) release of histamine and other vasoactive amines via sensitization with specific IgE antibodies. Most individual lesions develop and fade within 24 hours. Allergic skin diseases such as urticaria and angioedema as well as atopic dermatitis are not clearly defined as true allergic diseases. Urticaria and angioedema are both due to excessive mast cell activity in the skin. Chronic urticaria and angioedema are seldom due to a definable IgE mechanism (as is the case with all allergies) but, when determined, is generally due to a drug, food, or food additive.

V

vasodilation: Excessive relaxation or dilation of the blood vessel walls. The resulting low blood pressure causes an inadequate blood supply to body cells, which can result in shock (blood pressure too low to sustain life). Causes of excessive dilation include head injury, liver failure, poisoning, drug overdoses, and severe bacterial infection.

virus: A group of submicroscopic pathogens consisting essentially of a core of a single nucleic acid surrounded by a protein coat. The smallest known infectious organism. Characterized by their inability to reproduce outside of a living host cell. Viruses may subvert the host cells' normal functions, causing the cell to behave in a manner determined by the virus. They are unable to live or multiply outside of a host cell, since most do not possess the means to synthesize protein. Once inside a cell, a virus releases its DNA or RNA (the genetic code to produce more viruses) and takes over some aspects of the host cell's metabolism. The virus then uses its host to manufacture more virus particles. The virus either kills its host or alters it so that it divides abnormally, becoming cancerous. Viruses are usually cell- and, to a certain extent, species-specific. Defense against viruses includes the physical barriers of skin and mucous membranes as well as interferon, which is released by infected cells to increase the resistance of surrounding noninfected cells. The last line of defense are the various types of white blood cell. Immunity to a virus is produced by injecting a vaccine that resembles a virus, thus increasing the number of T- and B-cells that can recognize the virus.

vitamins: Chemicals essential in small quantities for good health. Some vitamins are not manufactured by the body, but adequate quantities are present in a normal diet. People whose diets are inadequate or who have digestive tract or liver disorders may need to take supplementary vitamins.

Chapter 68

Resources

For further assistance, this chapter lists in alphabetical order contact information for some of the government agencies, professional associations, and individual experts that conduct research, provide educational literature, and offer advice and support concerning asthma. Additionally, following each entry is a brief description of online asthma related products and services.

Allergy and Asthma Network—Mothers of Asthmatics, Inc.
2751 Prosperity Ave., Ste. 150, Fairfax, VA 22031
Phone: (703)641-9595, toll free: (800)878-4403
Fax: (703)573-7794
E-mail: aanma@aol.com
Internet: http://www.aanma.org

- news bulletins
- educational programs
- magazine, newsletter, discounts on asthma and allergy related products and services
- toll free hotline for asthma and allergy related questions
- directory of member physicians

American Academy of Allergy, Asthma, and Immunology
611 East Wells St., Milwaukee, WI 53202
Phone: (414)272-6071, toll free: (800)822-2762
Fax: (414)272-6070

American Academy of Allergy, Asthma, and Immunology, continued
E-mail: info@aaaai.org
Internet: http://www.aaaai.org

- news bulletins and advice
- publishes *Asthma and Allergy Advocate* newsletter
- order or download *The Allergy Report*; order asthma and allergy related videos
- local pollen/spore counts
- physician referral

American Academy of Pediatrics
141 Northwest Point Blvd., Elk Grove Village, IL 60007-1098
Phone: (847)434-4000, toll free: (800)433-9016
Fax: (847)434-8000
E-mail: kidsdocs@aap.org
Internet: http://www.aap.org

- conducts research in areas of child health, including asthma and allergies
- publishes *Pediatrics*
- order *Guide to Your Child's Allergies and Asthma*

American Association for Respiratory Care
11030 Ables Ln, Dallas, TX 75229-4593
Phone: (972)243-2272
Fax: (972)484-2720, (972)484-6010
E-mail: info@aarc.org
Internet: http://www.aarc.org

- health tips on asthma, allergies, and COPD
- Buyers' Guide of respiratory care products
- asthma I.Q. test
- publishes *AARC Times* magazine and *Respiratory Care Journal*

American College of Allergy, Asthma, and Immunology
85 West Algonquin Rd., Ste. 550, Arlington Heights, IL 60005
Phone: (847)427-1200, toll free: (800)842-7777
Fax: (847)427-1294
E-mail: mail@acaai.org
Internet: http://allergy.mcg.edu

- news bulletins and articles for patients, physicians, and employers

- information on free asthma screenings nationwide
- publishes *Annals of Allergy, Asthma and Immunology*

American College of Chest Physicians
3300 Dundee Rd., Northbrook, IL 60062-2348
Phone: (847)498-1400, toll free: (800)343-ACCP
Fax: (847)498-5460
E-mail: accp@chestnet.org
Internet: http://www.chestnet.org

- brochures: "Controlling Your Asthma," and "Getting Your Asthma under Control: A Self-Evaluation"
- online continuing education for medical professionals
- publishes *Chest*

American Lung Association
1740 Broadway, New York, NY 10019
Phone: (212)315-8700, toll free: (800)LUNG USA (For Nearest Chapter)
E-mail: info@lungusa.org
Internet: http://www.lungusa.org

- news and information about asthma and other lung diseases
- asthma statistics
- directory of children's asthma camps: http://www.lungusa.org/asthmacamps/index.html
- numerous publications including *Asthma Magazine*

American Pharmaceutical Association
2215 Constitution Ave. NW, Washington, DC 20037-2985
Phone: (202)628-4410
Fax: (202)783-2351
E-mail: webmaster@mail.aphanet.org
Internet: http://www.aphanet.org

- consumer information about pharmacists; taking medications
- brochure about drug interactions
- links to FDA Alerts and FDA Drug Recalls
- publishes *Pharmacy Today*

American Society of Health-System Pharmacists
7272 Wisconsin Ave., Bethesda, MD 20814
Phone: (301)657-3000

American Society of Health-System Pharmacists, continued
E-mail: www@ashp.org
Internet: http://www.ashp.org

- health care news
- order *Asthma Management Module*
- fact sheets on taking medications, alternative medicines, other health care tips
- shop at online 'superstore' for health care related books and software
- publishes *American Journal of Health System Pharmacy*

American Thoracic Society

1740 Broadway, New York, NY 10019
Phone: (212)315-8700
Fax: (212)315-6498
E-mail: jcorn@thoracic.org
Internet: http://www.thoracic.org

- conducts research on asthma and other lung diseases
- publishes *American Journal of Respiratory and Critical Care Medicine* and *American Journal of Respiratory Cell and Molecular Biology*
- links to other asthma and health related sites

Asthma and Allergy Foundation of America

1233 20th Street, NY, Suite 402, Washington, DC 20036
Phone: (202)466-7643, toll free: (800)727-8462
Fax: (202)466-8940
E-mail: info@aafa.org
Internet: http://www.aafa.org

- e-mail questions to board-certified allergist
- local pollen count
- 13 chapters and 130 educational support groups nationwide
- teen newsletter
- order publications from large Resource Catalogue

Louise H. Bethea, M.D., P.A.

17070 Red Oak Dr., Ste. 107, Houston, TX 77090
Phone: (281)580-6494
Fax: (281)580-2038

1001 Medical Plaza Dr., Ste. 240, The Woodlands, TX 77380
Phone: (281)364-0785
Fax: (281)292-3169
Internet: http://www.allergyasthma.com

- numerous articles on asthma and allergies by allergist/immunologist
- links to other asthma and allergy related sites

Center for Complementary and Alternative Medicine Research in Asthma
3150B Meyer Hall, University of California, Davis
One Shields Ave., Davis, CA 95616-8669
Phone: (530)752-6575
Fax: (530)752-1297
E-mail: camr@ucdavis.edu
Internet: http://www-camra.ucdavis.edu

- articles on research into alternative medical treatments for asthma and allergies
- links to other asthma and allergy related sites

The Food Allergy Network
10400 Eaton Pl., Ste. 107, Fairfax, VA 22030-2208
Phone: (703)691-3179, toll free: (800)929-4040
Fax: (703)691-2713
E-mail: fan@worldweb.net
Internet: http://www.foodallergy.org

- reports on food allergy research
- frequently asked questions about food allergies
- e-mails food product alerts free
- order pamphlets, videos, posters, and books on food allergy topics at online store

Healthy Kids: The Key to Basics
Eucational Planning for Students with Asthma
and Other Chronic Health Conditions
79 Elmore St., Newton, MA 02159-1137
Phone: (617)965-9637
Fax: (617)965-5407
E-mail: erg_hk@juno.com
Internet: http://www.information-engineer.com/kids//kidshp.htm

Healthy Kids: The Key to Basics, continued

- offers articles and workshops on schools' legal obligations to students with chronic or recurring health problems such as asthma (for parents, health professionals, and schools); topics include indoor air quality in the classroom

International Food Information Council Foundation
1100 Connecticut Ave. NW, Ste. 430, Washington, DC 20036
Phone: (202)296-6540
E-mail: foodinfo@ific.health.org
Internet: http://ificinfo.health.org

- food safety and nutrition information
- brochures: "Everything You Need to Know about Asthma and Food" and "Understanding Food Allergy;" also posters and videos
- publishes *Food Insight* newsletter
- links to other food safety, health, and government sites

JAMA Asthma Information Center
American Medical Association
515 N. State St., Chicago, IL 60610
Phone: (312)464-5000
E-mail: asthma@ama-assn.org
Internet: http://www.ama-assn.org/asthma

- news and statistics
- educational material for patients and parents
- articles from scholarly journals
- asthma treatment guidelines for medical professionals

National Association of School Nurses
P.O. Box 1300, Scarborough, ME 04070-1300
Phone: (207)883-2117
Fax: (207)883-2683
E-mail: nasn@nasn.org
Internet: http://www.nasn.org

- position statement on student use of asthma inhalers in the school
- numerous publications for school nurses on assessing child health including respiratory function
- links to more than 80 government and professional health care sites

National Center for Environmental Health (NCEH)
Centers for Disease Control and Prevention
Mail Stop F-29, 4770 Buford Hwy. NE, Atlanta, GA 30341-3724
Phone: (770)488-7020, toll free: (888)232-6789
E-mail: ncehinfo@cdc.gov
Internet: http://www.cdc.gov/nceh

- asthma statistics
- download "Asthma—A Speaker's Kit for Public Health Professionals" (includes asthma related information and graphics of 62 slides
- download "Asthma Prevention Program of the National Center for Environmental Health, Centers for Disease Control and Prevention, At a Glance 1999"
- links to other asthma related sites

National Heart, Lung, and Blood Institute Information Center (NHLBI)
P.O. Box 30105, Bethesda, MD 20824-0105
Toll Free: (800)575-WELL
Phone: (301)592-8573
Fax: (301)592-8563
E-mail: NHLBIinfo@rover.nhlbi.nih.gov
Internet: http://www.nhlbi.nih.gov

- information on asthma research, physician and patient education, discussion forums
- electronic library
- order or download *Expert Panel Report: Guidelines for the Diagnosis and Management of Asthma*
- articles include "How Asthma-Friendly Is Your School?", "Your Asthma Can Be Controlled: Expect Nothing Less," "Asthma and Physical Activity in the School," and others

National Institute for Occupational Safety and Health (NIOSH)
Information Resources Branch, 4676 Columbia Pkwy., Cincinnati, OH 45226
Phone: (513)533-8326, toll free: (800)356-4674
Fax: (513)533-8573
E-mail: pubstaff@cdc.gov
Internet: http://www.cdc.gov/niosh/homepage.html

- articles on latex allergy, indoor air quality, second-hand smoke, organic dust syndrome, etc.

National Institute of Allergy and Infectious Diseases (NIAID)

Office of Communications and Public Liaison, Bldg. 31, Rm. 7A-50
31 Center Dr. MSC2520, Bethesda, MD 20892-2520
Phone: (301)496-5717
E-mail: niaidoc@flash.niaid.nih.gov
Internet: http://www.niaid.nih.gov

- news and statistics
- fact sheets and brochures on asthma and allergies
- links to other asthma and allergy related sites

National Institute of Environmental Health Sciences (NIEHS)

Office of Communications, P.O. Box 12233, Research Triangle Park,
NC 27709
Phone: (919)541-3345
E-mail: webcenter@niehs.nih.gov
Internet: http://www.niehs.nih.gov

- information on the Environmental Genome Project; other research projects
- facts about environment related diseases (such as asthma) and health risks
- extensive electronic library
- publishes *Environmental Health Perspectives* magazine
- links to other environmental and health sites

National Jewish Medical and Research Center

1400 Jackson St., Denver, CO 80206
Phone: (303)388-4461, LUNG LINE® toll free: (800)222-LUNG (5864)
LUNG FACTS® toll free (taped info): (800)552-LUNG
E-mail: lungline@njc.org
Internet: http://www.njc.org

- phone in asthma and allergy related questions to trained nurses (LUNG LINE® toll free: see above)
- health news; medical scientific updates
- online newsletter
- fact sheets on asthma, allergies, emphysema, and COPD

U.S. Department of Education

Office for Civil Rights, Customer Service Team, Mary E. Switzer Bldg.
330 C St. SW, Washington, DC 20202-1328

Phone: (202)205-5413, toll free: (800)421-3481
Fax: (202)205-9862
E-mail: OCR@ED.Gov
Internet: http://www.ed.gov/offices/OCR

- information on the legal rights of students with disabilities

U.S. Department of Health and Human Services (HHS)
200 Independence Ave. SW, Washington, DC 20201
Phone: (202)619-0257, toll free: (877)696-6775
E-mail: hhsmail@os.dhhs.gov
E-mail: healthfinder@health.org
Internet: http://www.hhs.gov
Internet: http://www.healthfinder.gov

- search both Internet addresses for a multitude of publications and links to asthma and allergy related sites

U.S. Environmental Protection Agency (EPA)
Ariel Rios Bldg., 1200 Pennsylvania Ave. NW, Washington, DC 20460
Phone: (202)260-2090
Indoor Air Quality Information Clearinghouse
Phone toll free: (800)438-4318
E-mail: iaqinfo@aol.com
Internet: http://www.epa.gov/iaq/asthma/index.html
Internet: http://www.epa.gov/airnow/health.html

- first listed Internet address concerns indoor air quality; includes basic facts about asthma, asthma-in-the-home quiz, kid's page, and "IAQ [indoor air quality] Tools for Schools," article about asthma in the classroom, plus links to related sites
- second listed Internet address concerns outdoor air quality and several articles about air pollution; includes several articles: "Smog— Who Does It Hurt?", "Ozone and Your Health," and others

U.S. Food and Drug Administration (FDA)
5600 Fishers Lane, Rm 17-65, Rockville, MD 20857
Phone: (301)827-4420, toll free: (888)INFO-FDA (463-6332)
E-mail: webmail@oc.fda.gov
Internet: http://www.fda.gov

- health advisories
- drug recall bulletins

U.S. Food and Drug Administration (FDA), continued

- publishes *FDA Consumer* magazine (articles on asthma and allergies, food safety, cosmetics, drugs, etc.)

Index

Index

Page numbers followed by 'n' indicate a footnote. Page numbers in *italics* indicate a table or illustration.

A

AAAAI *see* American Academy of Allergy, Asthma and Immunology
AANMA *see* Allergy and Asthma Network-Mothers of Asthmatics, Inc.
AARC Times magazine 574
The ABCs of Safe and Healthy Child Care, "What You Should Know about...Asthma in the Child Care Setting" 481n
Accolate (zafirlukast) 7, 438
ACE inhibitors *see* angiotensin-converting enzyme inhibitors
acetaminophen 28
acetylethyltetramethyltetralin (AETT) 298
ACIP *see* Advisory Committee on Immunization Practices
ACS *see* American Cancer Society
acute, defined 549
acute cough 73
adenoidal hypertrophy 31
adenovirus 226
adrenal gland 549

adrenergics 411–14, 426
Advisory Committee on Immunization Practices (ACIP) 524, 525
aeroallergens 30, 142
Aerobid (flunisolide) 7, 389, 403
AETT *see* acetylethyltetramethyltetralin
African Americans
  asthma 4, 84, 196, 213–15
  asthma health care access 345–62
Afrin (oxymetazoline decongestant spray) 75
age factor
  air pollution 279
  asthma 147–49, 169–85, 423, 507–10
  cardiac asthma 43
  drug safety 379–85
  rhinitis treatment 39–40
agricultural allergens 317–27
Agricultural Research Service (ARS) 301, 302, 303
Air Conditioning, Heating and Refrigeration News, "Don't Force Your Lungs to Clean Your Home's Air" 513n
air pollution
  asthma triggers 6, 17, 86, 481
  respiratory health problems 266–70
  seasonal asthma hospitalizations 137
  vitamins 517–18

air quality index (AQI) 254–55
airway epithelium 16
airway hyperreactivity 217, 310
  see also bronchial hyperreactivity
airway hyperresponsiveness 73, 86, 97
airway inflammation 5, 10, 399
airways 549–50
  cough reflex 69
ALA see American Lung Association
Alabama
  asthma death statistics 122, 124
  self-reported asthma prevalence 134
Alaska
  asthma death statistics 123
  self-reported asthma prevalence
    135
albuterol 7, 19, 375, 376, 383, 407,
    414, 464, 541
  asthma study 223
  pregnancy 503
allele, defined 550
Allerest (oxymetazoline decongestant
    spray) 75
allergens
  allergic rhinitis 30
  asthma triggers 6, 85, 86, 137
  buildings 313
  defined 550
  described 555
  immunotherapy 39
  skin tests 33, 171–72
allergic alveolitis 321
allergic rhinitis 29–30
  defined 550
allergies
  asthma 221, 481, 541
  defined 550–51
  fragrances 297–300
  prevention 236
  symptoms 236
  tests 551
  see also animal allergies
allergists 41, 449
Allergy and Asthma Magazine, "Theophylline" (Gershwin) 397n
Allergy and Asthma Network-Mothers
  of Asthmatics, Inc. (AANMA)
  Asthma Clinical Genetics Network
    209n

Allergy and Asthma Network-Mothers
  of Asthmatics, Inc. (AANMA), continued
  contact information 211, 408, 510,
    573
  metered dose inhaler 407
The Allergy Report, video information
  574
Allergy Respiratory Institute, latex
  allergy 334
allergy shots 433–35
alternative treatments, allergies 435
Alupent (metaproterenol) 7, 414, 503
alupent syrup 384
alveolitis 321
AMA see American Medical Association
Amani, Paris 21
amantadine 526
Ambulatory Oxygen (Petty), chronic
  obstructive pulmonary diseases 50
American Academy of Allergy,
  Asthma and Immunology (AAAAI)
    435
  contact information 408, 510, 573–
    74
  exercise-induced asthma 16
  latex allergy 333
  metered dose inhaler 407
American Academy of Family Physicians, "Chronic Cough" 69n
American Academy of Pediatrics
  chickenpox vaccine 393
  contact information 574
  pediatric and geriatric drug safety
    382
American Association for Respiratory
  Care 50
  contact information 51, 408, 574
American Cancer Society (ACS)
  contact information 237
  energy policies 267
American College of Allergy, Asthma,
  and Immunology, contact information 408, 510, 574–75
American College of Chest Physicians
  contact information 408, 575
  cost-effective treatment 443
  Interleukin-11 and asthma 217n
  risk of asthma death 155n

American College of Chest Physicians, continued
seasonal variation of hospitalizations 137n
American Family Physician, "Chronic
Cough" (Philp) 69n
*American Journal of Health System
Pharmacy* 576
American Journal of Public Health,
asthma and race 213, 214
*American Journal of Respiratory and
Critical Care Medicine* 576
*American Journal of Respiratory Cell
and Molecular Biology* 576
American Lung Association (ALA)
asthma deaths 3–4
asthma sufferers 520
contact information 51, 237, 408,
510, 521, 575
energy policies 268, 269
metered dose inhaler 407
occupational asthma 188
symptom differences 169n
American Lung Association/American
Thoracic Society International Conference 518
American Lung Association of Oregon,
asthma surveillance 118
American Medical Association (AMA)
chronotherapy 479
JAMA Asthma Information Center,
contact information 578
American Medical Products, patented
technology 334
American Pharmaceutical Association,
contact information 409, 575
*American Review of Respiratory Dis-
ease*, asthma and race 213
American Society of Health-System
Pharmacists, contact information
409, 575–76
Americans with Disabilities Act
(1990), occupational asthma 315
American Thoracic Society (ATS)
asthma syndromes 223
contact information 409, 576
occupational asthma 308
spirometric testing 222
spirometry 171

amino acids, defined 551
amoxicillin 504
amoxicillin-clavulanate potassium 75
ampicillin 383
anaphylactic shock 550
anaphylaxis 437
defined 551
food allergy 339–40
latex allergy 330–31
Anderson, Chris 304
Anderson, Henry A. 83n, 94, 95
angioedema, defined 551
angiotensin-converting enzyme inhibitors (ACE inhibitors) 31, 71–73
anhydrous ammonia 310
animal allergies 241–42, 541
occupational asthma 309
pets 241–42, 433
asthma 215
cats 555
defined 567
rhinitis 35
animal studies
endotoxins 325–26
interleukin-11 219
*Annals of Allergy, Asthma, and Im-
munology* 34, 575
antibiotics
allergies 551
asthma 495
defined 551
pregnancy 426, 504
sinusitis 27
anticholinergics 73, 493, 504
asthma study 176
defined 551
rhinitis 38
antidepressants 385
antigens
cockroaches 298
defined 552
antihistamines
breastfeeding 505
combinations 74–75
cough treatment 73
defined 552
pregnancy 504
rhinitis 36
sinusitis 27–28

antihypertensive medications 31
antiinflammatory medications 7, 12, 86
  defined 552
  exercise-induced asthma 18
antileukotriene medications 7, 39
antioxidants 519–21
antipsychotics 385
antireflux barrier, described 54
antitussives 74
Anto, Josep M. 245n, 248
AQI *see* air quality index
arachidonic acid 438
Arden, Nancy 528
Argonne National Laboratory, Advanced Photon Source 198
Arizona
  asthma death statistics 123, 125
  self-reported asthma prevalence 135
Arkansas
  asthma death statistics 122, 124
  self-reported asthma prevalence 134
Arkansas Children's Hospital Research Institute, cockroach antigens 301
ARS *see* Agricultural Research Service
asbestiosis 187
Ashizawa, Annette 97n, 129
Asmacort (triamcinolone) 7, 389
aspartame 339
Aspen Publishers, Inc., asthma health care 345n
aspirin 28, 423
  rhinitis 31
Association of Occupational and Environmental Clinics, occupational asthma 191
astemizole 28, 36
asthma
  causes 195–231
  control programs 89–90
  defined 552
  described 3–4, 53, 84
  diagnosis 6, 11–12, 365–70
  education 367–68, 452–53, 489, 541, 543

asthma, continued
  exercise induced 15–23
  extrinsic 161
    defined 559
  genetic factors 85, 195–201, 203–7, 209–11
  immunologic 308–10
  infectious 221–31
  intervention programs 83–95
  intrinsic 161
    defined 564
  latex allergy 330
  management 443–510
    defined 552
    stepwise 415–27
  nonimmunologic 310
  prevalence 134–35, 151–53
  prevention 86–89
  'quiet part', described 5
  severity classification 417
  statistics 3–4, 83–192, 195, 446–48
  treatment 6–8, 9–13, 86–89, 371–439
"Asthma: A Concern for Minority Populations" 213n
Asthma and Allergy Advocate 574
Asthma and Allergy Foundation of America
  contact information 341, 409, 510, 576
  metered dose inhaler 407
"Asthma and Allergy Prevention" 235n
"Asthma and Physical Activity in the School" 579
"Asthma and the Elderly" (Bethea) 43n
"Asthma - A Speaker's Kit for Public Health Professionals" 579
Asthma Clinical Genetics Network, clinical tests for asthma 210
"Asthma Genetics: The Human Genome Project" 203n
AsthmaHaler 412, 414
Asthma in America 151, 153
"Asthma in America: Executive Summary" 151n
"Asthma in America: Missing the Mark" 151n
Asthma Magazine 575

Asthma Management Kit for Clinicians
"Check Your Asthma I.Q." 470
"Teach Your Patients about Asthma: A Clinician's Guide" 470
"Your Asthma Can Be Controlled: Expect Nothing Less" 470
Asthma Management Module 576
AsthmaNefrin 412, 414
"Asthma Prevention Program of the National Center for Environmental Health..." 579
asymptomatic, defined 552
athletes
exercised-induced asthma (EIA) 15–23
rhinitis 40
atopic dermatitis 157
atopy, defined 552
Atrovent (ipratropium) 73
ATS *see* American Thoracic Society
Augmentin (amoxicillin-clavulanate potassium) 75
auralgan otic solution 383
Axid (nizatidine) 58
azelastine 37
azole antifungals 36

B

"Backgrounder - Food Allergy/ Asthma" 337n
bacteria
defined 553
endotoxins 323
Bactrim (trimethorprim-sulfamethoxazole) 75
Ball, Lauren B. 97n, 129
Barbee, Robert A. 471
Bardana, Emil J., Jr. 307n, 315
barium enemas, latex allergy 330
barium esophogram, gastroesophageal reflux 57
bark stripper's disease 320, 321
Barrett's esophagus, gastroesophageal reflux 55
Bartsokas, Tom W. 21
Bartter, Thaddeus 443n
basophils, defined 553

Bassett, David 283
B-cells (B-lymphocytes), defined 553–54
Beatrix Children's Hospital (Netherlands) 210
Becklake, Margaret 190, 191, 322
beclomethasone dipropionate 20, 27, 38, 372, 389, 400–401, 421, 504
Beconase (beclomethasone) 27, 389
Beconase AQ (beclomethasone) 27, 504
Beeten, Bob 21
Behavioral Risk Factor Survey (BRFSS)
asthma studies 88, 118–20, 133
Benson, Veronica 147n
benzoates 339
beta-adrenergic receptor agonists, defined 554
beta-adrenergic receptors, chronic cough 73
beta agonists 403, 463, 464, 491–94, 541
asthma study 176
chronic bronchitis 74
chronic cough treatment 76
exercise-induced asthma 18–20
pregnancy 503
beta blockers 31, 73, 424
bethanechol 59
Bethea, Louise H. 43n, 44, 485n, 576–77
bile salts 54
biological rhythms 477–79
biomarkers, asthma 85
bitolterol 414, 464, 503
Blaese, Michael 200, 201
Blair, Joan 471
BLS *see* Bureau of Labor Statistics
Boodram, B. 131n, 136
Boothwyn Heating and Air Conditioning, home air cleaners 514
breastfeeding, allergies 505
breathing retraining 47, 533–35
breathing tests
flow volume loop 66
pulmonary function tests (PFT) 18, 74, 156–58, 222–23
see also tests
Brenner, Richard 302, 303, 305

Brethaire (terbutaline) 7, 414, 503
BRFSS *see* Behavioral Risk Factor Survey
Bricanyl (terbutaline) 503
Bridges, Betty 297n, 300
British Thoracic Society, death from asthma 446
brompheniramine 27, 426
bronchial hyperreactivity 399
  see also airway hyperreactivity
bronchioles, defined 554
bronchitis 17
  asthma 221
  chronic 73–74, 137, 321, 366
  chronic obstructive pulmonary disease 45
  defined 554
  hospitalizations 137–45
bronchodilators 158, 227, 314, 388, 521
  adrenergic 411–14
  asthma therapy 5, 310
  chronic bronchitis 73, 74
  chronic obstructive pulmonary disease 46–47
  defined 554
  side effects 413
bronchoprovocation 314
bronchospasm 218, 402
  described 5
  exercise induced 424
bronchus, defined 555
Bronkaid 412, 414
Bronkometer (isoetharine) 414
Brown, Clive M. 83n, 94, 95
budesonide 38, 372, 373, 400
Buist, A. Sonia 137n, 169n
Bureau of Labor Statistics (BLS), asthma in the workplace 187
Business News Publishing Co., home air cleaners 513n
Buxton, Ted 471
byssinosis 187, 320, 323–24

C

California
  asthma death statistics 123, 125
  self-reported asthma prevalence 135

Carafate (sucralfate) 76
carbon monoxide 269–70
cardiac asthma, emphysema 43–44
CARM *see* conservative anti-reflux measures
Castellan, Robert M. 319, 323, 324, 326
Castranova, Vincent 320, 321, 324, 325, 326
cat allergy *see* animal allergies
cationic molecules 218
causal factors, defined 555
causes of death
  asthma 4, 84, 112–15, 155–67, 195, 447–48
  childhood asthma 343–44
  latex allergy 330
  workplace 187
CDC *see* Centers for Disease Control and Prevention
Cell 197
Center for Biologics Evaluation and Research, cockroach antigens 303
Center for Environmental Health, asthma control program 89
Centers for Disease Control and Prevention (CDC)
  allergy receptor 197
  asthma control program 89
  asthma surveillance survey 84, 87, 97n, 117, 119
  breathing method 534
  child care setting 481n
  clinical guidelines 90
  flu vaccine 526
  health survey 147n
  latex allergy 330, 331
  Office on Smoking and Health, contact information 294
  prevalence by state 131
cephalosporin 75
cetirizine 36
CFC *see* chlorofluorocarbons
Chakravarti, Aravinda 200
"Challenges for Parents of Asthmatics: Barriers to Cooperation at School; Part 1" (Bethea) 485n
"The Changing Face of Respiratory Illness" (Minter) 187n

Check Your Asthma "I.Q". 470
chemicals, occupational asthma 309
Chest 575
　"Asthma: Better Outcome at Lower
　　Cost? The Role of the Expert in
　　the Care System" (Bartter, et
　　al.) 443n
　"Asthma-Associated Viruses Specifi-
　　cally Induce Lung Stromal Cells
　　to Produce Interleukin-11,
　　..."(Einarsson, et al.) 217n
　"Health-Care Reform and Pulmo-
　　nary/Critical Care Medicine: A
　　Revolution with or without
　　Data" (McDonald, et al.) 453
　latex allergy 334
　"Mortality and Markers of Risk of
　　Asthma Death among 1,075
　　Outpatients with Asthma"
　　(Ulrik, et al.) 155n
　"Periodicity of Asthma, Emphy-
　　sema, and Chronic Bronchitis in
　　a Northwest..."(Osborne, et al.)
　　137n
chest physiotherapy 47
chickenpox *see* varicella
children
　asthma 4, 84, 196
　　diagnosis 365–70
　　management 481–88
　　medications 372–73
　　risk factors 343–44
　　study 170–71, 214
　　treatment 418–19
　corticosteroids 393
　environmental tobacco smoke 286–
　　88, 291
　ozone levels 252
　rhinitis 35–36
　　treatment 39–40
　sinus passages 25
Children's Hospital of Wisconsin
　asthma surveillance 117
　latex allergy 330
Children's National Medical Center
　(Washington, DC), latex allergy 331
Chlamydia pneumoniae 226
chloramphenicol 380–81
chloride 310

chlorine 310
chlorofluorocarbons (CFC) 405–9
chlorpheniramine 27, 504
chlorpromazine 31
Chlor-Trimeton (chlorpheniramine)
　504
cholinergic hyperactivity 218
chronic, defined 555
chronic bronchitis 73–74, 137, 321, 366
　corticosteroids 388
　see also bronchitis
*The Chronic Bronchitis and Emphy-
　sema Handbook* (Haas) 50
chronic cough *see* coughing
chronic obstructive pulmonary dis-
　ease (COPD) 45–51, 141
　versus asthma 116, 179, 228
　corticosteroids 388
　symptoms 48–49
　treatment 45–48
chronotherapy 477–79
cigarette smoke *see* environmental to-
　bacco smoke
cimetidine 58
ciprofloxacin 36
　pregnancy 426
circadian rhythm 477
cisapride 59, 76
clarithromycin 36
Claritin (loratadine) 28
Clean Air Act (1970) 254, 266, 268, 271
Cliggott Publishing Co., rhinitis pub-
　lication 29n
coal worker's pneumoconiosis 187
Cockrell, G. 306
cockroaches 237–38, 301–6
　allergies 35, 541
　asthma 84, 86, 215
　see also insect allergens
Colorado
　asthma death statistics 123, 125
　self-reported asthma prevalence 135
congestive heart failure, chronic
　cough 70, 71, 74
Connecticut
　asthma death statistics 121, 124
　self-reported asthma prevalence 134
conservative anti-reflux measures
　(CARM) 57–58

Consultant
"Rhinitis Update: A Guide to Diagnosis" (Dykewicz) 29n
"Rhinitis Update: A Guide to Treatment" (Dykewicz) 29n
Consumer Product Safety Commission (CPSC), fragrances and health 299
Consumer Reports Books, chronic obstructive pulmonary diseases 50
contributing factors, defined 555
"Controlling Your Asthma" 575
Cookson, William 196
COPD *see* chronic obstructive pulmonary disease
Cornish, Katrina 334
corticosteroids 155, 314, 387–95, 463, 503
 asthma study 176
 cough treatment 76
 defined 555–56
 exercise-induced asthma 20
 listed 7
 rhinitis 36, 37
 rhinitis medicamentosa 40–41
 side effects 392–93
 sinusitis 26, 27
 see also steroids
cortisol 387
cotton dust 321–23, 327
coughing
 acute 73
 chronic 69–80
cough reflex, described 69
Council of State and Territorial Epidemiologists (CSTE), asthma surveillance survey 84, 87, 117
Council on Environmental Quality, energy policies 268
counseling, vocal cord dysfunction 66–67
CPSC *see* Consumer Product Safety Commission
Creer, Thomas 535
Creticos, Peter 21
cromolyn sodium 19–20, 38, 76, 176, 314, 374, 418, 419, 425–26, 463, 503, 540
crural diaphragm 54

CSTE *see* Council of State and Territorial Epidemiologists
Cunningham, Joan 214
"Current Estimates from the National Health Interview Survey, 1995" (Benson, et al.) 147n
Cushing's syndrome 560
cytokines 217, 323
 defined 556

D

dander 433, 541
 see also animal allergies
D'Andrea, Tom 514, 515
Danish Death Register 158
Danish National Board of Health
 death certificates 158
 published statistics 160
Danish Personal Identity Register 158
death certificates, asthma 155
decongestants
 defined 556
 pregnancy 426, 504
 rhinitis 37
 sinusitis 27
 see also antihistamines
Delaware
 asthma death statistics 122, 124
 self-reported asthma prevalence 134
Dennie-Morgan lines 33
deoxyribonucleic acid (DNA), defined 557
D'Epiro, Nancy Walsh 329n
dermatitis, latex allergy 332
desensitization therapy, defined 556
deviated septum 31
Dewey, Jackie 50
dexamethasone sodium phosphate 38
DHHS *see* US Department of Health and Human Services
diagnostic techniques, defined 556–57
diaphragmatic breathing 47
diet and nutrition, chronic obstructive pulmonary disease 46

Disabella, Vincent 537n, 545
District of Columbia (Washington, DC)
  asthma death statistics 122, 124
  self-reported asthma prevalence 134
diuretics 44
DNA *see* deoxyribonucleic acid
Dockery, Douglas W. 214, 215
DOE *see* US Department of Energy
dog allergy *see* animal allergies
Dowden Publishing Co. 221n
Drazen, Jeffrey 199, 201
Dristan (oxymetazoline decongestant spray) 75
drug abuse 313
drug allergy, defined 557
dry powder inhalers 19
Duke University Medical Center (Durham, NC) 210
dust 240
  agricultural 318–20
  defined 557
  gravimetric 324
  see also house dust; organic dust
dust mites 171–72, 238, 433, 541
  asthma 84, 86, 215
  defined 557
  rhinitis 34–35
  see also insect allergens
Dykewicz, Mark S. 29n, 41

E

eczema 157
edema, defined 557
education, asthma 367–68, 452–53, 489, 541, 543
Eggleston, P. 306
EIA *see* exercise-induced asthma
Einarsson, Oskar 217n, 220
Elias, Jack A. 217n, 220
emergency action plan
  asthma 496
  chronic obstructive pulmonary disease 49
emergency departments, asthma attacks 100, 102, 108–9, 444, 489–99

emphysema
  asthma 366
  cardiac asthma 43–44
  chronic obstructive pulmonary disease 45
  hospitalizations 137–45
endoscopy
  gastroesophageal reflux 57
  rhinitis diagnosis 33
endothelial cells 399
endotoxins 319, 323–26
  asthma 215
Energy Information Administration 271
energy policies, public health 265–83
Enjoying Life with Emphysema (Petty, et al.) 50
environmental control
  defined 557
  rhinitis treatment 34–35
environmental factors
  chronic bronchitis 74
  exercise-induced asthma 17
  genetic studies 85, 195
Environmental Genome Project 203, 204, 205, 207
"Environmental Genome Project Overview" 203n
Environmental Health Perspectives 580
  "Allergy Receptor Pictured" 195n
  "Asthma Gene Is Nothing to Sneeze At" 195n
  "Focus: Danger in the Dust" (Lang) 317n
  "Fragrances and Health" (Bridges) 297n
  "Genes and Ozone" 195n
  "Latex Allergies Stretch beyond Rubber Gloves" 329n
  "The Question of Asthma and Race" 213n
  "Working the Bugs Out of Asthma" (Potera) 301n
environmental response gene, defined 557
environmental tobacco smoke (ETS) 236–37, 481
  allergies 236–37
  asthma 17, 85, 86, 195, 312, 481
  see also tobacco use

eosinophils 30, 161, 218, 310, 399
    defined 558
    respiratory health effects 285–95
EPA *see* US Environmental Protection Agency
epinephrine 376, 412, 414, 423, 426
    defined 558
epitope, defined 558
erthromycin 36
Ervin, Christine A. 265n, 283
esophageal cancer, gastroesophageal reflux 55
esophageal manometry, gastroesophageal reflux 57
esophagus, gastroesophageal reflux 54
    see also gastroesophageal reflux
estrogen, asthma 529–31
ethnography, described 348
etiology, defined 558
ETS *see* environmental tobacco smoke
Etzel, Ruth A. 83n, 94, 95
European Federation of Asthma and Allergy Associations, contact information 409
"Everything You Need to Know about Asthma and Food" 337n, 578
exacerbation, defined 558
exercise
    chronic bronchitis 74
    ozone levels 256–57
exercise-induced asthma (EIA) 6, 15–23, 424, 481, 538–40
    diagnosis 18
    treatment 18–21
exercises, asthma 537–45
Expert Panel Report: Guidelines for the Diagnosis and Management of Asthma 579
Expert Panel Report 2: Guidelines for the Diagnosis and Management of Asthma 365n, 371n
    asthma management guidelines 470
    controlling asthma 489n
    management of symptoms 415n
    peak flow monitoring 473n
    "Practical and Effective Asthma Care" 9n

Expert Panel Report 2: Guidelines for the Diagnosis and Management of Asthma, continued
    recommendations 11–12
    role of the pharmacist 462
    use your inhaler effectively 429n
extrinsic asthma 161
    defined 559

F

Facts about Asthma 471
"Fact Sheet: Health and Environmental Effects of Ground-Level Ozone" 249n
Family and Community Health, "Access to Health Care: Perspectives of African American Families with...(Peterson, et al.) 345n
family issues, asthma 345–62
famotidine 58
farmer's lung disease 320, 321
farming allergies 317–27
fatigue, chronic obstructive pulmonary disease 48–49
FDA *see* US Food and Drug Administration
FDA Consumer 582
    "Controlling Asthma" (Flieger) 3n
    "How to Avoid the Flu" (Zamula) 523n
    "How to Take Your Medicines: Adrenergic Bronchodilators (Inhaled)" (Williams) 411n
    "Pediatric Drug Studies: Protecting Pint-Sized Patients" (Nordenberg) 379n
    "A Time to Heal: Chronotherapy Tunes in to Body's Rhythms" (Stehlin) 477n
FDA Modernization Act (1997) 382
Federal Register, pediatric and geriatric drug study 380
feline allergy *see* animal allergies
Ferrell, M. Craig 21
FEV *see* forced expiratory volume
fexofenadine 36, 40
financial concerns, asthma management 53, 443–59

Flieger, Ken 3n, 8
Florida
 asthma death statistics 122, 124
 self-reported asthma prevalence
  134
Flovent 7
fluconazole 36
Flumadine (rimantadine) 526–27
flunisolide 20, 27, 38, 372, 373, 389,
 402–3
fluticasone 38, 372, 373
fluticasone propionate 20
food allergies 238–39, 433
 asthma 337–41
 defined 559
 diagnosis 340
 latex allergy 332
 occupational asthma 309
Food Allergy Network, contact information 341, 577
Food Insight 578
food intolerance, defined 559
forced expiratory volume (FEV)
 endotoxins 324
 in one second (FEV_1) 16, 425, 445,
  495
  asthma diagnosis 366
  asthma studies 156–58, 161–63,
   174, 180, 224–26, 228
  chronic cough 75
forced vital capacity (FVC), chronic
 cough 75
Forest Pharmaceuticals, asthma inhalation therapy 403
Fragranced Products Information
 Network, web site 300
fragrances 297–300
Frederiksberg Hospital 156, 158
Frederiksen, Jens 155n
Fulwood, Robinson 471
Furukawa, Clifton T. 21
FVC *see* forced vital capacity

G

Ganley, Charles 384
Garman, Scott 197
gastric acid 54

gastroesophageal reflux (GER)
 asthma 53–63
 diagnosis 56–57
 symptoms 56
 treatment 57–60
"Gastroesophageal Reflux: A Common
 Exacerbating Factor in Adult
 Asthma" (Sullivan, et al.) 53n
gastrointestinal (GI), defined 559
gastrointestinal reflux disease
 (GERD)
 treatment 76
Geba, Gregory P. 217n, 220
gender factor, asthma 169–85
genes, defined 559
genetic, defined 560
genetic factors, asthma 85, 195–201,
 203–7, 209–11
genetic predisposition, defined 560
genome projects 203–7
Georgia
 asthma death statistics 122, 124
 self-reported asthma prevalence
  134
GER *see* gastroesophageal reflux
GERD *see* gastrointestinal reflux disease
Gergen, Peter 214
geriatric drug safety 384–85
Gershwin, M. Eric 397n, 398
"Getting Your Asthma under Control:
 A Self-Evaluation" 575
GI *see* gastrointestinal
Glaxo Wellcome
 Asthma Clinical Genetics Network
  209
 asthma patients survey 151n, 152
 clinical genetics network 211
 clinical tests for asthma 210
 exercise-induced asthma 22
Glindmeyer, Henry 321, 322
glucocorticoids 400, 541
 defined 560
glycoprotein, defined 560
Goldberg, Wendy 379, 381
Gould Medical Products, Inc. 222–23
grain fever 320
granulocyte colony-stimulating factor
 399, 556

grass pollens 239–40, 433
gravimetric dust 324
Groningen University Hospital
 (Netherlands) 210
*Guide to Your Child's Allergies and
 Asthma* 574

H

Haas, Francois 50
Haas, Sheila Sperber 50
Hahn, David L. 221n
hapten, defined 560
Harber, Philip 307n, 315
Harris, Gale 471
Harvard Medical School
 allergy receptor 197
 energy policies 267
Harvard School of Public Health, en-
 ergy policies 269, 278
Hatch, Gary 520
Hawaii
 asthma death statistics 123
 self-reported asthma prevalence
  135
health care workers
 latex allergy 329–30
HealthInfo Center 50
Healthline Publishing Inc. 397n
health maintenance organizations
 (HMO)
 asthma 346
 asthma study 170, 179
Healthy Kids: The Key to Basics, con-
 tact information 577–78
Healthy People 2000
 asthma surveillance 84
 National Health Promotion and
  Disease Prevention Objectives
  91
HEDIS, asthma studies 88
Helm, Ricki 304, 306
Helms, Peter 210
helper T-cells, defined 560
Hendeles, Leslie 471
Henry Ford Hospital (Detroit, MI) 330
HEPA *see* high-efficiency particulate
 arrestance

heredity
 asthma 209
 defined 560
 see also genetic factors
Hevea brasiliensis 329
HHS *see* US Department of Health
 and Human Services
hiatal hernia, gastroesophageal reflux 55, 57
high-efficiency particulate arrestance
 (HEPA) filters 514
Hipkins, Sharon 201
Hippokration General Hospital
 (Greece) 210
Hismanal (astemizole) 28
histamine antagonists 74–75
histamine-receptor antagonists 58
histamines
 asthma 338, 399
 defined 560–61
hives *see* urticaria
HMO *see* health maintenance organizations
Homa, David M. 97n, 129
home care
 air cleaners 513–15
 asthma attacks 489–99
Hopkin, Julian 196
hormones
 defined 561
 nonallergic rhinitis 31
hospitalizations
 asthma attacks 100, 102–3, 110–11,
  444, 489–99
  seasonal variations 137–45
 asthma study 176–77
 bronchitis 137–45
 emphysema 137–45
Hospital Practice (Martin) 478
house dust 240, 541
 see also dust; organic dust
house dust mites *see* dust mites
"How Asthma-Friendly Is Your
 School?" 485n, 579
Human Genome Project 203–4, 206
humidity levels 142, 541
hymenoptera, defined 561
hyperemia 16
hyperosmolarity 16

hypersensitivity, defined 561
hypersensitivity pneumonitis 321, 326
hypertrophy
  adenoidal 31
  tonsillar 33

I

IAQ INFO *see* Indoor Air Quality Information Clearinghouse
"IAQ (indoor air quality) Tools for Schools" 581
ibuprofen 28
ICD see *International Classification of Diseases*
Idaho
  asthma death statistics 123
  self-reported asthma prevalence 135
IgE *see* immunoglobulin E
IL-4 *see* interleukin-4
IL-11 *see* interleukin-11
Illinois
  asthma death statistics 121, 124
  self-reported asthma prevalence 134
imaging techniques, rhinitis diagnosis 33
immune globulin 393
immune system
  corticosteroids 393
  defined 561–62
  endotoxins 323
  sinuses 25
immunizations, chronic bronchitis 74
  see also vaccines
immunoglobulin E (IgE)
  asthma 195, 197–99, 338
  defined 562
  pulmonary function tests 157
  rhinitis 33
immunologic asthma 308–10
immunologists 41
Immunology and Allergy Clinics of North America 343n
immunotherapy 433–35, 541–42
  defined 562
  pregnancy 426, 504
  rhinitis 39

incidence, defined 562
income levels
  asthma 84, 147–49, 214
Indiana
  asthma death statistics 121, 124
  self-reported asthma prevalence 134
Indoor Air Quality Information Clearinghouse (IAQ INFO) 294
Industries of the Future program 274
infections
  asthma 142
  chronic obstructive pulmonary disease 46
infectious asthma 221–31
"Infectious Asthma: A Reemerging Clinical Entity?" (Hahn) 221n
inflammation, defined 562–63
inflammatory cells 399
influenza immunizations 74
influenza vaccine 504, 523–28
infradian rhythm 477
inhalation therapy 399–404
inhalers 7, 429–32
  exercise-induced asthma 19
  see also dry powder inhalers; metered dose inhalers
insect allergens 319
  rhinitis 35
insect sting allergy 433
  defined 563
Intal (cromolyn) 76, 314, 383, 503
interaction, defined 563
interferons 556
  defined 563
interleukin-4 (IL-4), asthma studies 215
interleukin-11 (IL-11), asthma 217–20
interleukins 399, 556
  defined 563–64
International Classification of Diseases
  ambulatory medical care 100
  asthma surveillance 117
  causes of death 158
  changes in codes 103, 116
  coding practices 164
  hospital discharge diagnosis 138
  mortality 101
  seasonal patterns 141

International Food Information
Council Foundation
contact information 578
food and asthma 337n
International Fragrance Association
298
International Pharmaceutical Aerosol
Consortium
contact information 409
metered dose inhaler 405n, 407
intrinsic asthma 161
defined 564
iodides, pregnancy 426
Iowa
asthma death statistics 121
self-reported asthma prevalence 134
ipratropium bromide 19–20, 73, 376,
541
isoetharine 414
"Isolation and characterization of a
clone encoding a major
allergen"...(Helm, et al.) 306
isoproterenol 170, 414
Isuprel (isoproterenol) 414
itraconazole 36

J

Jack, Elizabeth 97n, 129
JAMA Asthma Information Center,
contact information 578
Jardetzky, Theodore S. 197, 198, 199
Johnson, Carol A. 97n, 129
Joint Task Force on Practice Param-
eters in Allergy, Asthma, and Im-
munology 34
*Journal of Allergy and Clinical Im-
munology* 334
*Journal of Clinical Pharmacology
and Therapeutics* 5
Journal of Psychosomatic Medicine
535
Joyner, David M. 15n, 21, 23

K

Kaarsberg, Tina 283

Kaiser Permanente
seasonal variation of hospitaliza-
tions 138
symptom differences 170
Kang, David S. 97n, 129
Kansas
asthma death statistics 121, 124
self-reported asthma prevalence
134
Kattan, M. 306
Katz, Roger M. 21
Kelly, H. W. 5, 471
Kelly, Kevin J. 329, 330, 331, 332,
333
Kentucky
asthma death statistics 122, 124
self-reported asthma prevalence
134
Kinet, Jean-Pierre 197, 199
Kleeberger, Steven 200, 201
Knight, Kenneth 21
Koenig, Jane 517
Kotses, Harry 533, 534, 535
Kovner, David 283
Kruse, Roger 21

L

Lambert, Lark 299
Lancet Ltd., contact information 245n
Landry, George L. 21
Landry, Mary 217n, 220
Lang, Leslie 317n, 327
lansoprazole 59
laparoscope, gastroesophageal reflux
treatment 60
laryngoscopy, vocal cord dysfunction
66
latex, defined 564
latex allergy 329–36
defined 564
Lea & Febiger 50
legislation
Americans with Disabilities Act
(1990) 315
Clean Air Act (1970) 254, 266, 268,
271
FDA Modernization Act (1997) 382

legislation, continued
  Omnibus Budget and Reconciliation Act (1990) 462
  Rehabilitation Act 488
Lehtinen, John L. 21
Leikauf, George 200
Lenfant, Claude 461n
leukocytes (white blood cells), defined 564–65
  see also basophils; eosinophils; lymphocytes; neutrophils
leukotriene 375, 399, 437
  defined 565
  see also anti-leukotriene medications
Linton, Kathryn P. 169n
lipid A 323
Living Well with Chronic Asthma, Bronchitis, and Emphysema (Shayevitz) 50
"Living with Asthma: Special Concerns for Older Adults" 507n
Lockey, James E. 307n, 315
Lomax, Reuben 21
"Long-Term Hope for Asthma Sufferers Lies in Their Genes: Glaxo Wellcome Establishes Asthma Clinical Genetics Network" 209n
Lopez, Jean 21
loratadine 28, 36, 40
lotrinsone cream 383
Louisiana
  asthma death statistics 122, 125
  self-reported asthma prevalence 134
LUNG LINE
  contact information 51, 434, 580
  COPD resource 50
lymphocytes 321, 399
  defined 565
lymphokines 556
lysis 323

M

macrolides 36
macrophages 399
  defined 565

Maine
  asthma death statistics 121
  self-reported asthma prevalence 134
"Management of Chronic Obstructive Pulmonary Disease" 45n
Mannino, David M. 97n, 129
Marano, Marie A. 147n
marijuana 313
Martin, Richard 478
Maryland
  asthma death statistics 122, 125
  self-reported asthma prevalence 134
Massachusetts
  asthma death statistics 121, 124
  self-reported asthma prevalence 134
mast cells
  asthma 338, 399
  defined 565–66
Material Safety Data Sheets (MSDS) 313
Maxair (pirbuterol) 414, 503
McFadden, E. R., Jr. 21
McGraw-Hill Companies, Inc.
  asthma publication 15n
  exercise for asthma patients 537n
McRorie, Teresa 471
MDI *see* metered dose inhalers
"Med Facts: Adult Peak Flow Monitoring" 473n
"Med Facts: Asthma and Pregnancy" 501n
"Med Facts: Corticosteroids" 387n
"Med Facts: Immunotherapy (Allergy Shots)" 433n
"Med Facts: Sinusitis" 25n
"Med Facts: Use of the Chickenpox Vaccine in Children" 387n
mediator, defined 566
Medicaid
  asthma health care 347
  asthma studies 88
  asthma surveillance survey 88, 118
  clinical guidelines 91
Medical Devices Bureau, latex allergy 333
Medical Economics Publishing Co.
  estrogen fluctuation 529n
  latex allergy 329n
  occupational asthma 307n

Medical Sciences Bulletin
  "Asthma Inhalation Therapy" 399n
  "Focus on...New Receptor Antago-
    nists" 437n
Medicare, asthma surveillance 118
medications
  asthma treatment 6–8, 371–78
    pregnancy 502–4
  gastroesophageal reflux treatment
    58–59
  see also pharmacists
MediHaler-Epi 414
Medihaler-Iso (isoproterenol) 414
Medline 443
Medrol 7
Merchant, James 318, 322
Merck, leukotriene receptor 438
Metaprel (metaproterenol) 7, 503
metaproterenol 7, 19, 414, 503
metered dose inhalers (MDI) 19, 169,
  171, 177–78, 181–82, 401–4, 494
  bronchodilators 411
  children 418–19
  chlorofluorocarbons 405–9
  effective use 429–32, 465–67
methacholine 76, 219
methyldopa 31
methylprednisolone 374, 376
metoclopramide 59, 76
Meyer, Robert 5
Michigan
  asthma death statistics 121, 124
  self-reported asthma prevalence
    134
Michigan Department of Community
  Health, Michigan Inpatient Discharge Database 117
Michocki, Robert 384, 385
miconazole 36
mill fever 323
Minnesota
  asthma death statistics 121
  self-reported asthma prevalence
    134
Minter, Stephen G. 187n
Mississippi
  asthma death statistics 122, 125
  self-reported asthma prevalence
    134

Missouri
  asthma death statistics 121, 124
  self-reported asthma prevalence 134
*MMWR see Morbidity and Mortality
  Weekly Review*
mold, defined 566
mold allergy, defined 566
molds
  asthma 215, 491
  rhinitis 34
mold spores 240–41
mometasone 38
monoclonal antibodies, defined 566
Montaluo, David 21
Montana
  asthma death statistics 123
  self-reported asthma prevalence
    135
montelukast 7, 438
Montreal Protocol (1987)
  information 408
  metered dose inhaler 406
*Morbidity and Mortality Weekly Re-
  view* (MMWR)
  "Forecasted State-Specific Esti-
    mates of Self-Reported
    Asthma..." (Rappaport, et al.)
    131n
  "Surveillance for Asthma - United
    States, 1960-1995" (Mannino, et
    al.) 97n
Mosby Year Book 50
Moser, Kenneth M. 50
Mothers of Asthmatics 487
  see also Allergy and Asthma Net-
    work-Mothers of Asthmatics, Inc.
mucus
  asthma 5
  gastroesophageal reflux 54
  sinuses 25
mushroom worker's lung disease 321
musk compounds 298
Mycoplasma pneumoniae 226

N

NAEPP *see* National Asthma Education and Prevention Program

Nasacort (triamcinolone) 27
nasal congestion 29, 36
Nasalcrom (cromolyn) 76, 504
nasal cytology 33
Nasalide (flunisolide) 27
nasal polyps 31–32
nasal saline wash 26, 504
nasal sprays
  chronic cough treatment 75
  sinusitis 24, 27
National Advisory Environmental
  Health Sciences Council 204
National Association of School
  Nurses, contact information 409,
  578
National Asthma Education and Prevention Program (NAEPP)
  asthma and aging 507n
  asthma assessment 75
  contact information 409
  managing asthma at school 485n
  metered dose inhaler 405n, 407
  publications 470
  role of the pharmacist 461, 462
"National Asthma Education Panel
  Expert Report" 53
National Asthma Education Program
  chronic cough 75
  clinical guidelines 90
  Expert Panel Guidelines 171
National Cancer Institute (NCI), contact information 295
National Center for Environmental
  Health (NCEH), contact information 579
National Center for Health Statistics
  (NCHS)
  asthma surveillance 120
  genetics of asthma 197
  health survey 147n
  National Ambulatory Medical Care
    Survey (NAMCS) 99
    emergency departments 100
  National Health Interview Survey
    (NHIS) 99, 120
  National Hospital Discharge Survey
    100
    asthma 106
  prevalence by state 132, 134–35

National Center for Infectious Diseases 481n
National Health Interview Survey
  (NHIS) 131–32, 147, 148
National Heart, Lung, and Blood Institute (NHLBI)
  asthma
    aging 507n
    assessment and diagnosis 365n
    control 489n, 542
    genetic basis 215
    goals 153
    patients survey 152
    surveillance 85
  contact information 51, 295, 510,
    579
  inhaled medications 540
  inhaler use 429n
  management of systems 415n
  managing asthma at school 485n
  metered dose inhaler 405n
  National Asthma Education Pro-
    gram 90
  peak flow monitoring 473n
  "Practical and Effective Asthma
    Care" 9n
  role of the pharmacist 461n
National Hospital Discharge Survey
  141
National Institute for Occupational
  Safety and Health (NIOSH)
  agricultural allergens 320, 327
  contact information 295, 579
  dust diseases 191
  occupational asthma 192
National Institute of Allergy and Infectious Diseases (NIAID)
  allergy receptor 197
  contact information 580
  genetic basis of asthma 215
  genetics of asthma 196
National Institute of Environmental
  Health Sciences (NIEHS)
  agricultural allergens 317n
  asthma and race 213n
  cockroach antigens 301n
  contact information 580
  Environmental Genome Project
    203, 204, 205, 207

601

National Institute of Environmental Health Sciences (NIEHS), continued
fragrances and health 297n
genetics of asthma 195n
latex allergy 329n
targeting asthma triggers 235n
National Institutes of Health (NIH)
asthma patients survey 152
Environmental Genome Project 203
food and asthma 337
genetics of asthma 197
latex allergy 329n
National Jewish Medical and Research Center
allergy shots 433n
asthma and pregnancy 501n
chickenpox vaccine 393
chronic obstructive pulmonary diseases publications 50
chronic obstructive pulmonary disease treatment 45
chronotherapy 479
contact information 51, 510, 580
corticosteroid nasal spray 27
corticosteroid preparations 388, 390
corticosteroids 387n
corticosteroids research 394, 395
LUNG LINE information 50, 51, 434, 580
"Med Facts: Sinusitis 25n
peak flow monitoring 473n
sinusitis as trigger of asthma 28
sinusitis treatment 26
"Vocal Cord Dysfunction" 65n
vocal cord dysfunction research 67
National Jewish Medical and Research Center 47
National Research Council (NRC), passive smoking 286, 289, 290
Natural Resources Defense Counsel (NRDC), energy policies 267–68
Nature Genetics 196, 200
NCEH *see* National Center for Environmental Health
NCHS *see* National Center for Health Statistics
NCI *see* National Cancer Institute

Nebraska
asthma death statistics 121
self-reported asthma prevalence 134
nebulizers 406
children 419
nedocromil sodium 19–20, 374, 395, 418, 419, 425–26, 463, 503, 540
Nelson, Harold S. 21
Nett, Louise M. 50
neurotoxins *see* acetylethyltetramethyltetralin
neutrophils 321, 553
defined 566–67
Nevada
asthma death statistics 123
self-reported asthma prevalence 135
New England Journal of Medicine
cockroach antigens 304
"The role of cockroach allergy and exposure to cockroach allergen..." (Rosenstreich) 306
New Hampshire
asthma death statistics 121
self-reported asthma prevalence 134
New Jersey
asthma death statistics 121, 124
self-reported asthma prevalence 134
New Mexico
asthma death statistics 123
self-reported asthma prevalence 135
"New Training Method Helps Reduce Asthma Attacks" 533n
New York state
asthma death statistics 121, 124
self-reported asthma prevalence 134
NHIS *see* National Health Interview Survey
NHLBI *see* National Heart, Lung, and Blood Institute
NIAID *see* National Institute of Allergy and Infectious Diseases
Nicotine Anonymous, contact information 237
NIEHS *see* National Institute of Environmental Health Sciences

NIH *see* National Institutes of Health

NIOSH *see* National Institute for Occupational Safety and Health

NIOSH Alert

agricultural allergens 327

Preventing Allergic Reactions to Natural Rubber Latex in the Workplace" 329n

Nissen fundoplication 60

nitrates 339

nitrites 339

nitrogen dioxide, asthma 17, 245–48

"Nitrogen Dioxide and Allergic Asthma: Starting to Clarify an Obscure Association" (Anto, et al.) 245n

Nixon, Leah L. 97n, 129

nizatidine 58

nonallergic rhinitis

with eosinophilia syndrome (NARES) 30–31, 33

without eosinophilia 30

nonsteroidal anti-inflammatory drugs (NSAID) 385, 423

Nordenberg, Tamar 379n, 385

North Carolina

asthma death statistics 122, 125

self-reported asthma prevalence 134

North Dakota

asthma death statistics 121

self-reported asthma prevalence 134

Northwestern University, allergy receptor 197

Notorfrancesco, Christopher 513, 514, 515

Notorfrancesco, Donna 513, 514, 515

Notorfrancesco, James 513

NRC *see* National Research Council

NRDC *see* Natural Resources Defense Counsel

The Nurse Practitioner 53n

O

OAQPS *see* Office of Air Quality Planning and Standards

obstructive airway diseases, reversible 44

obstructive lung disease, diagnosis 75

occupational asthma 31, 188, 307–15

causes 309

occupational chronic cough 71

occupational respiratory disorders 187–88

Occupational Safety and Health Administration (OSHA), agricultural allergens 327

OCR *see* Office for Civil Rights

O'Donnell, Sean 21

ODTS *see* organic dust toxic syndrome

Office for Civil Rights (OCR), managing asthma at school 488

Office of Air Quality Planning and Standards (OAQPS) 249n

Office of Energy Efficiency and Renewable Energy (DOE) 272

Of Life and Breath (Dewey) 50

Ohio

asthma death statistics 121, 124

self-reported asthma prevalence 134

Ohio University, breathing method 534

Oklahoma

asthma death statistics 122, 125

self-reported asthma prevalence 134

Olenchock, Stephen A. 323

omeprazole 59

Omnibus Budget and Reconciliation Act (1990) 462

Ono Pharmaceutical, leukotriene receptor 438

oral contraceptives, rhinitis 31

Oregon

asthma death statistics 123

self-reported asthma prevalence 135

organic dust 318

see also dust; house dust

organic dust toxic syndrome (ODTS) 320–21

Osborne, Molly L. 137n, 169n

OSHA *see* Occupational Safety and Health Administration

osmolar theory 16
osteoporosis, corticosteroids 392
over-the-counter medications (OTC)
  asthma treatment 7–8, 412
  chronic cough treatment 75
  gastroesophageal reflux treatment 59
oxygen therapy
  asthma 490–91
  chronic obstructive pulmonary dis-
    ease 47
oxymetazoline 75, 504
ozone 17, 199–201, 245, 249–63, 268–69
  described 249–50
  metered dose inhalers 405
Ozone: Good Up High, Bad Nearby 250
"Ozone and Your Health" 581

P

pain relievers, sinusitis 28
pancreatic enzymes 54
Panuska, James R. 217n, 220
parainfluenza virus 217
parietal cell 59
particulates 17, 267–68
passive smoking *see* environmental
  tobacco smoke
Patient Care
  "Asthma in the ED: The Effect of
    Menstrual Phase" (Pinkowish)
    529n
  "Latex Allergy: Potentially Dis-
    abling" (D'Epiro) 329n
  "Occupational Asthma: Breathing
    Easier on the Job" (Bardana, et
    al.) 307n
peak expiratory flow (PEF)
  asthma 464
  chronic cough 567
  home monitored, defined 567
peak expiratory flow rate (PEFR)
  313–14, 467–69
peak flow meters 18, 425, 467–68,
  473–76
peanut allergy, defined 567
Pediapred 7

pediatric drug safety 379–84
Pediatrics
  asthma and race 213, 214
  information 574
Pediatrics for Parents 343n
PEF *see* peak expiratory flow
PEFR *see* peak expiratory flow rate
Pennsylvania
  asthma death statistics 121, 124
  self-reported asthma prevalence
    134
Penton Publishing Inc. 187n
Pepcid (famotidine) 58
pepsin 54
peptides, defined 567
perfumes 298
  see also fragrances
Pericak-Vance, Margaret 210
persistent cough *see* chronic cough
Pertowski, Carol A. 97n, 129
pesticides 319
pet allergies *see* animal allergies
Peter, Margaret 21
Peterson, Jane W. 345n, 362
Petty, Thomas L. 50
PFT *see* pulmonary function tests
phagocytes 323–24
Pharmaceutical Information Associates, Ltd.
  asthma inhalation therapy 399n
  leukotriene receptor 437n
pharmacists, asthma treatment 461–71
Pharmacy Today 575
phenergan 383
phenylephrine 37, 556
phenylpropanolamine 27, 37, 556
Philp, Elizabeth B. 69n, 80
phrenoesophageal ligament 54
PHS *see* US Public Health Service
The Physician and Sportsmedicine
  "Exercise for Asthma Patients:
    Little Risk, Big Rewards"
    (Disabella, et al.) 537n
  "Update on Exercise-Induced
    Asthma: A Report of the
    Olympic...(Storms, et al.) 15n
Pinkowish, Mary Desmond 529n
pirbuterol 414, 464, 503
pirbuterol acetate 19

placebo, defined 567
placebo effect, defined 567
platelet-activating factor 399, 556
Plaut, Marshall 196
pneumonia 226
  asthma 221
  coal workers 187
  vaccine 74
pobilukast 439
pollen allergy, defined 568
pollens 239–40, 242–43, 433
  defined 568
  rhinitis 34
pollution prevention 270–77
polypeptide, defined 568
postnasal drainage 29, 33, 74
potassium bisulfite 339
potassium metabisulfite 339
Potera, Carol 301n, 306
poverty, asthma 84
  see also income levels
PPI *see* proton pump inhibitors
*Practical Guide for the Diagnosis and
  Management of Asthma*
  "How to Use Your Metered-Dose In-
    haler the Right Way" 429n
  "Initial Assessment and Diagnosis
    of Asthma" 365n
  "Managing Asthma Exacerbations
    at Home, in the Emergency..."
    489n
  "Patients Handouts" 473n
  "Pharmacologic Therapy: Managing
    Asthma Long Term" 371n, 415n
  "Practical and Effective Asthma
    Care" 9n
pranlukast 438
Pratter, Melvin R. 443n
prazosin 31
precipitants, described 10
prednisolone 374, 376, 423
prednisone 374, 376, 560
pregnancy
  asthma 501–6
  rhinitis 40
Prelone 7
preservatives 339
Prevacid (lansoprazole) 59
prevalence, defined 568

preventive treatment, defined 568
Prilosec (omeprazole) 59
Primatene 412, 414
*Proceedings of the 1st International
  Conference on Insect Pests...* 305
prognosis, defined 568
prokinetic agents 59
prophylaxis, defined 568
Propulsid (cisapride) 59, 76
protein, defined 568
proton pump inhibitors (PPI) 59
Proventil (albuterol) 7, 414, 503
Provocholine (methacholine) 76
prozac 383
pruritus 29, 31
pseudoephedrine 27, 37, 504, 556
psychotropic medications 385
public health
  endotoxins 323
  energy policies 265–83
Public Health Reports
  "Asthma: The States' Challenge"
    (Brown, et al.) 83n
  "How Energy Policies Affect Public
    Health" (Romm, et al.) 265n
Pulmicort 7
pulmonary function tests (PFT) 18,
  156–58
  asthma 222–23
  chronic bronchitis 74
pulmonary rehabilitation, chronic obstructive pulmonary disease 47
pulmonologists 449
Purdue Frederick Co., chronotherapy
  478

Q

quality of life
  asthma 169, 177
  rhinitis 29
quanethidine 31

R

racial factor, asthma 4, 104–15, 213–
  15, 345–62

radioallergosorbent tests (RAST) 156
radon 294
RADS *see* reactive airway dysfunction syndrome
ragweed pollen 242
Ramazzini, Bernardo 319
Rand Child Health Status scale 171
ranitidine 58–59
Rappaport, S. 131n, 136
RAST *see* radioallrgosorbent tests
reactive airway dysfunction syndrome (RADS) 310
reagin response *see* atopy
Reasoner, John, Jr. 22
receptors, defined 568
"Recognizing Signs and Symptoms of Chronic Obstructive Pulmonary Disease" 45n
Reese, Troy V. 22
reflux, gastroesophageal 53–63
Reglan (metoclopramide) 59, 76
Regnery, Helen 528
Rehabilitation Act, managing asthma at school 488
Reisseissen, F. D. 519
Research Institute for Fragrance Materials 298
reserpine 31
"Resources for Chronic Obstructive Pulmonary Disease" 45n
Respiratory Care Journal 574
respiratory disorders
air pollution 266–70
environmental tobacco smoke 288–91
"Respiratory Health Effects of Passive Smoking: Lung Cancer and Other Disorders" 285n
respiratory heat loss 16
respiratory infections 17, 218, 422
acute cough 73
asthma 222
respiratory syncytial virus (RSV) 217, 226
respiratory system, defined 568
rhinitis 29–41, 157
defined 569
diagnosis 29–32
rhinitis medicamentosa 40–41

rhinoconjunctivitis, latex allergy 330
Rhinocort (budesonide) 400
rhinomanometry 33
rhinorrhea 29
rhinovirus 217
Rhode Island
asthma death statistics 121
self-reported asthma prevalence 134
Richardson, Denise 22
risk factors, defined 569
ritalin 384
Roberts, Rosemary 380, 381
"The Role of the Pharmacist in Improving Asthma Care" 461n
Romm, Joseph J. 265n, 283
Rosenstreich, D. L. 306
Roses, Allen 210
Royal Dutch/Shell 273
RSV *see* respiratory syncytial virus
rush immunotherapy, described 434–35

S

SAD *see* seasonal affective disorder
salmeterol 7, 19–20, 375, 540
Samuelson, Wayne M. 53n, 63
Sander, Nancy 151
SAS Institute *see* Statistical Analysis System
Schenker, Marc B. 317, 319, 326
Schulman, Ronca and Bucuvalas, Inc. (SRBI) 151
Schwartz, David A. 318, 319, 325
seasonal affective disorder (SAD) 477
Seaton, Anthony 453, 454
"Secondhand Smoke: What You Can Do about Secondhand Smoke as Parents, Decisionmakers, and Building Occupants" 285n
Seldane (terfenadine) 28
Self, Timothy 471
Septra (trimethorprim-sulfamethoxazole) 75
Serevent (salmeterol) 7
Shayevitz, Berton R. 50
Shayevitz, Myra B. 50
Sherman, Carl 537n, 545

Shortness of Breath: A Guide to Better Living and Breathing (Moser) 50
SIDS *see* sudden infant death syndrome
silicosis 187
silo unloader's syndrome 320
Silverman, Robert 530
Silvers, William S. 22
Singulair (montelukast) 7, 438
sinuses
  defined 569
  described 25
sinusitis 17, 25–28
  defined 569
  described 25–26
  diagnosis 26
  treatment 26–28
Skobeloff, Emil M. 529, 530
Slo-bid (theophylline) 504
SmithKline Beecham 438
"Smog—Who Does It Hurt?" 249n, 581
smoking cessation programs 46, 294
Smolensky, Michel 478
sodium bisulfite 339
sodium metabisulfite 339
sodium sulfite 339
South Carolina
  asthma death statistics 122, 125
  self-reported asthma prevalence 134
South Dakota
  asthma death statistics 121
  self-reported asthma prevalence 134
Speizer, Frank E. 214
sphincter, lower esophageal 54
Spiegel, William 513, 514, 515
spina bifida, latex allergy 331
spirometric tests 158, 171, 222, 366, 542
Springhouse Corporation 53
sputum, chronic obstructive pulmonary disease 48
Stanley, J. S. 306
states
  asthma death statistics 121–25
  asthma prevalence 134–35
  asthma programs 87–89

Statistical Analysis System (SAS), asthma study 98, 172
Stehlin, Isadora 477n, 479
Stein Funtional Status II-R scale 171
Sterling, Yvonne M. 345n, 362
steroids 372, 374, 389, 425, 491–93
  asthma study 176, 223
  breastfeeding 505
  chronic cough treatment 76
  cough treatment 73, 75, 76
  defined 569
  inhaled 20
  step down therapy 416
  step up therapy, described 417–18
  see also corticosteroids
Stire, Janis 383
Stone, Jenny 22
Storms, William W. 15n, 21, 23
Stout, Cynthia 535
stress
  asthma 481
  vocal cord dysfunction 67
strictures, gastroesophageal reflux 55
subthreshold exercise 18–19
sucralfate 76
Sudafed (pseudoephedrine) 504
sudden infant death syndrome (SIDS), environmental tobacco smoke 288
sulfanomides, pregnancy 426
sulfites 339
sulfur dioxide 17, 270, 310, 339
Sullivan, Carrie A. 53n, 63
Sunyer, Jordi 245n, 248
surgical procedures
  gastroesophageal reflux treatment 60
  sinusitis 28
Symmetrel (amantadine) 526
systemic, defined 569

T

tachykinin production 218
Tagemet (cimetidine) 58
Taggart, Virginia Silver 471
T-cells (T-lymphocytes)
  defined 570
  helper, defined 560

Teach Your Patients about Asthma: A Clinician's Guide 471

Tennessee
  asthma death statistics 122, 125
  self-reported asthma prevalence 134
terbutaline 7, 19, 376, 414, 464, 503, 541
terfenadine 28, 36
tests
  allergies 33
    listed 551
  asthma 542
  asthma diagnosis 366, 368
  chronic cough 77
  cockroach antigens 304
  food allergies 340
  gastroesophageal reflux 57
  human immunodeficiency virus 526
  latex allergy 331–32
  pulmonary function 18, 74, 156–58, 222–23
  rhinitis 33
  skin allergens 33, 171–72
  spirometry 158, 171
  tuberculosis 74
  vocal cord dysfunction 66
tetracycline, pregnancy 426
Texas
  asthma death statistics 122, 125
  self-reported asthma prevalence 134
TH1 cells, defined 570
TH2 cells, defined 570
Theo-24 (theophylline anhydrous) 7
Theo-dur (theophylline) 504
Theolair (theophylline) 504
theophylline 20, 59, 375, 397–98, 423, 463, 494
  asthma study 176
  breastfeeding 505
  defined 570
  pregnancy 503–4
theophylline anhydrous 7
thermal expenditure theory 16
Thieme-Stratton 50
Tilade (nedocromil sodium) 503
Tinkelman, David 22
T-killer cells, defined 570

tobacco use
  asthma 85
  asthma study 157, 161
  chronic bronchitis 73–74
  chronic cough 69–71
  chronic obstructive pulmonary disease 46, 141
  endotoxins 326
  farmers 319
  see also environmental tobacco smoke
tomelukast 439
Tornalate (bitolterol) 414, 503
Traveling with Oxygen 50
tree pollen 242–43, 433
Trenga, Carol 517, 518
triamcinolone acetonide 20, 27, 38, 372, 373, 389
triggers
  asthma 6, 85, 86, 137, 235–43, 338–39, 502
  defined 570
  listed 5
  peak flow meters 475
  rhinitis 34–35
  vocal cord dysfunction 66
trimethoprim-sulfamethoxazole 75
tropelennamine 504
tuberculin skin test 74
Tufts University Diet & Nutrition Letter 519n
tumor necrosis factor 55, 200–201
Tylenol (acetaminophen) 28

U

Ulrik, Charlotte Suppli 155n
Ultair (pranlukast) 438
ultradian rhythm 477
"Understanding Food Allergy" 578
UNDP *see* United Nations Development Programme
Uniphyl (theophylline) 504
United Nations Development Program (UNDP), asthma health care 346
University of Aberdeen, Medical School (Scotland) 210

University of California
  Center for Complementary and Alternative Medicine Research in Asthma 517n, 533n
  contact information 577
University of Leicester, Department of Child Health (England) 210
University of Sheffield, Medical School (England) 210
Urecholine (bethanechol) 59
urticaria (hives) 157
  defined 570–71
  latex allergy 330
US Bureau of Census
  asthma surveillance 98
  prevalence by state 132
US Conference of Mayors, energy policies 275
USDA *see* US Department of Agriculture
US Department of Agriculture (USDA)
  cockroach antigens 301, 302
  latex allergy 334
  occupational asthma 192
US Department of Education, contact information 580–81
US Department of Energy (DOE)
  energy policies 265, 266, 272–73, 274, 275, 276, 277
  managing asthma at school 488
US Department of Health and Human Services (HHS)
  asthma assessment and diagnosis 365n
  asthma surveillance 83n
  contact information 581
  controlling asthma 489n
  energy policies 265
  latex allergy 329n
  management of systems 415n
  peak flow monitoring 473n
  "Practical and Effective Asthma Care" 9n
  use your inhaler effectively 429n
US Environmental Protection Agency (EPA)
  Agenda 2020 274
  air quality colors 255
  contact information 409, 581

US Environmental Protection Agency (EPA), continued
  energy policies 265, 268, 278
  environmental tobacco smoke 285n, 286, 291
  fragrances and health 299
  metered dose inhaler 407
  ozone and your health 249n, 250, 253, 254, 256, 262
US Food and Drug Administration (FDA)
  adrenergic bronchodilators 411n
  asthma deaths 4
  asthma inhalation therapy 403
  chronotherapy 477n, 478
  cockroach antigens 301
  contact information 409, 581–82
  "Controlling Asthma" 3n
  flu vaccine 523n, 526
    license 524
  fragrances and health 298
  latex allergy 331
  leukotriene receptor 437, 438
  metered dose inhaler 406, 407, 408
  pediatric and geriatric drug safety 379, 380, 382, 384
  Vaccines and Related Biologicals Advisory Committee 527, 528
  Voluntary Cosmetic Registration Program 299
USOC *see* US Olympic Committee
US Olympic Committee (USOC)
  banning of corticosteroids 40
  Drug Referral Hotline 425
  Sports Medicine Division 15
US Public Health Service (PHS)
  agricultural allergens 323
  environmental tobacco smoke 286
  flu vaccine 524
Utah
  asthma death statistics 123
  self-reported asthma prevalence 135

V

vaccines
  chronic obstructive pulmonary disease 46

vaccines, continued
  influenza 504, 523–28
  pregnancy 426, 504
  varicella 392–93
  see also immunizations
Vancenase (beclomethasone) 27
Vancenase AQ (beclomethasone) 27, 504
Vanceril (beclomethasone) 7, 389, 400
varicella (chickenpox), corticosteroids 392–93
vasodilation, defined 571
vasomotor rhinitis 30, 40
VCD *see* vocal cord dysfunction
Ventolin (albuterol) 7, 414, 503
verlukast 439
Vermont
  asthma death statistics 121
  self-reported asthma prevalence 134
vertical elutriator, described 324
Virginia
  asthma death statistics 122, 125
  self-reported asthma prevalence 134
virus, defined 571
vitamins
  asthma treatment 419, 517–21
  defined 571–72
"Vitamin Supplements May Help Asthmatics Cope with Air Pollution" 517n
vocal cord dysfunction (VCD) 65–67
Vokestoppen Children's Asthma and Allergy Centre (Norway) 210
volatile organic compounds 265
Vollmer, William M. 137n, 169n

W

Wagener, Diane 197
Wagner, Gregory 187, 188, 189, 191, 192
Ward, Robert M. 380, 382
Warner Books 50
Washington, DC *see* District of Columbia

Washington state
  asthma death statistics 123, 125
  self-reported asthma prevalence 135
Washington University School of Medicine (St. Louis, MO) 343
Weekes, DeLois P. 345n, 362
Weiler, John M. 22
Weiss, Scott 152
Westmoreland, Timothy 381, 382
West Virginia
  asthma death statistics 122, 125
  self-reported asthma prevalence 134
wheals 172
wheezing 97, 214, 223, 310, 366
white blood cells *see* leukocytes
WHO *see* World Health Organization
Wiley 50
Williams, Brock 334
Williams, Dennis 471
Williams, Rebecca D. 411n, 414
Wisconsin
  asthma death statistics 121, 124
  self-reported asthma prevalence 134
wood smoke 17, 541
workplace
  asthma 187–92
    see also occupational asthma
  environmental tobacco smoke 291–93
"Work-Related Lung Disease Surveillance Report (1994)" 189–90
World Health Organization (WHO)
  cause of death 158
  formulating the vaccine 527
Wyoming
  asthma death statistics 123
  self-reported asthma prevalence 135

X

x-rays
  cardiac asthma 44
  sinuses 26

Y

yarn manufacturing 322

Your Asthma Can Be Controlled: Expect Nothing Less 471, 579

"Your Metered-Dose Inhaler Will Be Changing...Here Are the Facts" 405n

Z

zafirlukast 7, 375, 438

Zamula, Evelyn 523n, 528

Zantac (ranitidine) 58

Zhu, Zhou 217n, 220

zileuton 7, 375, 438

zoloft 384

Zyflo (zileuton) 7, 438

Health Reference Series
COMPLETE CATALOG

AIDS Sourcebook, 1st Edition

Basic Information about AIDS and HIV Infection, Featuring Historical and Statistical Data, Current Research, Prevention, and Other Special Topics of Interest for Persons Living with AIDS

Along with Source Listings for Further Assistance

Edited by Karen Bellenir and Peter D. Dresser. 831 pages. 1995. 0-7808-0031-1. $78.

"One strength of this book is its practical emphasis. The intended audience is the lay reader . . . useful as an educational tool for health care providers who work with AIDS patients. Recommended for public libraries as well as hospital or academic libraries that collect consumer materials."
— *Bulletin of the Medical Library Association, Jan '96*

"This is the most comprehensive volume of its kind on an important medical topic. Highly recommended for all libraries." — *Reference Book Review, '96*

"Very useful reference for all libraries."
— *Choice, Association of College and Research Libraries, Oct '95*

"There is a wealth of information here that can provide much educational assistance. It is a must book for all libraries and should be on the desk of each and every congressional leader. Highly recommended."
— *AIDS Book Review Journal, Aug '95*

"Recommended for most collections."
— *Library Journal, Jul '95*

■

AIDS Sourcebook, 2nd Edition

Basic Consumer Health Information about Acquired Immune Deficiency Syndrome (AIDS) and Human Immunodeficiency Virus (HIV) Infection, Featuring Updated Statistical Data, Reports on Recent Research and Prevention Initiatives, and Other Special Topics of Interest for Persons Living with AIDS, Including New Antiretroviral Treatment Options, Strategies for Combating Opportunistic Infections, Information about Clinical Trials, and More

Along with a Glossary of Important Terms and Resource Listings for Further Help and Information

Edited by Karen Bellenir. 751 pages. 1999. 0-7808-0225-X. $78.

"Highly recommended."
— *American Reference Books Annual, 2000*

"Excellent sourcebook. This continues to be a highly recommended book. There is no other book that provides as much information as this book provides."
— *AIDS Book Review Journal, Dec-Jan 2000*

"Recommended reference source."
— *Booklist, American Library Association, Dec '99*

"A solid text for college-level health libraries."
— *The Bookwatch, Aug '99*

Cited in *Reference Sources for Small and Medium-Sized Libraries, American Library Association, 1999*

■

Alcoholism Sourcebook

Basic Consumer Health Information about the Physical and Mental Consequences of Alcohol Abuse, Including Liver Disease, Pancreatitis, Wernicke-Korsakoff Syndrome (Alcoholic Dementia), Fetal Alcohol Syndrome, Heart Disease, Kidney Disorders, Gastrointestinal Problems, and Immune System Compromise and Featuring Facts about Addiction, Detoxification, Alcohol Withdrawal, Recovery, and the Maintenance of Sobriety

Along with a Glossary and Directories of Resources for Further Help and Information

Edited by Karen Bellenir. 635 pages. 2000. 0-7808-0325-6. $78.

SEE ALSO *Drug Abuse Sourcebook, Substance Abuse Sourcebook*

■

Allergies Sourcebook

Basic Information about Major Forms and Mechanisms of Common Allergic Reactions, Sensitivities, and Intolerances, Including Anaphylaxis, Asthma, Hives and Other Dermatologic Symptoms, Rhinitis, and Sinusitis

Along with Their Usual Triggers Like Animal Fur, Chemicals, Drugs, Dust, Foods, Insects, Latex, Pollen, and Poison Ivy, Oak, and Sumac; Plus Information on Prevention, Identification, and Treatment

Edited by Allan R. Cook. 611 pages. 1997. 0-7808-0036-2. $78.

■

Alternative Medicine Sourcebook

Basic Consumer Health Information about Alternatives to Conventional Medicine, Including Acupressure, Acupuncture, Aromatherapy, Ayurveda, Bioelectromagnetics, Environmental Medicine, Essence Therapy, Food and Nutrition Therapy, Herbal Therapy, Homeopathy, Imaging, Massage, Naturopathy, Reflexology, Relaxation and Meditation, Sound Therapy, Vitamin and Mineral Therapy, and Yoga, and More

Edited by Allan R. Cook. 737 pages. 1999. 0-7808-0200-4. $78.

"Recommended reference source."
— *Booklist, American Library Association, Feb '00*

■

Alzheimer's, Stroke & 29 Other Neurological Disorders Sourcebook, 1st Edition

Basic Information for the Layperson on 31 Diseases or Disorders Affecting the Brain and Nervous System, First Describing the Illness, Then Listing Symptoms, Diagnostic Methods, and Treatment Options, and Including Statistics on Incidences and Causes

Edited by Frank E. Bair. 579 pages. 1993. 1-55888-748-2. $78.

SEE ALSO *Brain Disorders Sourcebook*

■

Alzheimer's Disease Sourcebook, 2nd Edition

Basic Consumer Health Information about Alzheimer's Disease, Related Disorders, and Other Dementias, Including Multi-Infarct Dementia, AIDS-Related Dementia, Alcoholic Dementia, Huntington's Disease, Delirium, and Confusional States

Along with Reports Detailing Current Research Efforts in Prevention and Treatment, Long-Term Care Issues, and Listings of Sources for Additional Help and Information

Edited by Karen Bellenir. 524 pages. 1999. 0-7808-0223-3. $78.

Arthritis Sourcebook

Basic Consumer Health Information about Specific Forms of Arthritis and Related Disorders, Including Rheumatoid Arthritis, Osteoarthritis, Gout, Polymyalgia Rheumatica, Psoriatic Arthritis, Spondyloarthropathies, Juvenile Rheumatoid Arthritis, and Juvenile Ankylosing Spondylitis

Along with Information about Medical, Surgical, and Alternative Treatment Options, and Including Strategies for Coping with Pain, Fatigue, and Stress

Edited by Allan R. Cook. 550 pages. 1998. 0-7808-0201-2. $78.

■

Asthma Sourcebook

Basic Consumer Health Information about Asthma, Including Symptoms, Traditional and Nontraditional Remedies, Treatment Advances, Quality-of-Life Aids, Medical Research Updates, and the Role of Allergies, Exercise, Age, the Environment, and Genetics in the Development of Asthma

Along with Statistical Data, a Glossary, and Directories of Support Groups, and Other Resources for Further Information

Edited by Annemarie S. Muth. 628 pages. 2000. 0-7808-0381-7. $78.

■

Back & Neck Disorders Sourcebook

Basic Information about Disorders and Injuries of the Spinal Cord and Vertebrae, Including Facts on Chiropractic Treatment, Surgical Interventions, Paralysis, and Rehabilitation

Along with Advice for Preventing Back Trouble

Edited by Karen Bellenir. 548 pages. 1997. 0-7808-0202-0. $78.

■

Blood & Circulatory Disorders Sourcebook

Basic Information about Blood and Its Components, Anemias, Leukemias, Bleeding Disorders, and Circulatory Disorders, Including Aplastic Anemia, Thalassemia, Sickle-Cell Disease, Hemochromatosis, Hemophilia, Von Willebrand Disease, and Vascular Diseases

Along with a Special Section on Blood Transfusions and Blood Supply Safety, a Glossary, and Source Listings for Further Help and Information

Edited by Karen Bellenir and Linda M. Shin. 554 pages. 1998. 0-7808-0203-9. $78.

Brain Disorders Sourcebook

Basic Consumer Health Information about Strokes, Epilepsy, Amyotrophic Lateral Sclerosis (ALS/Lou Gehrig's Disease), Parkinson's Disease, Brain Tumors, Cerebral Palsy, Headache, Tourette Syndrome, and More

Along with Statistical Data, Treatment and Rehabilitation Options, Coping Strategies, Reports on Current Research Initiatives, a Glossary, and Resource Listings for Additional Help and Information

Edited by Karen Bellenir. 481 pages. 1999. 0-7808-0229-2. $78.

SEE ALSO *Alzheimer's, Stroke & 29 Other Neurological Disorders Sourcebook, 1st Edition*

Breast Cancer Sourcebook

Basic Consumer Health Information about Breast Cancer, Including Diagnostic Methods, Treatment Options, Alternative Therapies, Help and Self-Help Information, Related Health Concerns, Statistical and Demographic Data, and Facts for Men with Breast Cancer

Along with Reports on Current Research Initiatives, a Glossary of Related Medical Terms, and a Directory of Sources for Further Help and Information

Edited by Edward J. Prucha. 600 pages. 2000. 0-7808-0244-6. $78.

SEE ALSO *Cancer Sourcebook for Women, 1st and 2nd Editions, Women's Health Concerns Sourcebook*

Burns Sourcebook

Basic Consumer Health Information about Various Types of Burns and Scalds, Including Flame, Heat, Cold, Electrical, Chemical, and Sun Burns

Along with Information on Short-Term and Long-Term Treatments, Tissue Reconstruction, Plastic Surgery, Prevention Suggestions, and First Aid

Edited by Allan R. Cook. 604 pages. 1999. 0-7808-0204-7. $78.

SEE ALSO *Skin Disorders Sourcebook*

Cancer Sourcebook, 1st Edition

Basic Information on Cancer Types, Symptoms, Diagnostic Methods, and Treatments, Including Statistics on Cancer Occurrences Worldwide and the Risks Associated with Known Carcinogens and Activities

Edited by Frank E. Bair. 932 pages. 1990. 1-55888-888-8. $78.

New Cancer Sourcebook, 2nd Edition

Basic Information about Major Forms and Stages of Cancer, Featuring Facts about Primary and Secondary Tumors of the Respiratory, Nervous, Lymphatic, Circulatory, Skeletal, and Gastrointestinal Systems, and Specific Organs; Statistical and Demographic Data; Treatment Options; and Strategies for Coping

Edited by Allan R. Cook. 1,313 pages. 1996. 0-7808-0041-9. $78.

"The amount of factual and useful information is extensive. The writing is very clear, geared to general readers. Recommended for all levels."
— *Choice, Association of College and Research Libraries, Jan '97*

■

Cancer Sourcebook, 3rd Edition

Basic Consumer Health Information about Major Forms and Stages of Cancer, Featuring Facts about Primary and Secondary Tumors of the Respiratory, Nervous, Lymphatic, Circulatory, Skeletal, and Gastrointestinal Systems, and Specific Organs

Along with Statistical and Demographic Data, Treatment Options, Strategies for Coping, a Glossary, and a Directory of Sources for Additional Help and Information

Edited by Edward J. Prucha. 1,069 pages. 2000. 0-7808-0227-6. $78.

■

Cancer Sourcebook for Women, 1st Edition

Basic Information about Specific Forms of Cancer That Affect Women, Featuring Facts about Breast Cancer, Cervical Cancer, Ovarian Cancer, Cancer of the Uterus and Uterine Sarcoma, Cancer of the Vagina, and Cancer of the Vulva; Statistical and Demographic Data; Treatments, Self-Help Management Suggestions, and Current Research Initiatives

Edited by Allan R. Cook and Peter D. Dresser. 524 pages. 1996. 0-7808-0076-1. $78.

"... written in easily understandable, non-technical language. Recommended for public libraries or hospital and academic libraries that collect patient education or consumer health materials."
— *Medical Reference Services Quarterly, Spring '97*

"Would be of value in a consumer health library.... written with the health care consumer in mind. Medical jargon is at a minimum, and medical terms are explained in clear, understandable sentences."
— *Bulletin of the Medical Library Association, Oct '96*

"The availability under one cover of all these pertinent publications, grouped under cohesive headings, makes this certainly a most useful sourcebook."
— *Choice, Association of College and Research Libraries, Jun '96*

"Presents a comprehensive knowledge base for general readers. Men and women both benefit from the gold mine of information nestled between the two covers of this book. Recommended."
— *Academic Library Book Review, Summer '96*

"This timely book is highly recommended for consumer health and patient education collections in all libraries." — *Library Journal, Apr '96*

SEE ALSO *Breast Cancer Sourcebook, Women's Health Concerns Sourcebook*

Cancer Sourcebook for Women, 2nd Edition

Basic Consumer Health Information about Specific Forms of Cancer That Affect Women, Including Cervical Cancer, Ovarian Cancer, Endometrial Cancer, Uterine Sarcoma, Vaginal Cancer, Vulvar Cancer, and Gestational Trophoblastic Tumor; and Featuring Statistical Information, Facts about Tests and Treatments, a Glossary of Cancer Terms, and an Extensive List of Additional Resources

Edited by Edward J. Prucha. 600 pages. 2000. 0-7808-0226-8. $78.

SEE ALSO *Breast Cancer Sourcebook, Women's Health Concerns Sourcebook*

■

Cardiovascular Diseases & Disorders Sourcebook, 1st Edition

Basic Information about Cardiovascular Diseases and Disorders, Featuring Facts about the Cardiovascular System, Demographic and Statistical Data, Descriptions of Pharmacological and Surgical Interventions, Lifestyle Modifications, and a Special Section Focusing on Heart Disorders in Children

Edited by Karen Bellenir and Peter D. Dresser. 683 pages. 1995. 0-7808-0032-X. $78.

"... comprehensive format provides an extensive overview on this subject."
— *Choice, Association of College and Research Libraries, Jun '96*

"... an easily understood, complete, up-to-date resource. This well executed public health tool will make valuable information available to those that need it most, patients and their families. The typeface, sturdy non-reflective paper, and library binding add a feel of quality found wanting in other publications. Highly recommended for academic and general libraries. "
— *Academic Library Book Review, Summer '96*

SEE ALSO *Healthy Heart Sourcebook for Women, Heart Diseases & Disorders Sourcebook, 2nd Edition*

■

Communication Disorders Sourcebook

Basic Information about Deafness and Hearing Loss, Speech and Language Disorders, Voice Disorders, Balance and Vestibular Disorders, and Disorders of Smell, Taste, and Touch

Edited by Linda M. Ross. 533 pages. 1996. 0-7808-0077-X. $78.

"This is skillfully edited and is a welcome resource for the layperson. It should be found in every public and medical library." — *Booklist Health Sciences Supplement, American Library Association, Oct '97*

Congenital Disorders Sourcebook

Basic Information about Disorders Acquired during Gestation, Including Spina Bifida, Hydrocephalus, Cerebral Palsy, Heart Defects, Craniofacial Abnormalities, Fetal Alcohol Syndrome, and More

Along with Current Treatment Options and Statistical Data

Edited by Karen Bellenir. 607 pages. 1997. 0-7808-0205-5. $78.

"**Recommended reference source.**"
— Booklist, American Library Association, Oct '97

SEE ALSO *Pregnancy & Birth Sourcebook*

■

Consumer Issues in Health Care Sourcebook

Basic Information about Health Care Fundamentals and Related Consumer Issues, Including Exams and Screening Tests, Physician Specialties, Choosing a Doctor, Using Prescription and Over-the-Counter Medications Safely, Avoiding Health Scams, Managing Common Health Risks in the Home, Care Options for Chronically or Terminally Ill Patients, and a List of Resources for Obtaining Help and Further Information

Edited by Karen Bellenir. 618 pages. 1998. 0-7808-0221-7. $78.

"**Both public and academic libraries will want to have a copy in their collection for readers who are interested in self-education on health issues.**"
— American Reference Books Annual, 2000

"**The editor has researched the literature from government agencies and others, saving readers the time and effort of having to do the research themselves. Recommended for public libraries.**"
— Reference and User Services Quarterly, American Library Association, Spring '99

"**Recommended reference source.**"
— Booklist, American Library Association, Dec '98

■

Contagious & Non-Contagious Infectious Diseases Sourcebook

Basic Information about Contagious Diseases like Measles, Polio, Hepatitis B, and Infectious Mononucleosis, and Non-Contagious Infectious Diseases like Tetanus and Toxic Shock Syndrome, and Diseases Occurring as Secondary Infections Such as Shingles and Reye Syndrome

Along with Vaccination, Prevention, and Treatment Information, and a Section Describing Emerging Infectious Disease Threats

Edited by Karen Bellenir and Peter D. Dresser. 566 pages. 1996. 0-7808-0075-3. $78.

Death & Dying Sourcebook

Basic Consumer Health Information for the Layperson about End-of-Life Care and Related Ethical and Legal Issues, Including Chief Causes of Death, Autopsies, Pain Management for the Terminally Ill, Life Support Systems, Insurance, Euthanasia, Assisted Suicide, Hospice Programs, Living Wills, Funeral Planning, Counseling, Mourning, Organ Donation, and Physician Training

Along with Statistical Data, a Glossary, and Listings of Sources for Further Help and Information

Edited by Annemarie S. Muth. 641 pages. 1999. 0-7808-0230-6. $78.

"**This book is a definite must for all those involved in end-of-life care.**"
— Doody's Review Service, 2000

■

Diabetes Sourcebook, 1st Edition

Basic Information about Insulin-Dependent and Non-insulin-Dependent Diabetes Mellitus, Gestational Diabetes, and Diabetic Complications, Symptoms, Treatment, and Research Results, Including Statistics on Prevalence, Morbidity, and Mortality

Along with Source Listings for Further Help and Information

Edited by Karen Bellenir and Peter D. Dresser. 827 pages. 1994. 1-55888-751-2. $78.

"**. . . very informative and understandable for the layperson without being simplistic. It provides a comprehensive overview for laypersons who want a general understanding of the disease or who want to focus on various aspects of the disease.**"
— Bulletin of the Medical Library Association, Jan '96

■

Diabetes Sourcebook, 2nd Edition

Basic Consumer Health Information about Type 1 Diabetes (Insulin-Dependent or Juvenile-Onset Diabetes), Type 2 (Noninsulin-Dependent or Adult-Onset Diabetes), Gestational Diabetes, and Related Disorders, Including Diabetes Prevalence Data, Management Issues, the Role of Diet and Exercise in Controlling Diabetes, Insulin and Other Diabetes Medicines, and Complications of Diabetes Such as Eye Diseases, Periodontal Disease, Amputation, and End-Stage Renal Disease

Along with Reports on Current Research Initiatives, a Glossary, and Resource Listings for Further Help and Information

Edited by Karen Bellenir. 688 pages. 1998. 0-7808-0224-1. $78.

"**This comprehensive book is an excellent addition for high school, academic, medical, and public libraries. This volume is highly recommended.**"
— American Reference Books Annual, 2000

"**An invaluable reference.**" *— Library Journal, May '00*

Selected as one of the 250 "Best Health Sciences Books of 1999." — *Doody's Rating Service, Mar-Apr 2000*

"Recommended reference source."
— *Booklist, American Library Association, Feb '99*

". . . provides reliable mainstream medical information . . . belongs on the shelves of any library with a consumer health collection." — *E-Streams, Sep '99*

"Provides useful information for the general public."
— *Healthlines, University of Michigan Health Management Research Center, Sep/Oct '99*

■

Diet & Nutrition Sourcebook, 1st Edition

Basic Information about Nutrition, Including the Dietary Guidelines for Americans, the Food Guide Pyramid, and Their Applications in Daily Diet, Nutritional Advice for Specific Age Groups, Current Nutritional Issues and Controversies, the New Food Label and How to Use It to Promote Healthy Eating, and Recent Developments in Nutritional Research

Edited by Dan R. Harris. 662 pages. 1996. 0-7808-0084-2. $78.

"Useful reference as a food and nutrition sourcebook for the general consumer." — *Booklist Health Sciences Supplement, American Library Association, Oct '97*

"Recommended for public libraries and medical libraries that receive general information requests on nutrition. It is readable and will appeal to those interested in learning more about healthy dietary practices." — *Medical Reference Services Quarterly, Fall '97*

"An abundance of medical and social statistics is translated into readable information geared toward the general reader." — *Bookwatch, Mar '97*

"With dozens of questionable diet books on the market, it is so refreshing to find a reliable and factual reference book. Recommended to aspiring professionals, librarians, and others seeking and giving reliable dietary advice. An excellent compilation." — *Choice, Association of College and Research Libraries, Feb '97*

SEE ALSO *Digestive Diseases & Disorders Sourcebook, Gastrointestinal Diseases & Disorders Sourcebook*

■

Diet & Nutrition Sourcebook, 2nd Edition

Basic Consumer Health Information about Dietary Guidelines, Recommended Daily Intake Values, Vitamins, Minerals, Fiber, Fat, Weight Control, Dietary Supplements, and Food Additives

Along with Special Sections on Nutrition Needs throughout Life and Nutrition for People with Such Specific Medical Concerns as Allergies, High Blood Cholesterol, Hypertension, Diabetes, Celiac Disease, Seizure Disorders, Phenylketonuria (PKU), Cancer, and Eating Disorders, and Including Reports on Current Nutrition Research and Source Listings for Additional Help and Information

Edited by Karen Bellenir. 650 pages. 1999. 0-7808-0228-4. $78.

"This reference document should be in any public library, but it would be a very good guide for beginning students in the health sciences. If the other books in this publisher's series are as good as this, they should all be in the health sciences collections."
— *American Reference Books Annual, 2000*

"Recommended reference source."
— *Booklist, American Library Association, Dec '99*

SEE ALSO *Digestive Diseases & Disorders Sourcebook, Gastrointestinal Diseases & Disorders Sourcebook*

■

Digestive Diseases & Disorders Sourcebook

Basic Consumer Health Information about Diseases and Disorders that Impact the Upper and Lower Digestive System, Including Celiac Disease, Constipation, Crohn's Disease, Cyclic Vomiting Syndrome, Diarrhea, Diverticulosis and Diverticulitis, Gallstones, Heartburn, Hemorrhoids, Hernias, Indigestion (Dyspepsia), Irritable Bowel Syndrome, Lactose Intolerance, Ulcers, and More

Along with Information about Medications and Other Treatments, Tips for Maintaining a Healthy Digestive Tract, a Glossary, and Directory of Digestive Diseases Organizations

Edited by Karen Bellenir. 335 pages. 1999. 0-7808-0327-2. $48.

"Recommended reference source."
— *Booklist, American Library Association, May '00*

SEE ALSO *Diet & Nutrition Sourcebook, 1st and 2nd Editions, Gastrointestinal Diseases & Disorders Sourcebook*

■

Disabilities Sourcebook

Basic Consumer Health Information about Physical and Psychiatric Disabilities, Including Descriptions of Major Causes of Disability, Assistive and Adaptive Aids, Workplace Issues, and Accessibility Concerns

Along with Information about the Americans with Disabilities Act, a Glossary, and Resources for Additional Help and Information

Edited by Dawn D. Matthews. 616 pages. 2000. 0-7808-0389-2. $78.

"Recommended reference source."
— *Booklist, American Library Association, Jul '00*

"An involving, invaluable handbook."
— *The Bookwatch, May '00*

Domestic Violence & Child Abuse Sourcebook

Basic Consumer Health Information about Spousal/ Partner, Child, Sibling, Parent, and Elder Abuse, Covering Physical, Emotional, and Sexual Abuse, Teen Dating Violence, and Stalking; Includes Information about Hotlines, Safe Houses, Safety Plans, and Other Resources for Support and Assistance, Community Initiatives, and Reports on Current Directions in Research and Treatment

Along with a Glossary, Sources for Further Reading, and Governmental and Non-Governmental Organizations Contact Information

Edited by Helene Henderson. 600 pages. 2000. 0-7808-0235-7. $78.

■

Drug Abuse Sourcebook

Basic Consumer Health Information about Illicit Substances of Abuse and the Diversion of Prescription Medications, Including Depressants, Hallucinogens, Inhalants, Marijuana, Narcotics, Stimulants, and Anabolic Steroids

Along with Facts about Related Health Risks, Treatment Issues, and Substance Abuse Prevention Programs, a Glossary of Terms, Statistical Data, and Directories of Hotline Services, Self-Help Groups, and Organizations Able to Provide Further Information

Edited by Karen Bellenir. 629 pages. 2000. 0-7808-0242-X. $78.

SEE ALSO Alcoholism Sourcebook, Substance Abuse Sourcebook

■

Ear, Nose & Throat Disorders Sourcebook

Basic Information about Disorders of the Ears, Nose, Sinus Cavities, Pharynx, and Larynx, Including Ear Infections, Tinnitus, Vestibular Disorders, Allergic and Non-Allergic Rhinitis, Sore Throats, Tonsillitis, and Cancers That Affect the Ears, Nose, Sinuses, and Throat

Along with Reports on Current Research Initiatives, a Glossary of Related Medical Terms, and a Directory of Sources for Further Help and Information

Edited by Karen Bellenir and Linda M. Shin. 576 pages. 1998. 0-7808-0206-3. $78.

"Overall, this sourcebook is helpful for the consumer seeking information on ENT issues. It is recommended for public libraries."
    —*American Reference Books Annual, 1999*

"Recommended reference source."
    —*Booklist, American Library Association, Dec '98*

Endocrine & Metabolic Disorders Sourcebook

Basic Information for the Layperson about Pancreatic and Insulin-Related Disorders Such as Pancreatitis, Diabetes, and Hypoglycemia; Adrenal Gland Disorders Such as Cushing's Syndrome, Addison's Disease, and Congenital Adrenal Hyperplasia; Pituitary Gland Disorders Such as Growth Hormone Deficiency, Acromegaly, and Pituitary Tumors; Thyroid Disorders Such as Hypothyroidism, Graves' Disease, Hashimoto's Disease, and Goiter; Hyperparathyroidism; and Other Diseases and Syndromes of Hormone Imbalance or Metabolic Dysfunction

Along with Reports on Current Research Initiatives

Edited by Linda M. Shin. 574 pages. 1998. 0-7808-0207-1. $78.

"Omnigraphics has produced another needed resource for health information consumers."
    —*American Reference Books Annual, 2000*

"Recommended reference source."
    —*Booklist, American Library Association, Dec '98*

■

Environmentally Induced Disorders Sourcebook

Basic Information about Diseases and Syndromes Linked to Exposure to Pollutants and Other Substances in Outdoor and Indoor Environments Such as Lead, Asbestos, Formaldehyde, Mercury, Emissions, Noise, and More

Edited by Allan R. Cook. 620 pages. 1997. 0-7808-0083-4. $78.

"Recommended reference source."
    —*Booklist, American Library Association, Sep '98*

"This book will be a useful addition to anyone's library."   —*Choice Health Sciences Supplement, Association of College and Research Libraries, May '98*

". . . a good survey of numerous environmentally induced physical disorders . . . a useful addition to anyone's library."
    —*Doody's Health Sciences Book Reviews, Jan '98*

". . . provide[s] introductory information from the best authorities around. Since this volume covers topics that potentially affect everyone, it will surely be one of the most frequently consulted volumes in the *Health Reference Series*."   —*Rettig on Reference, Nov '97*

■

Ethnic Diseases Sourcebook

Basic Consumer Health Information for Ethnic and Racial Minority Groups in the United States, Including General Health Indicators and Behaviors, Ethnic Diseases, Genetic Testing, the Impact of Chronic Diseases, Women's Health, Mental Health Issues, and Preventive Health Care Service

Along with a Glossary and a Listing of Additional Resources

Edited by Joyce Brennfleck Shannon. 600 pages. 2001. 0-7808-0336-1. $78.

Family Planning Sourcebook

Basic Consumer Health Information about Planning for Pregacy and Contraception, Including Traditional Methods, Barrier Methods, Hormonal Methods, Permanent Methods, Future Methods, Emergency Contraception, and Birth Control Choices for Women at Each Stage of Life

Along with Statistics, a Glossary, and Sources of Additional Information

Edited by Amy Marcaccio Keyzer. 600 pages. 2000. 0-7808-0379-5. $78.

SEE ALSO *Pregnancy & Birth Sourcebook*

■

Fitness & Exercise Sourcebook

Basic Information on Fitness and Exercise, Including Fitness Activities for Specific Age Groups, Exercise for People with Specific Medical Conditions, How to Begin a Fitness Program in Running, Walking, Swimming, Cycling, and Other Athletic Activities, and Recent Research in Fitness and Exercise

Edited by Dan R. Harris. 663 pages. 1996. 0-7808-0186-5. $78.

"A good resource for general readers."
— *Choice, Association of College and Research Libraries, Nov '97*

"The perennial popularity of the topic . . . make this an appealing selection for public libraries."
— *Rettig on Reference, Jun/Jul '97*

■

Food & Animal Borne Diseases Sourcebook

Basic Information about Diseases That Can Be Spread to Humans through the Ingestion of Contaminated Food or Water or by Contact with Infected Animals and Insects, Such as Botulism, E. Coli, Hepatitis A, Trichinosis, Lyme Disease, and Rabies

Along with Information Regarding Prevention and Treatment Methods, and Including a Special Section for International Travelers Describing Diseases Such as Cholera, Malaria, Travelers' Diarrhea, and Yellow Fever, and Offering Recommendations for Avoiding Illness

Edited by Karen Bellenir and Peter D. Dresser. 535 pages. 1995. 0-7808-0033-8. $78.

"Targeting general readers and providing them with a single, comprehensive source of information on selected topics, this book continues, with the excellent caliber of its predecessors, to catalog topical information on health matters of general interest. Readable and thorough, this valuable resource is highly recommended for all libraries."
— *Academic Library Book Review, Summer '96*

"A comprehensive collection of authoritative information." — *Emergency Medical Services, Oct '95*

Food Safety Sourcebook

Basic Consumer Health Information about the Safe Handling of Meat, Poultry, Seafood, Eggs, Fruit Juices, and Other Food Items, and Facts about Pesticides, Drinking Water, Food Safety Overseas, and the Onset, Duration, and Symptoms of Foodborne Illnesses, Including Types of Pathogenic Bacteria, Parasitic Protozoa, Worms, Viruses, and Natural Toxins

Along with the Role of the Consumer, the Food Handler, and the Government in Food Safety; a Glossary, and Resources for Additional Help and Information

Edited by Dawn D. Matthews. 339 pages. 1999. 0-7808-0326-4. $48.

"This book takes the complex issues of food safety and foodborne pathogens and presents them in an easily understood manner. [It does] an excellent job of covering a large and often confusing topic."
— *American Reference Books Annual, 2000*

"Recommended reference source."
— *Booklist, American Library Association, May '00*

■

Forensic Medicine Sourcebook

Basic Consumer Information for the Layperson about Forensic Medicine, Including Crime Scene Investigation, Evidence Collection and Analysis, Expert Testimony, Computer-Aided Criminal Identification, Digital Imaging in the Courtroom, DNA Profiling, Accident Reconstruction, Autopsies, Ballistics, Drugs and Explosives Detection, Latent Fingerprints, Product Tampering, and Questioned Document Examination

Along with Statistical Data, a Glossary of Forensics Terminology, and Listings of Sources for Further Help and Information

Edited by Annemarie S. Muth. 574 pages. 1999. 0-7808-0232-2. $78.

"There are several items that make this book attractive to consumers who are seeking certain forensic data. . . . This is a useful current source for those seeking general forensic medical answers."
— *American Reference Books Annual, 2000*

"Recommended for public libraries."
— *Reference & User Services Quarterly, American Library Association, Spring 2000*

"Recommended reference source."
— *Booklist, American Library Association, Feb '00*

"A wealth of information, useful statistics, references are up-to-date and extremely complete. This wonderful collection of data will help students who are interested in a career in any type of forensic field. It is a great resource for attorneys who need information about types of expert witnesses needed in a particular case. It also offers useful information for fiction and nonfiction writers whose work involves a crime. A fascinating compilation. All levels."
— *Choice, Association of College and Research Libraries, Jan 2000*

Gastrointestinal Diseases & Disorders Sourcebook

Basic Information about Gastroesophageal Reflux Disease (Heartburn), Ulcers, Diverticulosis, Irritable Bowel Syndrome, Crohn's Disease, Ulcerative Colitis, Diarrhea, Constipation, Lactose Intolerance, Hemorrhoids, Hepatitis, Cirrhosis, and Other Digestive Problems, Featuring Statistics, Descriptions of Symptoms, and Current Treatment Methods of Interest for Persons Living with Upper and Lower Gastrointestinal Maladies

Edited by Linda M. Ross. 413 pages. 1996. 0-7808-0078-8. $78.

". . . very readable form. The successful editorial work that brought this material together into a useful and understandable reference makes accessible to all readers information that can help them more effectively understand and obtain help for digestive tract problems."
—*Choice, Association of College and Research Libraries, Feb '97*

SEE ALSO *Diet & Nutrition Sourcebook, 1st and 2nd Editions, Digestive Diseases & Disorders Sourcebook*

Genetic Disorders Sourcebook, 1st Edition

Basic Information about Heritable Diseases and Disorders Such as Down Syndrome, PKU, Hemophilia, Von Willebrand Disease, Gaucher Disease, Tay-Sachs Disease, and Sickle-Cell Disease, Along with Information about Genetic Screening, Gene Therapy, Home Care, and Including Source Listings for Further Help and Information on More Than 300 Disorders

Edited by Karen Bellenir. 642 pages. 1996. 0-7808-0034-6. $78.

"Recommended for undergraduate libraries or libraries that serve the public."
—*Science & Technology Libraries, Vol. 18, No. 1, '99*

"Provides essential medical information to both the general public and those diagnosed with a serious or fatal genetic disease or disorder."
—*Choice, Association of College and Research Libraries, Jan '97*

"Geared toward the lay public. It would be well placed in all public libraries and in those hospital and medical libraries in which access to genetic references is limited." —*Doody's Health Sciences Book Review, Oct '96*

Genetic Disorders Sourcebook, 2nd Edition

Basic Consumer Health Information about Hereditary Diseases and Disorders, Including Cystic Fibrosis, Down Syndrome, Hemophilia, Huntington's Disease, Sickle Cell Anemia, and More; Facts about Genes, Gene Research and Therapy, Genetic Screening, Ethics of Gene Testing, Genetic Counseling, and Advice on Coping and Caring

Along with a Glossary of Genetic Terminology and a Resource List for Help, Support, and Further Information

Edited by Kathy Massimini. 650 pages. 2000. 0-7808-0241-1. $78.

Head Trauma Sourcebook

Basic Information for the Layperson about Open-Head and Closed-Head Injuries, Treatment Advances, Recovery, and Rehabilitation

Along with Reports on Current Research Initiatives

Edited by Karen Bellenir. 414 pages. 1997. 0-7808-0208-X. $78.

Health Insurance Sourcebook

Basic Information about Managed Care Organizations, Traditional Fee-for-Service Insurance, Insurance Portability and Pre-Existing Conditions Clauses, Medicare, Medicaid, Social Security, and Military Health Care

Along with Information about Insurance Fraud

Edited by Wendy Wilcox. 530 pages. 1997. 0-7808-0222-5. $78.

"Particularly useful because it brings much of this information together in one volume. This book will be a handy reference source in the health sciences library, hospital library, college and university library, and medium to large public library."
—*Medical Reference Services Quarterly, Fall '98*

Awarded "Books of the Year Award"
—*American Journal of Nursing, 1997*

"The layout of the book is particularly helpful as it provides easy access to reference material. A most useful addition to the vast amount of information about health insurance. The use of data from U.S. government agencies is most commendable. Useful in a library or learning center for healthcare professional students."
—*Doody's Health Sciences Book Reviews, Nov '97*

Healthy Aging Sourcebook

Basic Consumer Health Information about Maintaining Health through the Aging Process, Including Advice on Nutrition, Exercise, and Sleep, Help in Making Decisions about Midlife Issues and Retirement, and Guidance Concerning Practical and Informed Choices in Health Consumerism

Along with Data Concerning the Theories of Aging, Different Experiences in Aging by Minority Groups, and Facts about Aging Now and Aging in the Future; and Featuring a Glossary, a Guide to Consumer Help, Additional Suggested Reading, and Practical Resource Directory

Edited by Jenifer Swanson. 536 pages. 1999. 0-7808-0390-6. $78.

"Recommended reference source."
—*Booklist, American Library Association, Feb '00*

SEE ALSO *Physical & Mental Issues in Aging Sourcebook*

Healthy Heart Sourcebook for Women

Basic Consumer Health Information about Cardiac Issues Specific to Women, Including Facts about Major Risk Factors and Prevention, Treatment and Control Strategies, and Important Dietary Issues

Along with a Special Section Regarding the Pros and Cons of Hormone Replacement Therapy and Its Impact on Heart Health, and Additional Help, Including Recipes, a Glossary, and a Directory of Resources

Edited by Dawn D. Matthews. 336 pages. 2000. 0-7808-0329-9. $48.

SEE ALSO *Cardiovascular Diseases & Disorders Sourcebook, 1st Edition, Heart Diseases & Disorders Sourcebook, 2nd Edition, Women's Health Concerns Sourcebook*

Heart Diseases & Disorders Sourcebook, 2nd Edition

Basic Consumer Health Information about Heart Attacks, Angina, Rhythm Disorders, Heart Failure, Valve Disease, Congenital Heart Disorders, and More, Including Descriptions of Surgical Procedures and Other Interventions, Medications, Cardiac Rehabilitation, Risk Identification, and Prevention Tips

Along with Statistical Data, Reports on Current Research Initiatives, a Glossary of Cardiovascular Terms, and Resource Directory

Edited by Karen Bellenir. 612 pages. 2000. 0-7808-0238-1. $78.

SEE ALSO *Cardiovascular Diseases & Disorders Sourcebook, 1st Edition, Healthy Heart Sourcebook for Women*

Immune System Disorders Sourcebook

Basic Information about Lupus, Multiple Sclerosis, Guillain-Barré Syndrome, Chronic Granulomatous Disease, and More

Along with Statistical and Demographic Data and Reports on Current Research Initiatives

Edited by Allan R. Cook. 608 pages. 1997. 0-7808-0209-8. $78.

Infant & Toddler Health Sourcebook

Basic Consumer Health Information about the Physical and Mental Development of Newborns, Infants, and Toddlers, Including Neonatal Concerns, Nutrition Recommendations, Immunization Schedules, Common Pediatric Disorders, Assessments and Milestones, Safety Tips, and Advice for Parents and Other Caregivers

Along with a Glossary of Terms and Resource Listings for Additional Help

Edited by Jenifer Swanson. 585 pages. 2000. 0-7808-0246-2. $78.

Kidney & Urinary Tract Diseases & Disorders Sourcebook

Basic Information about Kidney Stones, Urinary Incontinence, Bladder Disease, End Stage Renal Disease, Dialysis, and More

Along with Statistical and Demographic Data and Reports on Current Research Initiatives

Edited by Linda M. Ross. 602 pages. 1997. 0-7808-0079-6. $78.

Learning Disabilities Sourcebook

Basic Information about Disorders Such as Dyslexia, Visual and Auditory Processing Deficits, Attention Deficit/Hyperactivity Disorder, and Autism

Along with Statistical and Demographic Data, Reports on Current Research Initiatives, an Explanation of the Assessment Process, and a Special Section for Adults with Learning Disabilities

Edited by Linda M. Shin. 579 pages. 1998. 0-7808-0210-1. $78.

Named "Oustanding Reference Book of 1999."
— New York Public Library, Feb 2000

"An excellent candidate for inclusion in a public library reference section. It's a great source of information. Teachers will also find the book useful. Definitely worth reading."
— Journal of Adolescent & Adult Literacy, Feb 2000

"Readable . . . provides a solid base of information regarding successful techniques used with individuals who have learning disabilities, as well as practical suggestions for educators and family members. Clear language, concise descriptions, and pertinent information for contacting multiple resources add to the strength of this book as a useful tool."
— Choice, Association of College and Research Libraries, Feb '99

"Recommended reference source."
— Booklist, American Library Association, Sep '98

"This is a useful resource for libraries and for those who don't have the time to identify and locate the individual publications."
— Disability Resources Monthly, Sep '98

Liver Disorders Sourcebook

Basic Consumer Health Information about the Liver and How It Works; Liver Diseases, Including Cancer, Cirrhosis, Hepatitis, and Toxic and Drug Related Diseases; Tips for Maintaining a Healthy Liver; Laboratory Tests, Radiology Tests, and Facts about Liver Transplantation

Along with a Section on Support Groups, a Glossary, and Resource Listings

Edited by Joyce Brennfleck Shannon. 591 pages. 2000. 0-7808-0383-3. $78.

"Recommended reference source."
— Booklist, American Library Association, Jun '00

Medical Tests Sourcebook

Basic Consumer Health Information about Medical Tests, Including Periodic Health Exams, General Screening Tests, Tests You Can Do at Home, Findings of the U.S. Preventive Services Task Force, X-ray and Radiology Tests, Electrical Tests, Tests of Blood and Other Body Fluids and Tissues, Scope Tests, Lung Tests, Genetic Tests, Pregnancy Tests, Newborn Screening Tests, Sexually Transmitted Disease Tests, and Computer Aided Diagnoses

Along with a Section on Paying for Medical Tests, a Glossary, and Resource Listings

Edited by Joyce Brennfleck Shannon. 691 pages. 1999. 0-7808-0243-8. $78.

"A valuable reference guide."
— *American Reference Books Annual, 2000*

"Recommended for hospital and health sciences libraries with consumer health collections."
— *E-Streams, Mar '00*

"This is an overall excellent reference with a wealth of general knowledge that may aid those who are reluctant to get vital tests performed."
— *Today's Librarian, Jan 2000*

■

Men's Health Concerns Sourcebook

Basic Information about Health Issues That Affect Men, Featuring Facts about the Top Causes of Death in Men, Including Heart Disease, Stroke, Cancers, Prostate Disorders, Chronic Obstructive Pulmonary Disease, Pneumonia and Influenza, Human Immunodeficiency Virus and Acquired Immune Deficiency Syndrome, Diabetes Mellitus, Stress, Suicide, Accidents and Homicides; and Facts about Common Concerns for Men, Including Impotence, Contraception, Circumcision, Sleep Disorders, Snoring, Hair Loss, Diet, Nutrition, Exercise, Kidney and Urological Disorders, and Backaches

Edited by Allan R. Cook. 738 pages. 1998. 0-7808-0212-8. $78.

"This comprehensive resource and the series are highly recommended."
— *American Reference Books Annual, 2000*

"Recommended reference source."
— *Booklist, American Library Association, Dec '98*

■

Mental Health Disorders Sourcebook, 1st Edition

Basic Information about Schizophrenia, Depression, Bipolar Disorder, Panic Disorder, Obsessive-Compulsive Disorder, Phobias and Other Anxiety Disorders, Paranoia and Other Personality Disorders, Eating Disorders, and Sleep Disorders

Along with Information about Treatment and Therapies

Edited by Karen Bellenir. 548 pages. 1995. 0-7808-0040-0. $78.

"This is an excellent new book . . . written in easy-to-understand language." — *Booklist Health Sciences Supplement, American Library Association, Oct '97*

". . . useful for public and academic libraries and consumer health collections."
— *Medical Reference Services Quarterly, Spring '97*

"The great strengths of the book are its readability and its inclusion of places to find more information. Especially recommended." — *Reference Quarterly, American Library Association, Winter '96*

". . . a good resource for a consumer health library."
— *Bulletin of the Medical Library Association, Oct '96*

"The information is data-based and couched in brief, concise language that avoids jargon. . . . a useful reference source." — *Readings, Sep '96*

"The text is well organized and adequately written for its target audience." — *Choice, Association of College and Research Libraries, Jun '96*

". . . provides information on a wide range of mental disorders, presented in nontechnical language."
— *Exceptional Child Education Resources, Spring '96*

"Recommended for public and academic libraries."
— *Reference Book Review, 1996*

■

Mental Health Disorders Sourcebook, 2nd Edition

Basic Consumer Health Information about Anxiety Disorders, Depression and Other Mood Disorders, Eating Disorders, Personality Disorders, Schizophrenia, and More, Including Disease Descriptions, Treatment Options, and Reports on Current Research Initiatives

Along with Statistical Data, Tips for Maintaining Mental Health, a Glossary, and Directory of Sources for Additional Help and Information

Edited by Karen Bellenir. 605 pages. 2000. 0-7808-0240-3. $78.

■

Mental Retardation Sourcebook

Basic Consumer Health Information about Mental Retardation and Its Causes, Including Down Syndrome, Fetal Alcohol Syndrome, Fragile X Syndrome, Genetic Conditions, Injury, and Environmental Sources

Along with Preventive Strategies, Parenting Issues, Educational Implications, Health Care Needs, Employment and Economic Matters, Legal Issues, a Glossary, and a Resource Listing for Additional Help and Information

Edited by Joyce Brennfleck Shannon. 642 pages. 2000. 0-7808-0377-9. $78.

"From preventing retardation to parenting and family challenges, this covers health, social and legal issues and will prove an invaluable overview."
— *Reviewer's Bookwatch, Jul '00*

Obesity Sourcebook

Basic Consumer Health Information about Diseases and Other Problems Associated with Obesity, and Including Facts about Risk Factors, Prevention Issues, and Management Approaches

Along with Statistical and Demographic Data, Information about Special Populations, Research Updates, a Glossary, and Source Listings for Further Help and Information

Edited by Wilma Caldwell and Chad T. Kimball. 400 pages. 2000. 0-7808-0333-7. $48.

Ophthalmic Disorders Sourcebook

Basic Information about Glaucoma, Cataracts, Macular Degeneration, Strabismus, Refractive Disorders, and More

Along with Statistical and Demographic Data and Reports on Current Research Initiatives

Edited by Linda M. Ross. 631 pages. 1996. 0-7808-0081-8. $78.

Oral Health Sourcebook

Basic Information about Diseases and Conditions Affecting Oral Health, Including Cavities, Gum Disease, Dry Mouth, Oral Cancers, Fever Blisters, Canker Sores, Oral Thrush, Bad Breath, Temporomandibular Disorders, and other Craniofacial Syndromes

Along with Statistical Data on the Oral Health of Americans, Oral Hygiene, Emergency First Aid, Information on Treatment Procedures and Methods of Replacing Lost Teeth

Edited by Allan R. Cook. 558 pages. 1997. 0-7808-0082-6. $78.

"Unique source whi: h will fill a gap in dental sources for patients and the lay public. A valuable reference tool even in a library with thousands of books on dentistry. Comprehensive, clear, inexpensive, and easy to read and use. It fills an enormous gap in the health care literature." — *Reference and User Services Quarterly, American Library Association, Summer '98*

"Recommended reference source."
— *Booklist, American Library Association, Dec '97*

Osteoporosis Sourcebook

Basic Consumer Health Information about Primary and Secondary Osteoporosis, Juvenile Osteoporosis, Related Conditions, and Other Such Bone Disorders as Fibrous Dysplasia, Myeloma, Osteogenesis Imperfecta, Osteopetrosis, and Paget's Disease

Along with Information about Risk Factors, Treatments, Traditional and Non-Traditional Pain Management, and Including a Glossary and Resource Directory

Edited by Allan R. Cook. 600 pages. 2000. 0-7808-0239-X. $78.

SEE ALSO *Women's Health Concerns Sourcebook*

Pain Sourcebook

Basic Information about Specific Forms of Acute and Chronic Pain, Including Headaches, Back Pain, Muscular Pain, Neuralgia, Surgical Pain, and Cancer Pain

Along with Pain Relief Options Such as Analgesics, Narcotics, Nerve Blocks, Transcutaneous Nerve Stimulation, and Alternative Forms of Pain Control, Including Biofeedback, Imaging, Behavior Modification, and Relaxation Techniques

Edited by Allan R. Cook. 667 pages. 1997. 0-7808-0213-6. $78.

"The text is readable, easily understood, and well indexed. This excellent volume belongs in all patient education libraries, consumer health sections of public libraries, and many personal collections."
— *American Reference Books Annual, 1999*

"A beneficial reference." — *Booklist Health Sciences Supplement, American Library Association, Oct '98*

"The information is basic in terms of scholarship and is appropriate for general readers. Written in journalistic style ... intended for non-professionals. Quite thorough in its coverage of different pain conditions and summarizes the latest clinical information regarding pain treatment."
— *Choice, Association of College and Research Libraries, Jun '98*

"Recommended reference source."
— *Booklist, American Library Association, Mar '98*

Pediatric Cancer Sourcebook

Basic Consumer Health Information about Leukemias, Brain Tumors, Sarcomas, Lymphomas, and Other Cancers in Infants, Children, and Adolescents, Including Descriptions of Cancers, Treatments, and Coping Strategies

Along with Suggestions for Parents, Caregivers, and Concerned Relatives, a Glossary of Cancer Terms, and Resource Listings

Edited by Edward J. Prucha. 587 pages. 1999. 0-7808-0245-4. $78.

"A valuable addition to all libraries specializing in health services and many public libraries."
— *American Reference Books Annual, 2000*

"Recommended reference source."
— *Booklist, American Library Association, Feb '00*

"An excellent source of information. Recommended for public, hospital, and health science libraries with consumer health collections." — *E-Stream, Jun '00*

Physical & Mental Issues in Aging Sourcebook

Basic Consumer Health Information on Physical and Mental Disorders Associated with the Aging Process, Including Concerns about Cardiovascular Disease, Pulmonary Disease, Oral Health, Digestive Disorders, Musculoskeletal and Skin Disorders, Metabolic

Changes, Sexual and Reproductive Issues, and Changes in Vision, Hearing, and Other Senses

Along with Data about Longevity and Causes of Death, Information on Acute and Chronic Pain, Descriptions of Mental Concerns, a Glossary of Terms, and Resource Listings for Additional Help

Edited by Jenifer Swanson. 660 pages. 1999. 0-7808-0233-0. $78.

"Recommended for public libraries."
—American Reference Books Annual, 2000

"This is a treasure of health information for the layperson."
— Choice Health Sciences Supplement, Association of College & Research Libraries, May 2000

"Recommended reference source."
—Booklist, American Library Association, Oct '99

SEE ALSO Healthy Aging Sourcebook

■

Reconstructive & Cosmetic Surgery Sourcebook

Basic Consumer Health Information on Cosmetic and Reconstructive Plastic Surgery, Including Statistical Information about Different Surgical Procedures, Things to Consider Prior to Surgery, Plastic Surgery Techniques and Tools, Emotional and Psychological Considerations, and Procedure-Specific Information

Along with a Glossary of Terms and a Listing of Resources for Additional Help and Information

Edited by M. Lisa Weatherford. 400 pages. 2000. 0-7808-0214-4. $48.

■

Podiatry Sourcebook

Basic Consumer Health Information about Foot Conditions, Diseases, and Injuries, Including Bunions, Corns, Calluses, Athlete's Foot, Plantar Warts, Hammertoes and Clawtoes, Club Foot, Heel Pain, Gout, and More

Along with Facts about Foot Care, Disease Prevention, Foot Safety, Choosing a Foot Care Specialist, a Glossary of Terms, and Resource Listings for Additional Information

Edited by M. Lisa Weatherford. 600 pages. 2000. 0-7808-0215-2. $78.

■

Pregnancy & Birth Sourcebook

Basic Information about Planning for Pregnancy, Maternal Health, Fetal Growth and Development, Labor and Delivery, Postpartum and Perinatal Care, Pregnancy in Mothers with Special Concerns, and Disorders of Pregnancy, Including Genetic Counseling, Nutrition and Exercise, Obstetrical Tests, Pregnancy Discomfort, Multiple Births, Cesarean Sections, Medical Testing of Newborns, Breastfeeding, Gestational Diabetes, and Ectopic Pregnancy

Edited by Heather E. Aldred. 737 pages. 1997. 0-7808-0216-0. $78.

"A well-organized handbook. Recommended."
— Choice, Association of College and Research Libraries, Apr '98

"Reecommended reference source."
—Booklist, American Library Association, Mar '98

"Recommended for public libraries."
—American Reference Books Annual, 1998

SEE ALSO Congenital Disorders Sourcebook, Family Planning Sourcebook

■

Public Health Sourcebook

Basic Information about Government Health Agencies, Including National Health Statistics and Trends, Healthy People 2000 Program Goals and Objectives, the Centers for Disease Control and Prevention, the Food and Drug Administration, and the National Institutes of Health

Along with Full Contact Information for Each Agency

Edited by Wendy Wilcox. 698 pages. 1998. 0-7808-0220-9. $78.

"Recommended reference source."
—Booklist, American Library Association, Sep '98

"This consumer guide provides welcome assistance in navigating the maze of federal health agencies and their data on public health concerns."
—SciTech Book News, Sep '98

■

Rehabilitation Sourcebook

Basic Consumer Health Information about Rehabilitation for People Recovering from Heart Surgery, Spinal Cord Injury, Stroke, Orthopedic Impairments, Amputation, Pulmonary Impairments, Traumatic Injury, and More, Including Physical Therapy, Occupational Therapy, Speech/ Language Therapy, Massage Therapy, Dance Therapy, Art Therapy, and Recreational Therapy

Along with Information on Assistive and Adaptive Devices, a Glossary, and Resources for Additional Help and Information

Edited by Dawn D. Matthews. 531 pages. 1999. 0-7808-0236-5. $78.

"Recommended reference source."
—Booklist, American Library Association, May '00

■

Respiratory Diseases & Disorders Sourcebook

Basic Information about Respiratory Diseases and Disorders, Including Asthma, Cystic Fibrosis, Pneumonia, the Common Cold, Influenza, and Others, Featuring Facts about the Respiratory System, Statistical and Demographic Data, Treatments, Self-Help Management Suggestions, and Current Research Initiatives

Edited by Allan R. Cook and Peter D. Dresser. 771 pages. 1995. 0-7808-0037-0. $78.

"Designed for the layperson and for patients and their families coping with respiratory illness. . . . an extensive array of information on diagnosis, treatment, management, and prevention of respiratory illnesses for the general reader."
— *Choice, Association of College and Research Libraries, Jun '96*

"A highly recommended text for all collections. It is a comforting reminder of the power of knowledge that good books carry between their covers."
— *Academic Library Book Review, Spring '96*

"A comprehensive collection of authoritative information presented in a nontechnical, humanitarian style for patients, families, and caregivers."
— *Association of Operating Room Nurses, Sep/Oct '95*

Sexually Transmitted Diseases Sourcebook

Basic Information about Herpes, Chlamydia, Gonorrhea, Hepatitis, Nongonoccocal Urethritis, Pelvic Inflammatory Disease, Syphilis, AIDS, and More

Along with Current Data on Treatments and Preventions

Edited by Linda M. Ross. 550 pages. 1997. 0-7808-0217-9. $78.

Sexually Transmitted Diseases Sourcebook, 2nd Edition

Basic Consumer Health Information about Sexually Transmitted Diseases, Including Information on the Diagnosis and Treatment of Chlamydia, Gonorrhea, Hepatitis, Herpes, HIV, Mononucleosis, Syphilis, and Others

Along with Information on Prevention, Such as Condom Use, Vaccines, and STD Education; And Featuring a Section on Issues Related to Youth and Adolescents, a Glossary, and Resources for Additional Help and Information

Edited by Dawn D. Matthews. 600 pages. 2000. 0-7808-0249-7. $78.

Skin Disorders Sourcebook

Basic Information about Common Skin and Scalp Conditions Caused by Aging, Allergies, Immune Reactions, Sun Exposure, Infectious Organisms, Parasites, Cosmetics, and Skin Traumas, Including Abrasions, Cuts, and Pressure Sores

Along with Information on Prevention and Treatment

Edited by Allan R. Cook. 647 pages. 1997. 0-7808-0080-X. $78.

". . . comprehensive, easily read reference book."
— *Doody's Health Sciences Book Reviews, Oct '97*

SEE ALSO *Burns Sourcebook*

Sleep Disorders Sourcebook

Basic Consumer Health Information about Sleep and Its Disorders, Including Insomnia, Sleepwalking, Sleep Apnea, Restless Leg Syndrome, and Narcolepsy

Along with Data about Shiftwork and Its Effects, Information on the Societal Costs of Sleep Deprivation, Descriptions of Treatment Options, a Glossary of Terms, and Resource Listings for Additional Help

Edited by Jenifer Swanson. 439 pages. 1998. 0-7808-0234-9. $78.

"This text will complement any home or medical library. It is user-friendly and ideal for the adult reader."
— *American Reference Books Annual, 2000*

"Recommended reference source."
— *Booklist, American Library Association, Feb '99*

"A useful resource that provides accurate, relevant, and accessible information on sleep to the general public. Health care providers who deal with sleep disorders patients may also find it helpful in being prepared to answer some of the questions patients ask."
— *Respiratory Care, Jul '99*

Sports Injuries Sourcebook

Basic Consumer Health Information about Common Sports Injuries, Prevention of Injury in Specific Sports, Tips for Training, and Rehabilitation from Injury

Along with Information about Special Concerns for Children, Young Girls in Athletic Training Programs, Senior Athletes, and Women Athletes, and a Directory of Resources for Further Help and Information

Edited by Heather E. Aldred. 624 pages. 1999. 0-7808-0218-7. $78.

"Public libraries and undergraduate academic libraries will find this book useful for its nontechnical language."
— *American Reference Books Annual, 2000*

"While this easy-to-read book is recommended for all libraries, it should prove to be especially useful for public, high school, and academic libraries; certainly it should be on the bookshelf of every school gymnasium."
— *E-Streams, Mar '00*

Substance Abuse Sourcebook

Basic Health-Related Information about the Abuse of Legal and Illegal Substances Such as Alcohol, Tobacco, Prescription Drugs, Marijuana, Cocaine, and Heroin; and Including Facts about Substance Abuse Prevention Strategies, Intervention Methods, Treatment and Recovery Programs, and a Section Addressing the Special Problems Related to Substance Abuse during Pregnancy

Edited by Karen Bellenir. 573 pages. 1996. 0-7808-0038-9. $78.

"A valuable addition to any health reference section. Highly recommended."
— *The Book Report, Mar/Apr '97*

"... a comprehensive collection of substance abuse information that's both highly readable and compact. Families and caregivers of substance abusers will find the information enlightening and helpful, while teachers, social workers and journalists should benefit from the concise format. Recommended."
— *Drug Abuse Update, Winter '96/'97*

SEE ALSO Alcoholism Sourcebook, Drug Abuse Sourcebook

■

Traveler's Health Sourcebook

Basic Consumer Health Information for Travelers, Including Physical and Medical Preparations, Transportation Health and Safety, Essential Information about Food and Water, Sun Exposure, Insect and Snake Bites, Camping and Wilderness Medicine, and Travel with Physical or Medical Disabilities

Along with International Travel Tips, Vaccination Recommendations, Geographical Health Issues, Disease Risks, a Glossary, and a Listing of Additional Resources

Edited by Joyce Brennfleck Shannon. 613 pages. 2000. 0-7808-0384-1. $78.

■

Women's Health Concerns Sourcebook

Basic Information about Health Issues That Affect Women, Featuring Facts about Menstruation and Other Gynecological Concerns, Including Endometriosis, Fibroids, Menopause, and Vaginitis; Reproductive Concerns, Including Birth Control, Infertility, and Abortion; and Facts about Additional Physical, Emotional, and Mental Health Concerns Prevalent among Women Such as Osteoporosis, Urinary Tract Disorders, Eating Disorders, and Depression

Along with Tips for Maintaining a Healthy Lifestyle

Edited by Heather E. Aldred. 567 pages. 1997. 0-7808-0219-5. $78.

"Handy compilation. There is an impressive range of diseases, devices, disorders, procedures, and other physical and emotional issues covered . . . well organized, illustrated, and indexed."   — *Choice, Association of College and Research Libraries, Jan '98*

SEE ALSO Breast Cancer Sourcebook, Cancer Sourcebook for Women, 1st and 2nd Editions, Healthy Heart Sourcebook for Women, Osteoporosis Sourcebook

Workplace Health & Safety Sourcebook

Basic Consumer Health Information about Workplace Health and Safety, Including the Effect of Workplace Hazards on the Lungs, Skin, Heart, Ears, Eyes, Brain, Reproductive Organs, Musculoskeletal System, and Other Organs and Body Parts

Along with Information about Occupational Cancer, Personal Protective Equipment, Toxic and Hazardous Chemicals, Child Labor, Stress, and Workplace Violence

Edited by Chad T. Kimball. 626 pages. 2000. 0-7808-0231-4. $78.

■

Worldwide Health Sourcebook

Basic Information about Global Health Issues, Including Malnutrition, Reproductive Health, Disease Dispersion and Prevention, Emerging Diseases, Risky Health Behaviors, and the Leading Causes of Death

Along with Global Health Concerns for Children, Women, and the Elderly, Mental Health Issues, Research and Technology Advancements, and Economic, Environmental, and Political Health Implications, a Glossary, and a Resource Listing for Additional Help and Information

Edited by Joyce Brennfleck Shannon. 500 pages. 2000. 0-7808-0330-2. $78.

■

Health Reference Series Cumulative Index 1999

A Comprehensive Index to the Individual Volumes of the Health Reference Series, Including a Subject Index, Name Index, Organization Index, and Publication Index;

Along with a Master List of Acronyms and Abbreviations

Edited by Edward J. Prucha, Anne Holmes, and Robert Rudnick. 990 pages. 2000. 0-7808-0382-5. $78.

627